Student Activity Manual to Accompany
The Professional Medical Assistant

Sharon Eagle, RN, MSN
Former Director, Medical Assisting Program
Nursing Faculty
Wenatchee Valley College
Wenatchee, WA

Candy Dailey, RN, MSN, CMA (AAMA)
Medical Assistant Program Director and Instructor
Nicolet Area Community College
Rhinelander, WI

Cheri Goretti, MA, MT(ASCP), CMA (AAMA)
Professor and Medical Assisting Program Director
Quinebaug Valley Community College
Danielson, CT

Cindi Brassington, MS, CMA (AAMA)
Professor of Allied Health
Quinebaug Valley Community College
Danielson, CT

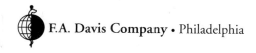
F.A. Davis Company • Philadelphia

F. A. Davis Company
1915 Arch Street
Philadelphia, PA 19103
www.fadavis.com

Printed in the United States of America

ISBN 10: 0-8036-1672-4
ISBN 13: 978-0-8036-1672-1

Last digit indicates print number: 10 9 8 7 6 5 4 3 2 1

Senior Acquisitions Editor: Andy McPhee
Manager of Content Development: George W. Lang
Developmental Editor: Karen Lynn Carter
Art and Design Manager: Carolyn O'Brien

As new scientific information becomes available through basic and clinical research, recommended treatments and drug therapies undergo changes. The author(s) and publisher have done everything possible to make this book accurate, up to date, and in accord with accepted standards at the time of publication. The author(s), editors, and publisher are not responsible for errors or omissions or for consequences from application of the book, and make no warranty, expressed or implied, in regard to the contents of the book. Any practice described in this book should be applied by the reader in accordance with professional standards of care used in regard to the unique circumstances that may apply in each situation. The reader is advised always to check product information (package inserts) for changes and new information regarding dose and contraindications before administering any drug. Caution is especially urged when using new or infrequently ordered drugs.

Reviewers

Darlene Kaye Acton, CMA (AAMA)
Director
Medical Assisting Department
Alamance Community College
Graham, NC

Carmen Carpenter, RN, MS, CMA (AAMA)
Chair
Allied Health and Medical Assisting
South University
West Palm Beach, FL

Mary Ann Crandall, RN, BS, MS
Instructor
Extended Campus Programs
Southern Oregon University
Ashland, OR

Marilyn M. Turner, RN, CMA (AAMA)
Director
Medical Assisting Program
Ogeechee Technical College
Statesboro, GA

Contents

UNIT I

General-Transdisciplinary

Critical Thinking

1. Jenna Delgado, a student in the sixth grade, is in for her annual physical exam. You ask her how school is going and she tells you she has to do a report on a famous person in medicine. She asks you for your input. Who would you recommend, and why?

_____

_____

_____

_____

2. As you are performing an interview on a new patient, she calls you "nurse." When you respond that you are not a nurse, she says, "Oh, you doctor's office staff are all the same." How would you respond to this patient?

_____

_____

_____

_____

Teamwork Exercises

1. Upon graduation, many medical assisting students continue their formal education. Divide into groups of two or three. Your instructor will assign each group one of the following health-care professions:

- Medical technologist
- Medical technician
- Registered nurse
- Physical therapist

- Pharmacist
- Physical therapist
- Physician assistant
- Medical coder

As a group, research the colleges in your area that may have these programs. Provide the following information in report format:

a. name of school or college

b. admissions requirements

c. curriculum

d. how your medical assisting curriculum complements these other programs

Office Project

As a class, research the local physician offices in your area. Are most of the offices single practitioners or are there more group practices? After researching at least 10 different practices in your area, have a discussion on the benefits and disadvantages of both types.

Therapeutic Communication

Key Term Review   *Define the following key terms:*

1. passive — Quality of submitting or yielding w/out offering resistance.

2. channels — Mode of conveying a message, including vision, hearing and touch.

3. feedback — Message returned by a reciever as a response to the senders message.

4. repression — Psychological response in which a person eliminates from concious thought traumatic experients or certain impulses that the person believes is unacceptable.

5. denial — Psychological response by which a person refuses to acknowledge the reality of something that is obvious to others.

6. assertive — Quality of advocating for ones owns rights while respeching the rights of others.

7. rationalization — psychological response in which a person makes excuses to justify innapropriate behaviors.

8. norms — Unwritten rules of socially acceptable behaviors.

9. projection — psychological response in which a person accuses others of that persons own feelings, attitudes, or behaviors.

10. passive–aggressive — Manipulative behavior that appears initially passive but seeks to control by retaliation in the form of procrastination, stubborness and forgetfullness.

11. sender — person who delivers a message.

12. compensation — psychological response in which a person offsets feelings of inadequacy in one aspect of that persons life by achievement in another aspect.

Key Term Review *cont.*

13.   receiver   <u>person who recieves a message and decodes it.</u>

14.   boundary   <u>physical or psychological space that indicates the limit of</u>
<u>appropriate versus inappropriate behaviors.</u>

Review Questions

1. Discuss the importance of a medical assistant possessing and using effective communications skills.

   _____

   _____

   _____

   _____

2. Discuss and define each feature of the communication cycle:

   a. referent:

   _____

   _____

   _____

   _____

   b. sender:

   _____

   _____

   _____

   _____

   c. receiver:

   _____

   _____

   _____

   _____

d. message:

_____

_____

_____

_____

e. channels:

_____

_____

_____

_____

f. feedback:

_____

_____

_____

_____

g. interpersonal variables:

_____

_____

_____

_____

h. environment:

_____

_____

_____

_____

3. What are some factors that can affect meaning during verbal communication?

_____

_____

_____

_____

4. List five effective verbal communication techniques a medical assistant can use when speaking to patients.

_____

_____

_____

_____

5. What is body language?

_____

_____

_____

6. List five positive body language messages.

_____

_____

_____

_____

7. List five negative body language messages.

_____

_____

_____

_____

8. Discuss the importance of understanding proxemics and how it relates to proper communication.

_____

_____

_____

_____

Critical Thinking

1. You are performing the initial patient interview and recording of the chief complaint. Develop some open-ended questions for the following scenarios:

a. 43-year-old patient who is complaining of back pain:
- What's the pain feel like
- How long have you had pain
- What activities you've done that could have caused it?
- Are you taking anything for it?

b. 27-year-old patient who has a red rash all over his body:
- How long have you had it?
- Does it hurt, itch, or bother you?
- Any new products being used, been in new areas?
- Where did it origionate?

c. A teenager who limps into the examination room:
- How long have you been limping?
- What caused the injury? Have you taken anything for it?
- Does anything else hurt? knee, back
- Does anything make it better? Ice pack hotpack?

d. A 5-year-old child who is complaining of a "bellyache." The child's dad is also in the room:
- When was the last BM or bathroom use?
- What things they've ate lately?
- Any other symptoms? fever?
- How long has it been hurting, how often?

2. You are a CMA working as the clinical supervisor in a general practitioner's office. You find that one of your CMAs, Holly, has a tendency of not performing the required weight determination on every patient's visit. When questioned why she does not do the procedure, she remarks to you, "There is no need to perform a weight every time a patient comes in, and it just gets them upset anyway." You respond that you understand what she is saying but that it is a requirement of the practice. The next day, when a physician asks Holly why she did not perform a weight measurement on another patient, she responds "Oh, sorry. I just forgot." How would you deal with Holly's passive–aggressive nature?

3. As a medical assistant, you will have patients who come from different heritages and cultures. Research various heritages such as Indian, Russian, African, Japanese, and Jewish and come up with some techniques for communicating effectively with these various cultures.

_____

_____

_____

_____

Teamwork Exercises

1. In groups of two, each student will take turns playing the medical assistant and one of the following patients in the following scenarios:

   a. The patient who is angry about the length of time she has been waiting to see the physician

   b. The geriatric patient who appears confused

   c. The 4-year-old patient who is scared to be at the doctor's office

   d. The patient who constantly interrupts you

   e. The patient who is upset over her bill and feels she was overcharged for her last visit

2. List the various cultures that are in your community. Divide into groups of two or three and have each group select one of the cultures on the list. Each group will research its culture and the language associated. Develop some basic phrases in your assigned culture's language that may help you as a medical assistant in your community.

Office Project

Invite various culturally diverse members of your community to come speak to your class about their heritage. Have the class create a list of questions to ask the guest speaker.

11. Describe the purpose of a durable power of attorney and a living will.

_____

_____

_____

_____

12. Describe patient release of information and how it is obtained.

_____

_____

_____

_____

13. List the circumstances in which patient authorization of release of information is not necessary.

_____

_____

_____

_____

14. Describe reporting requirements for child and elder abuse.

_____

_____

_____

_____

Critical Thinking

1. Jose Jimenez has been suffering from sleep apnea for many years. His physician recommends an uvulectomy to increase his ability to breathe in a supine position. The surgeon explains the risks and benefits of the procedure, and Jose agrees to the surgery. While performing the operation, the surgeon mistakenly cuts one of Jose's tonsils. Unable to stop the bleeding, the surgeon must remove the tonsil. While tonsils are commonly removed in the case of chronic infection, Jose did not consent to a tonsillectomy prior to the surgical procedure. Using the "four D's" of medical malpractice, is the surgeon guilty or not guilty of negligence? Discuss your reasoning with classmates.

_____

_____

_____

_____

2. You are the site supervisor for the medical assisting students who extern at your office. Your latest student, Josh, consistently asks to perform procedures that he has not been approved to do. You decide to sit down with him and have a discussion on the medical assistant's scope of practice. What do you say to Josh?

_____

_____

_____

_____

Teamwork Exercises

1. Divide the class into three groups. Your instructor will assign one of the following topics: elder abuse, child abuse, or domestic abuse. Create an abuse awareness brochure based on your individual topic. Research your local area for resources and contacts and include that information in your brochure. Discuss your brochure with the other groups.

2. Divide the classroom into groups of two or three students. Using the Internet, each group will research at least three malpractice cases. So that students don't research the same cases, the instructor may provide groups with a certain state in which each must find its case. Each group will write a summary of each case (what the lawsuit consisted of, how the case was decided, any awards granted, etc.) they researched and then present their findings. As a class, discuss each case and your opinions on how the case was settled.

Office Project

Invite a lawyer or a professional in health-care risk management to speak to your class on the topic of risk management. The class should come up with questions ahead of time to ask the guest speaker.

HIPAA and a Patient's Rights

Key Term Review   *Define the following key terms:*

1. data use agreement
2. authorization

3. individually identifiable health information (IIHI)
4. protected health information (PHI)
5. termination policy

6. privacy standard

7. Notice of Privacy Practices
8. business associate

9. de-identified information
10. disclosure

11. TPO

Key Term Review *cont.*

12. health-care operations _____

_____

13. transaction code sets (TCS) _____

_____

14. business associate contract _____

_____

Review Questions

1. What is the purpose of the HIPAA Act of 1996?

_____

_____

_____

_____

2. Discuss the two components of the HIPAA Public Law 104-191.

_____

_____

_____

_____

3. What are the three components of the security standard?

_____

_____

_____

_____

4. Describe who may be listed as a "covered entity," and list the responsibilities of the various entities.

_____

_____

_____

_____

5. Describe what treatment, payment, and operations (TPO) are.

_____

_____

_____

_____

6. Describe how to obtain consent to disclose protected health information (PHI) for TPO.

_____

_____

_____

_____

7. What are the patient's rights to PHI, and how is it obtained?

_____

_____

_____

_____

8. What is the PHI that a patient does not have a right to access?

_____

_____

_____

_____

9. List at least four safeguards of PHI in each category.

_____

_____

_____

_____

10. List the required privacy policy documents and their purposes.

_____

_____

_____

_____

11. What are some examples of PHI that can be verbally disclosed?

_____

_____

_____

_____

12. Discuss the penalties of failing to comply with HIPAA guidelines.

_____

_____

_____

_____

13. Discuss the three categories of the electronic transaction data sets.

_____

_____

_____

_____

14. What guidelines must be in place when a medical office uses a billing company to file electronic health-care claims?

_____

_____

_____

_____

15. List six types of information transactions that may occur between a medical office and its billing office.

_____

_____

_____

_____

16. Discuss confidentiality, integrity, and availability as they relate to PHI.

_____

_____

_____

_____

17. List some rights the patient has regarding his or her access to information.

Make an appointment to view whole medical chart w
someone present. Has the right to obtain, access, inspect
copy of their medical records. May be a charge.
Right to access: health info, amendment of PHI, additional restriction
of info, alternative means of communication, health info, accounting of
request medical record in writing, must be fulfilled in 30 days, disclosures of PHI.

18. List some exceptions to access of information under the HIPAA regulations.

_____

_____

_____

_____

19. What are some responsibilities of a HIPAA compliance officer?

_____

_____

_____

_____

20. Discuss some administrative safeguards a medical assistant can take to maintain confidentiality.

_____

_____

_____

_____

Critical Thinking

1. Charlene Lilly, a new physician assistant (PA), has just joined Dr. Miarecki's office. As the billing coordinator, you notice that claims are being denied on services provided by Charlene, due to the PA being identified as a nonparticipating provider for many of your patients'

insurance companies. When you bring this to the attention of your office manager, she tells you to put Dr. Miarecki's provider identification number on the claims. What do you do?

_____

_____

_____

_____

2. The primary care physician that Stella Wrona has gone to for the past 5 years has retired. She personally obtained her medical record to bring to her first appointment at your office. When she hands you her record, she claims that there are some inconsistencies in the record and requests the information be amended. How do you handle her request?

Make an appointment w/ new doctor to go over medical history. Have a titer done to see past labs. When she tells inconsistancies, try hardest to find accurate info. Ask doctor, have in writting what she requests to be amended

3. You are the compliance officer for your office. Two new medical assistants have joined your health-care team: One is a new graduate, and the other has 5 years of medical office experience. You are responsible for training employees on the office's HIPAA policies. Develop a plan for specialized training based on each employee's background.

_____

_____

_____

_____

Teamwork Exercises

1. Using the guidelines on page xxx for developing a Privacy Policy Procedure Manual, work in small groups to develop the suggested documents for your office.

2. In groups of two or three, role-play various scenarios that relate to the situations contained in "Disclosure: What Can I Say" on pages 75–76 in the textbook. You can take turns being the medical assistant and the person looking for information. After each scenario, have a discussion on the reasons for or against releasing the specific information.

PROCEDURE 7-1 – RELEASE OF PHI FOR NON-TPO PURPOSES

Name _____   Date _____   Score _____

Instructor _____

Task
Ensure that protected health information (PHI) released for purposes other than treatment, payment, or operations (TPO) is performed with proper patient authorization.

Conditions
Authorization to Release PHI form
Patient's medical record
Pen

Time _____

Standard
In the time specified and within the scoring parameters determined by the instructor, the student will successfully perform a release of PHI for non-TPO purposes.

Points assigned reflect importance of step to meeting the task

Important = 1 pt.
Essential = 5 pts.
Critical = 15 pts.

Automatic failure results if any of the **CRITICAL TASKS** are omitted or performed incorrectly.

(To use a pass/fail system, instructors can record "P" or "F" in the "points earned (pass/fail)" column.)

PERFORMANCE STANDARDS	PTS	PTS EARNED (Pass/Fail)	COMMENTS
1. Checked the Authorization to Release form's information for completeness, including:	15	_____	_____
a. patient's name, date of birth, and Social Security number			_____
b. patient's initials next to the notice of the right to revoke permission to disclose			_____
c. patient's or legal guardian's signature (original, not a photocopied or faxed signature)			_____
d. date signed			_____
e. information requested for reasonable length of time (for example, not entire record spanning 54 years)			_____
f. HIV, mental health, and substance abuse information specifically requested by the patient (separately indicated with initials or signature)			_____

PERFORMANCE STANDARDS (cont.)	PTS	PTS EARNED (Pass/Fail)	COMMENTS
g. indication of recipient of information, including name, address, and other contact information			_____ _____
2. Retrieved the patient's medical record.	1	_____	_____ _____
3. Photocopied the documentation requested.	1	_____	_____ _____
4. Rechecked the authorization and photocopied documentation to ensure that only the information requested and authorized is released.	5	_____	_____ _____
5. If a courier is picking up the information, checked the identification of the courier.	5	_____	_____ _____
6. Documented the release of information in the patient's medical record.	15	_____	_____ _____
7. Filed the Authorization to Release form in the patient's medical record or designated file.	5	_____	_____ _____

TOTAL POINTS	47		

DOCUMENTATION

COMMENTS

PROCEDURE 7-2 – PROVIDING, EXPLAINING, AND OBTAINING ACKNOWLEDGMENT OF NPP

Name _____   Date _____   Score _____

Instructor _____

Task

Use the Notice of Privacy Practices (NPP) to ensure that a patient understands his right to protected health information (PHI) and how the office will use the information for treatment, payment, and operations (TPO) and obtain the patient's signature on the acknowledgment form.

Conditions

Notice of Privacy Practices
Acknowledgment of receipt of NPP form
Patient's medical record
Pen

Time _____

Standards

In the time specified and within the scoring parameters determined by the instructor, the student will successfully provide and explain the NPP and obtain the patient's signature on the acknowledgment form.

Points assigned reflect importance of step to meeting the task

Important = 1 pt.
Essential = 5 pts.
Critical = 15 pts.

Automatic failure results if any of the **CRITICAL TASKS** are omitted or performed incorrectly.

(To use a pass/fail system, instructors can record "P" or "F" in the "points earned (pass/fail)" column.)

PERFORMANCE STANDARDS	PTS	PTS EARNED (Pass/Fail)	COMMENTS
1. Gave the patient the Notice of Privacy Practices (NPP) along with the new patient registration forms.	5	_____	
2. Asked the patient to read the NPP and answered any questions that he may have had.	1	_____	
3. Asked the patient to sign the acknowledgment of receipt and understanding of NPP.	1	_____	
4. Filed the acknowledgement in the patient's medical record	5	_____	

TOTAL POINTS	12		

DOCUMENTATION

COMMENTS

4. Compare and contrast the utilitarian and deontological theories.

_____

_____

_____

_____

5. Discuss the purpose of a code of ethics.

_____

_____

_____

_____

6. Explain the purpose of an ethics committee.

_____

_____

_____

_____

7. What are the features of an ethical dilemma?

_____

_____

_____

_____

8. Discuss the importance of the AAMA Code of Ethics.

_____

_____

_____

_____

Critical Thinking

1. What are the seven ethical principles for health care? Provide specific ways you can apply them to your career as a medical assistant.

   _____

   _____

   _____

   _____

2. As the medical assisting program coordinator, you are meeting with the site supervisor at the local women's clinic, where your student is doing her medical assisting externship. The site supervisor states that the student's skills are very good, but there's been some issues with the student's ethical conduct related to confidentiality, where in one instance the student told the staff how she went home the night before and told her husband that she saw two of her former high school classmates at the clinic, and actually identified them by name. The site supervisor spoke to the student, but as the program coordinator, how do you handle this situation?

   _____

   _____

   _____

   _____

3. For the following scenarios, describe how you would use the ethical reasoning process to identify a potential solution or course of action.

   a. A student observes another student cheating on an examination. What should she do?

   _____

   _____

   _____

   _____

   b. During the clinical externship, you grab a laboratory report off of the fax machine at your preceptor's request. As you glance at the report, you notice that it reveals the patient has tested positive for HIV. Then you recognize the patient's name as your new brother-in-law.

You feel grave concern for your sister's health and well-being but are aware that this is HIPAA-protected information. What should you do?

_____

_____

_____

_____

c. You are a new medical assistant recently hired to work in a family practice clinic. You observe at different times several different coworkers placing office supplies in their purses and taking them home. When you comment about it one day, the response is, "Oh, everyone does it. Get used to it." What will you do?

_____

_____

_____

d. A patient has a chronic foot ulcer due to poorly controlled diabetes. She has been advised by her physician to undergo an amputation of her foot. She isn't sure she wants to go through with the surgery. List as many ethical reasons as you can think of for her to (a) have the surgery and (b) not have the surgery.

_____

_____

_____

e. A geriatric woman has been providing care for her 10-year-old grandson since he was born. His mother died in a car accident. His father has never been involved in his life. He has severe physical and mental disabilities that have resulted in the need for total personal care. He will never be able to live independently. The woman's health is failing and she is worried about her ability to continue providing adequate care but feels sure that her daughter would never have wanted him to be institutionalized. What should she do?

_____

_____

_____

_____

f. A donor liver has become available. There are two people who are suitable matches and are in desperate need. Decide which one gets the liver. List all criteria that you will consider in this decision:

A 25-year-old single woman whose body is rejecting her second transplanted liver

_____

_____

_____

_____

A 40-year-old mother of three whose liver failure is due to alcoholism (she quit drinking 1 year ago)

_____

_____

_____

_____

Teamwork Exercises

1. Divide into groups of three or four students. Have a discussion of your personal and professional ethics and morals. When discussing, be respectful of each other's opinions, morals, beliefs, etc. After the discussion, each student will write up a summary of his or her personal and professional ethics and morals and how they related to the rest of the group's. How did they differ? Include in your summary how you would continue to relate to people who may have different morals and ethics than yours.

2. Divide into teams of three to five students. Select one of the projects listed below. Be prepared to present your results to the rest of the class at a time designated by your instructor.

   a. Nonmaleficence versus beneficence: A patient has been diagnosed with cancer. Describe the potential benefits and risks that may be associated with this client's various treatment options.

   b. Veracity: Discuss whether the truth should always be told 100% of the time and why. If your team allows for "little white lies," list at least five examples of situations in which such a lie might be acceptable.

c. Fidelity: Make a list of the type of obligations your patients might reasonably expect you to keep. Make a list of unreasonable expectations you believe your patients may have.

d. Autonomy: Discuss the "rights" that your team thinks should be guaranteed to all people. Now make a list of the "rights" that some people seem to think they should have but that you disagree with.

e. Distributive justice: Discuss among your team members the notion that all individuals are entitled to unlimited health care regardless of their ability to pay. Assuming that you all agree with this statement, how do you think such care should be financed? Now consider the possibility that health-care resources are scarce. Your team must recommend a system for determining who gets what.

f. Paternalism: Describe at least five different scenarios in which paternalism might occur. Give specific examples.

3. Divide into teams of three to five students. Each team must identify an issue that is somewhat controversial. Then design an argument for or against the issue based on one of the ethical philosophies. Describe the argument and explain why it adheres to one ethical philosophy or the other.

Office Project

Review the Medical Assisting Code of Ethics developed by the AAMA as well as the Medical Assistant's Creed. As a class, develop a poster for the AAMA's Code of Ethics and the Medical Assistant's Creed. Publicize both posters on the Medical Assistant Bulletin Board or in the classroom.

Teamwork Exercises

1. Divide into groups of two. Each student will research a medical condition or medical procedure and then explain it to his or her partner in understandable terms. Use teaching strategies learned in the chapter for ensuring that the classmate has understood what was explained.

2. Given the same topic (either the group can chose a topic or the instructor will assign one), each group will chose one of the following methods to teach the same information to the rest of the class on the topic:

   - Lecture

   - PowerPoint

   - Reading assignment

   - Poster presentation

   - Demonstration

   After all students' teaching presentations are completed, have a discussion about how effective each teaching method was.

Office Project

As a class, create a public bulletin board, either in your classroom or in a hallway at your school. Provide public interest fact sheets on various health and wellness issues. Post these fact sheets on the bulletin board for others to read.

UNIT II

Administrative

5. Describe how to contact emergency services by phone and direct them to the caller's location.

_____

_____

_____

_____

6. What is the purpose of an automatic routing unit?

_____

_____

_____

_____

Critical Thinking

1. A geriatric gentleman, identifying himself as Dr. Brine, is calling for the laboratory results on Nancy Chambers. You do not recognize the name of this physician as a local provider. How do you handle this call?

_____

_____

_____

_____

2. For the following phone calls, provide the action to be taken as well as who may handle the call (medical assistant – MA; nurse – RN; office manager – OM; doctor – DR): EXAMPLE: Patient looking for results of her throat culture: (Answer) Provide results, if available, to patient (MA, RN, DR).

   a. patient asking to speak with the doctor but will not leave his name

   _____

   _____

   _____

   _____

b. physician's husband calling to speak with her

_____

_____

_____

_____

c. patient calling for a refill on her Ventolin

_____

_____

_____

_____

d. patient calling for an appointment

_____

_____

_____

_____

e. patient calling about her bill

_____

_____

_____

_____

f. pharmaceutical representative calling to speak with the physician

_____

_____

_____

_____

g. hospital administrator calling to speak with the physician

_____

_____

_____

_____

h. insurance company calling with a question on a claim

_____

_____

_____

_____

i. hematology laboratory calling with a critical result on a patient

_____

_____

_____

_____

Teamwork Exercises

1. In groups of two, using telephones if possible, role-play the following scenarios.

   • A patient calls looking for the results of blood work that was just drawn that morning.

   • The medical assistant from Dr. Barry's office is calling looking for more information on a patient that your office referred them to.

   • The microbiology supervisor is calling to give the physician a STAT result from a cerebral spinal fluid analysis.

   • A new patient is calling for an appointment.

2. In groups of two or three, discuss some proper and improper phone answering greetings. Each student should explain why he or she thinks the greeting is appropriate or not appropriate.

Instructions for Procedure 11-1

Using the following scenarios for evaluation of Procedure 11-1, or scenarios supplied by your instructor, role-play with another student following the proper telephone techniques as discussed in the textbook:

   • Janice Bellows had just seen the physician this morning and forgot what the doctor told her about her medication and would like to speak with her. Janice is currently at work and can be reached at 306-541-8850.

- Vinny Cardoza, 306-541-6193, is returning a call the nurse practitioner left on his voice mail.

- Daiske Matsuzaka, 306-398-9915, is calling to speak with the billing coordinator to discuss a bill she received for a visit last month. The billing coordinator is not in today.

- The physician is at lunch when the hospital laboratory calls with a question regarding a blood work order on Anna Fleming.

- Gina Lafay, CMA, is currently in an examination room with a patient when her daughter's school calls. The guidance counselor would like to speak with Gina when she becomes available.

- T. J. Malone calls and asks to speak with Dr. Wong. He appears very agitated.

PROCEDURE 11-1 – DEMONSTRATING TELEPHONE TECHNIQUES

Name _____   Date _____   Score _____

Instructor _____

Task
Demonstrate proper telephone answering, screening, and message-taking techniques.

Conditions
Telephone
Message pad
Appointment schedule
Appropriate patient chart
Pen or pencil

Time: _____

Standards
In the time specified and in the scoring parameters of the instructor, the student will demonstrate proper telephone techniques by answering incoming calls, performing patient screening, and taking messages, all in an efficient and professional manner.

Points assigned reflect importance of step to meeting the task

> Important = 1 pt.
> Essential = 5 pts.
> Critical = 15 pts.

Automatic failure results if any of the **CRITICAL TASKS** are omitted or performed incorrectly.

(To use a pass/fail system, instructors can record "P" or "F" in the "points earned (pass/fail)" column.)

PERFORMANCE STANDARDS	PTS	PTS EARNED (Pass/Fail)	COMMENTS
1. Gathers all necessary supplies and have them handy near the telephone area.	5	_____	_____
2. Promptly answers the telephone on third ring.	5	_____	_____
3. Greets caller by identifying office and herself.	15	_____	_____
4. Proceeds to listen to caller, obtains caller's name and reason for the call.	15	_____	_____
5. Directs caller to appropriate person if available; obtain chart if caller is a patient.	5	_____	_____

PERFORMANCE STANDARDS *(cont.)*	PTS	PTS EARNED (Pass/Fail)	COMMENTS
6. Takes message if caller wishes to speak with a person who is not available at the time of the call; taking the following information: Person's/patient's name and contact phone number(s) Date and time of call Detailed message Name or initials of person taking message	15	_____	_____
7. Tells caller that he/she will be giving the message to the appropriate person and explains the office's policy for return calls, if appropriate.	15	_____	_____
8. If call is one that is appropriate for medical assistant to take, the medical assistant performs screening, asking appropriate questions to ensure proper answers.	5	_____	_____
9. If appropriate, asks to put caller on hold, waiting for the caller's answer.	5	_____	_____
10. Obtains answer to caller's question, takes caller off hold, and provides caller with requested information.	5	_____	_____
11. Properly identifies and responds to issues of confidentiality during entire telephone conversation.	5	_____	_____
12. Performs within legal and ethical boundaries during entire telephone conversation.	5	_____	_____
13. If call is patient related, documents phone call in patients chart as necessary.	5	_____	_____
TOTAL POINTS	**105**		

DOCUMENTATION

COMMENTS

Please use the materials below to complete Procedure 11-1.

Phone Message

For: Date: Time:

Name:
Contact information
Phone: ☐ home ☐ work ☐ cell
Fax:
Email:

Message:
_____
_____
_____
_____
_____
_____

Call taken by:
Date: Time :

Phone Message

For: Date: Time:

Name:
Contact information
Phone: ☐ home ☐ work ☐ cell
Fax:
Email:

Message:
_____
_____
_____
_____
_____
_____

Call taken by:
Date: Time :

Phone Message

For: Date: Time:

Name:
Contact information
Phone: ☐ home ☐ work ☐ cell
Fax:
Email:

Message:

_____
_____
_____
_____
_____
_____

Call taken by:
Date: Time :

Phone Message

For: Date: Time:

Name:
Contact information
Phone: ☐ home ☐ work ☐ cell
Fax:
Email:

Message:

_____
_____
_____
_____
_____
_____

Call taken by:
Date: Time :

Phone Message

For: Date: Time:

Name:
Contact information
Phone: ☐home ☐work ☐cell
Fax:
Email:

Message:

_____
_____
_____
_____
_____
_____

Call taken by:
Date: Time :

Phone Message

For: Date: Time:

Name:
Contact information
Phone: ☐home ☐work ☐cell
Fax:
Email:

Message:

_____
_____
_____
_____
_____
_____

Call taken by:
Date: Time :

Appointment Scheduling

Key Term Review

Define the following key terms:

1. triage _____
_____

2. modified wave _____
_____

3. stream scheduling _____
_____

4. cluster booking _____
_____

5. matrix _____
_____

6. catch-up time _____
_____

7. double booking _____
_____

8. wave scheduling _____
_____

9. no-show _____
_____

10. practice-based scheduling _____
_____

Review Questions

1. Discuss the importance that proper scheduling techniques have on quality patient care.

   _____

   _____

   _____

   _____

2. Explain the various types of scheduling methods:

   a. practice based:

   _____

   _____

   _____

   _____

   b. stream:

   _____

   _____

   _____

   _____

   c. cluster booking:

   _____

   _____

   _____

   _____

   d. double booking:

   _____

   _____

   _____

   _____

   e. wave:

   _____

   _____

   _____

   _____

f. modified wave:

_____

_____

_____

_____

g. open hours:

_____

_____

_____

_____

3. Discuss the importance of catch-up time.

_____

_____

_____

_____

4. Describe six considerations in scheduling appointments.

_____

_____

_____

_____

5. Discuss the importance of triage in scheduling appointments.

_____

_____

_____

_____

6. List some questions you would ask when triaging a patient calling for an appointment.

_____

_____

_____

_____

7. List and describe the various scheduling supplies needed in a office.

_____

_____

_____

_____

8. Discuss the importance of printing out a daily appointment worksheet.

_____

_____

_____

_____

9. What are some benefits of computerized scheduling software?

_____

_____

_____

_____

10. What are some reasons patients cancel their appointments? How can you help decrease the rate of cancellations?

_____

_____

_____

_____

11. Describe the appropriate way to handle a patient who has been a "no-show" his last three appointments.

_____

_____

_____

_____

12. Describe the medical assistant's role in processing referral forms.

_____

_____

_____

_____

Critical Thinking

1. Erica Stanhope is the new medical assistant in your office. As the office manager, you have assigned Erica to the reception area, which also includes answering the phones and making appointments. As a patient approaches the reception area, you overhear Erica say to the patient, "Well, how did you manage to get this appointment? We don't normally schedule this procedure at this time of day." How would you handle this situation?

_____

_____

_____

_____

2. As a front office medical assistant responsible for the scheduling, how would you handle the following situations:

   a. Juanita Prezario is calling to cancel her appointment for her physical exam for the second time.

   _____

   _____

   _____

   _____

   b. Donnie Gilrein has not shown up for his 2:15 p.m. appointment.

   _____

   _____

   _____

   _____

   c. Kye Dumas is demanding to switch her appointment from Friday at 3 p.m. to Tuesday at 9 a.m. since she has to work on Friday.

   _____

   _____

   _____

   _____

Teamwork Exercises

Create an appointment matrix and reminder cards for a blood pressure screening at your school. Discuss with your group how many patients can be seen per 15-minute time slot.

Divide the class into three or four teams. Give each team a medical specialty and have them come up with a plan for the optimum way to schedule the types of visits common to each specialty. The groups may have to research their specialty to understand typical procedures and/or patient groups seen by this specialty.

- Pediatrics
- Obstetrics and gynecology
- Orthopedics
- Family practice
- Neurology
- Cardiology
- Dermatology

PROCEDURE 12-1 – CREATING APPOINTMENT CARDS

Name _____   Date _____   Score _____

                                                                 Instructor _____

Task
Create appointment cards and give to five patients at the front desk after scheduling.

Conditions
Computer
Card stock
Scissors or paper cutter
Pen

Time: _____

Standard
In the time specified and within the scoring parameters determined by the instructor, the student will successfully create appointment cards to give to patients during appointment scheduling.

Points assigned reflect importance of step to meeting the task

Important = 1 pt.
Essential = 5 pts.
Critical = 15 pts.

Automatic failure results if any of the **CRITICAL TASKS** are omitted or performed incorrectly.

(To use a pass/fail system, instructors can record "P" or "F" in the "points earned (pass/fail)" column.)

PERFORMANCE STANDARDS	PTS	PTS EARNED (Pass/Fail)	COMMENTS
1. Using the computer, card stock, and scissors, created appointment cards that are the size of a business card.	5	_____	_____ _____
2. Included the following information on each appointment card: **a.** name and telephone number of the practice **b.** line for the patient's name **c.** line to write in the date and time of the appointment	15	_____	_____ _____ _____ _____ _____ _____
3. Printed appointment cards.	5	_____	_____ _____

PERFORMANCE STANDARDS (cont.)	PTS	PTS EARNED (Pass/Fail)	COMMENTS
4. Wrote out an appointment card for patient standing at desk and gave it to the patient.	15	_____	_____ _____

TOTAL POINTS	**40**		

DOCUMENTATION

COMMENTS

To the instructor: This project is created for use with a manual appointment matrix. Instructors can chose to use this project with any computer-based appointment scheduling software. Competency check-off evaluation sheet is available in student workbook as well as editable competency document on the instructor's resource disk. The student-completed appointment matrix and reminder cards are considered work products and should be attached to the competency check-off sheet.

COMPETENCY CHECKLIST

PROCEDURE 12-2 – CREATING AN APPOINTMENT MATRIX AND SCHEDULING APPOINTMENTS USING THE RULES OF TRIAGE

Name _____

Date _____ Score _____

Instructor _____

Task
Create an appointment matrix and manage appointments.

Conditions
Computer and printer
Pen

Time: _____

Standards
In the time specified and within the scoring parameters determined by the instructor, the student will successfully create an appointment matrix and perform scheduling procedures as instructed.

Points assigned reflect importance of step to meeting the task

Important = 1 pt.
Essential = 5 pts.
Critical = 15 pts.

Automatic failure results if any of the **CRITICAL TASKS** are omitted or performed incorrectly.

(To use a pass/fail system, instructors can record "P" or "F" in the "points earned (pass/fail)" column.)

PERFORMANCE STANDARDS	PTS	PTS EARNED (Pass/Fail)	COMMENTS
1. Created an appointment matrix for Drs. Greer, Rodriquez, Wilson, Lee, and Sharon Piecek, APRN, for Monday, Tuesday, and Wednesday. Took all of the appointment requests on Monday. There were appointments already made for Monday. Used the following information when creating the matrix:	15	_____	_____
a. The office is open from 8:30 a.m. to 6 p.m. on Monday, Tuesday, and Thursday.			

PERFORMANCE STANDARDS (cont.)	PTS	PTS EARNED (Pass/Fail)	COMMENTS
b. The office is open from 8:30 a.m. to 4:00 p.m. on Wednesday and Friday.			
c. Create the matrix in 15-minute intervals. Appointments are based on 15-, 30-, 45-, and 60-minute appointments.			
2. Blocked out 1 hour for lunch for each provider.	1	_____	
3. Printed the appointment matrix to use at the front desk.	5	_____	
With role-playing, practiced telephone procedures by taking the following five appointments over the phone.			
1. Candace Burns: flulike symptoms. Prefers to see the nurse practitioner. Wants to come in today.	15	_____	
2. John Howard: new patient, will see any provider. Available mornings, any day.	15	_____	
Took down the following information required for new patients:	15	_____	
Full name Date of birth Daytime phone number or cell phone number Complete address Source of referral (if any) Reason for appointment Insurance coverage			
3. Lynn Littel: sore throat. Patient of Dr. Greer's. Wants to be seen today.	15	_____	
4. Gary O'Neil: new patient, smoking cessation. Patient of Dr. Wilson's. Wants Tuesday afternoon appt.	15	_____	

PERFORMANCE STANDARDS *(cont.)*	PTS	PTS EARNED (Pass/Fail)	COMMENTS
5. Jeff Ramierz: suture removal. Patient of Dr. Rodriguez	15	_____	_____
Role-played using students as five patients at the front desk. Scheduled appointments and created reminder cards, which included the following information:			
Name of provider patient is seeing **Phone number of practice** **Name of patient** **Date and time of appointment**			
1. Cindy Panterella: adult PE. Patient of Sharon Piecek, APRN. Prefers morning appointment.	15	_____	_____
2. Hannah Collins: BP check. Patient of Dr. Lee's. Wants first appointment after lunch physician's lunch hour.	15	_____	_____
3. Sadie Hernandez: cast removal. Patient of Dr. Wilson's.	15	_____	_____
4. Christopher Evans: sports PE, patient of Dr. Greer's.	15	_____	_____
5. Jill Evans: sports PE, patient of Dr. Greer's. Mother wants both appointments on same day.	15	_____	_____
Scheduled phone appointments for the following patients without role-playing:			
1. Habid Bahb: saw physician on Monday for BP medication change, not feeling good, wants to see physician on Wednesday.	15	_____	_____
2. Lilly Miarecki: lower back pain. Patient of Dr. Lee, wants a Tuesday appointment after work.	15	_____	_____
3. Sandro Valencia: follow-up with Dr. Rodriguez, wants a Tuesday appointment.	15	_____	_____

PERFORMANCE STANDARDS (cont.)	PTS	PTS EARNED (Pass/Fail)	COMMENTS
4. Michail Brennan: soccer injury, wants to be seen today (Monday). Patient of nurse practitioner.	15	_____	_____ _____
5. Mia Gowan: fever and swollen glands. Patient of Dr. Wilson's.	15	_____	_____ _____

TOTAL POINTS	261		

DOCUMENTATION

COMMENTS

Monday

Time	Greer	Wilson	Rodriguez	Lee	Piecek
8:00 a.m.					
8:15					
8:30	Sr. Janet Mayes—F/U	OFF	Cheryl Pearl—PE	Alana Nalski—vomiting X3 days	Chuck DeLise— NP PE
8:45	Marc Blais—NP PE			Cathie Nunes—blood work	
9:00 a.m.					
9:15					
9:30					
9:45					
10:00 a.m.					Paul Gomes— glucose check
10:15			Dave Plano – EKG		
10:30					Shakir Vishnu sigmoidoscopy
10:45					
11:00 a.m.	Habid Bahd—BP check				
11:15			J. C. Pastor— dressing change		
11:30					
11:45					
12:00 p.m.					

continued

Monday—*cont'd*

Time	Greer	Wilson	Rodriguez	Lee	Piecek
12:15					
12:30					
12:45					
1:00 p.m.	Qui Lui—blood work			Surgical procedure at hospital	
1:15					
1:30					
1:45					
2:00 p.m.					
2:15					
2:30					
2:45					
3:00 p.m.					
3:15					
3:30					
3:45					
4:00 p.m.					
4:15					
4:30					

Student Activity Manual to Accompany The Professional Medical Assistant

Time	Greer	Wilson	Rodriguez	Lee	Piecek
Monday—*cont'd*					
4:45					
5:00 p.m.					
5:15					
5:30					
5:45					
6:00 p.m.					

Time	Greer	Wilson	Rodriguez	Lee	Piecek
8:00 a.m.					
8:15					
8:30	OFF	Roman Alves—blood work	Darcy Stills—PE	Alicia Commins—medication check	Shayla Nieves—NP PE
8:45		Clint Poui—fever, malaise			
9:00 a.m.		Jay Inez—EKG			
9:15					
9:30					
9:45					
10:00 a.m.					
10:15					
10:30					
10:45					
11:00 a.m.					
11:15					
11:30					
11:45					
12:00 p.m.					
12:15					

Tuesday

Student Activity Manual to Accompany The Professional Medical Assistant

Time	Greer	Wilson	Rodriguez	Lee	Piecek
12:30					
12:45					
1:00 p.m.					
1:15					
1:30					
1:45					
2:00 p.m.					
2:15					
2:30					
2:45					
3:00 p.m.		Brandi Hodgson—post-op check			
3:15					
3:30					
3:45					
4:00 p.m.					
4:15					
4:30					
4:45					

Table title: Tuesday—*cont'd*

continued

Tuesday—*cont'd*					
Time	**Greer**	**Wilson**	**Rodriguez**	**Lee**	**Piecek**
5:00 p.m.					
5:15					
5:30					
5:45					
6:00 p.m.					

Time	Greer	Wilson	Rodriguez	Lee	Piecek
8:00 a.m.					
8:15					
8:30			OFF		Zoe Clarke—PE
8:45	Bryn Viens—NP PE				
9:00 a.m.					
9:15					
9:30					
9:45					
10:00 a.m.		Jamie Choinard—sigmoidoscopy			
10:15					
10:30					
10:45					
11:00 a.m.	Joseph Burke—BP check				
11:15					
11:30					
11:45					
12:00 p.m.					
12:15					

Wednesday

continued

Wednesday—*cont'd*

Time	Greer	Wilson	Rodriguez	Lee	Piecek
12:30					
12:45					
1:00 p.m.					
1:15					
1:30					
1:45					
2:00 p.m.					
2:15					
2:30					
2:45					
3:00 p.m.					
3:15					
3:30					
3:45					
4:00 p.m.					
4:15					
4:30					
4:45					

Wednesday—*cont'd*					
Time	**Greer**	**Wilson**	**Rodriguez**	**Lee**	**Piecek**
5:00 p.m.					
5:15					
5:30					
5:45					
6:00 p.m.					

Appointment Reminder
_____

Has an appointment with
_____

at
_____

If unable to keep this appt., please call:
_____

Appointment Reminder
_____

Has an appointment with
_____

at
_____

If unable to keep this appt., please call:
_____

Appointment Reminder
_____

Has an appointment with
_____

at
_____

If unable to keep this appt., please call:
_____

Appointment Reminder
_____

Has an appointment with
_____

at
_____

If unable to keep this appt., please call:
_____

Appointment Reminder
_____

Has an appointment with
_____

at
_____

If unable to keep this appt., please call:
_____

PROCEDURE 12-3 – DOCUMENTING APPOINTMENT CANCELLATIONS AND NO-SHOWS AND RESCHEDULING APPOINTMENTS

Name _____   Date _____   Score _____

Instructor _____

Task
Document cancellations and no-shows and reschedule appointments.

Conditions
Appointment matrix created for Competency 12-2
Pen

Time: _____

Standards
In the time specified and within the scoring parameters determined by the instructor, the student will successfully document three cancelled appointments and reschedule these appointments and document a no-show appointment in the appointment matrix and call the no-show patient to reschedule.

Points assigned reflect importance of step to meeting the task

Important = 1 pt.
Essential = 5 pts.
Critical = 15 pts.

Automatic failure results if any of the **CRITICAL TASKS** are omitted or performed incorrectly.

(To use a pass/fail system, instructors can record "P" or "F" in the "points earned (pass/fail)" column.)

PERFORMANCE STANDARDS	PTS	PTS EARNED (Pass/Fail)	COMMENTS
Telephone role-played the following scenarios and documented schedule changes on appointment matrix created for Competency 12-2.			
Scenario 1. Lynn Littel needed to reschedule her Monday appointment for a Wednesday afternoon appointment.			
1. Marked Ms. Littel's appointment as cancelled in the appointment matrix and rescheduled her appointment.	15	_____	
2. Repeated the new date and time of the appointment to Ms. Littel.	5	_____	

PERFORMANCE STANDARDS _(cont.)_	PTS	PTS EARNED (Pass/Fail)	COMMENTS
Scenario 2. Shakir Vishnu called to reschedule his sigmoidoscopy with the nurse practitioner. He wanted to reschedule it for Wednesday afternoon.			_____ _____ _____
3. Marked Mr. Vishnu's appointment as cancelled in the appointment matrix and rescheduled his appointment.	15	_____	_____ _____
4. Repeated the new date and time of the appointment to Mr. Vishnu.	5	_____	_____ _____
Scenario 3. J. C. Pastor did not show up for his dressing change scheduled for Monday at 11:15 a.m. with Dr. Rodriguez.			_____ _____ _____
5. Called Mr. Pastor and identified yourself and the practice. Told him that he had an appointment on the date and at the time specified in your appointment matrix.	15	_____	_____ _____ _____
6. Asked him to reschedule. If he chose to do so, rescheduled the appointment.	5	_____	_____ _____
7. Informed him of the no-show policy of the office (if a charge applied to no-show appointments).	15	_____	_____ _____
8. If he chose not to reschedule, told him to call in the future if he needs care from the office.	5	_____	_____ _____
9. Marked the no-show appointment in the matrix.	15	_____	_____ _____
10. Marked the new appointment for Mr. Pastor (if necessary) and added the new patient information for the new appointment.	15	_____	_____ _____

TOTAL POINTS	110		

DOCUMENTATION

_____ | _____
_____ | _____
_____ | _____
_____ | _____

COMMENTS

_____
_____
_____
_____

PROCEDURE 12-4 – SCHEDULING INPATIENT AND OUTPATIENT PROCEDURES

Name _____   Date _____   Score _____

Instructor _____

Tasks
Schedule a patient for one inpatient and two outpatient procedures using the physician's orders and obtain proper precertification and referrals.

Conditions
Physician's orders
Two copies of a blank referral form
Hospital precertification form
Patient's medical record (office notes)
Reminder card
Pen

Time: _____

Standards
In the time specified and within the scoring parameters determined by the instructor, the student will successfully complete a referral form for hospital admission precertification and outpatient specialty referrals and schedule related procedures.

Points assigned reflect importance of step to meeting the task

Important = 1 pt.
Essential = 5 pts.
Critical = 15 pts.

Automatic failure results if any of the **CRITICAL TASKS** are omitted or performed incorrectly.

(To use a pass/fail system, instructors can record "P" or "F" in the "points earned (pass/fail)" column.)

PERFORMANCE STANDARDS	PTS	PTS EARNED (Pass/Fail)	COMMENTS
1. Made an extra copy of the blank referral.	1	_____	_____ _____
MRI referral			_____
2. Called the patient's insurance carrier for referral approval and a referral number.	15	_____	_____ _____
3. Using the information gathered from the order, the photocopy of her insurance card, the patient's office notes, and the insurance phone call, completed the referral form for an MRI scan.	15	_____	_____ _____ _____ _____
4. Checked the referral for spelling and completeness.	5	_____	_____ _____

PERFORMANCE STANDARDS (cont.)	PTS	PTS EARNED (Pass/Fail)	COMMENTS
5. Called the MRI scheduler with the patient at the desk and coordinated between the hospital's schedule and the patient.	5	_____	_____ _____
6. Gave patient a reminder card with the scheduled appointment.	1	_____	_____ _____
7. Asked patient if she needed directions to the MRI facility and provided them as needed.	1	_____	_____ _____ _____
Arthroscopic surgery precertification			
8. Referred to treatment notes from 10/03/08.	5	_____	_____ _____
9. Called the patient's insurance carrier for precertification.	15	_____	_____ _____
10. Using the necessary documentation, completed the hospital precertification for surgery, being sure to include a precertification number.	15	_____	_____ _____ _____
11. Checked the precertification for completeness and accuracy.	5	_____	_____ _____
12. Scheduled the surgery with the patient and the hospital scheduler.	5	_____	_____ _____
Physical therapy referral			
13. Referred to the patient's office notes from 10/14/08, postsurgical check up.	5	_____	_____ _____
14. Referred to the second outpatient services referral form for the patient's postsurgical care.	5	_____	_____ _____ _____
15. Using the physician's orders, operative notes, and treatment notes, completed the referral form for physical therapy, being sure to check for completeness and accuracy.	15	_____	_____ _____ _____ _____

PERFORMANCE STANDARDS (cont.)	PTS	PTS EARNED (Pass/Fail)	COMMENTS
16. Called the PT office to schedule the first PT visit while the patient is present.	5	_____	_____ _____
17. Documented all procedures and field forms in patient's chart	15	_____	_____ _____

TOTAL POINTS	133		

DOCUMENTATION

COMMENTS

Written Office Communications and Mail

Key Term Review   *Define the following key terms:*

1.   dictation   _____

_____

2.   transcription   _____

_____

3.   business letter   _____

_____

4. internal marketing   _____

_____

5.   proofreading   _____

_____

6.   summary of care   _____

_____

Review Questions

1. Describe three reasons why a medical assistant may need to write a professional letter.

_____

_____

_____

_____

2. List and describe the four basic letter styles that may be used in the medical office.

_____

_____

_____

_____

3. Besides patient letters, what other types of letters might a medical office send?

_____

_____

_____

_____

4. Provide the purpose of the following parts to a professional letter:

a. salutation

_____

_____

_____

_____

b. body

_____

_____

_____

_____

c. attention line

_____

_____

_____

_____

d. enclosure notation

_____

_____

_____

_____

e. reference notation

_____

_____

_____

_____

5. Provide the correct abbreviations for the following states:

a. Alaska

_____

_____

_____

_____

b. Montana

_____

_____

_____

_____

c. New York

_____

_____

_____

_____

d. Vermont

_____

_____

_____

_____

e. Utah

_____

_____

_____

_____

f. Maryland

_____
_____
_____
_____

g. Maine

_____
_____
_____
_____

h. Hawaii

_____
_____
_____
_____

6. For which office communication circumstances are a postcard appropriate?

_____
_____
_____
_____

7. What are some important things to take into consideration when faxing medical documents?

_____
_____
_____
_____

8. Discuss the importance of internal marketing for a medical office.

_____
_____
_____
_____

9. What are some important guidelines to consider when sending emails?

_____

_____

_____

_____

10. List and describe eight types of incoming mail that the medical assistant may handle.

_____

_____

_____

_____

11. Compare and contrast certified, registered, and restricted delivery mail.

_____

_____

_____

_____

12. What is the difference between first-, second-, third-, and fourth-class mail. Give an example of each type.

_____

_____

_____

_____

13. Identify with a "c" which of the following words are spelled correctly and an "i" for the words that are spelled incorrectly. For the words spelled incorrectly, write the correct spelling.

   a. ischimum

_____

_____

_____

_____

b. vaccine

_____

_____

_____

_____

c. capillary

_____

_____

_____

_____

d. abcess

_____

_____

_____

_____

e. anurysm

_____

_____

_____

_____

f. chancre

_____

_____

_____

_____

g. epididimis

_____

_____

_____

_____

h. occlusion

_____

_____

_____

_____

i. hemorrhoid

_____

_____

_____

_____

j. asthma

_____

_____

_____

_____

k. benign

_____

_____

_____

_____

l. dessication

_____

_____

_____

_____

m. parenteral

_____

_____

_____

_____

n. humurus

_____

_____

_____

_____

o. dissect

_____

_____

_____

_____

Critical Thinking

1. Sophia Ivanov is a new medical assistant in your office. With English as her second language, she is having a difficult time with her work emails and is often confused by responses sent back to her. What advice can you give Sophia regarding tone and impressions made from electronic communication?

_____

_____

_____

_____

2. Proofread the following letter for grammatical and format errors as well as professionalism. On a separate piece of paper, rewrite the letter making the proper corrections.

_____

_____

_____

_____

BAYBRIDGE ORTHOPEDIC GROUP
213 HAMILTON ROAD, OXFORD, MA 01540

Dr. Robert Giordano, MD
100 South Street
Webster, MA 01570

January 23,2009

Dear Bob,

I'd like to thank you very very much for your consideration in refering Maggie D'Toro to the Baybbridge Orthopedic Group. It was confirmed via MRI that Maggie has torn her ACL and is scheduled to undergo reconstruction surgery to be scheduled on February 2, 2009.

Upon post-operative, follow-up care provided by me, I told Maggie to return to your care as her primery care provider.

Thank you again for your referral. I look forward to seeing you on the golf course soon!

Cheryl

Cheryl Baker, MD

Teamwork Exercises

1. Divide the class into teams of three or four. Each team will chose a different office specialty and then develop various ideas for marketing their office. Based on the ideas developed, each team will create one marketing piece to share with the class.

2. Pair up with a fellow student. Take turns listening to transcription tapes and transcribing what is being said. Proofread each other's transcribed documents and make corrections, suggestions, as needed.

Instructions for Procedure 13-1

Using the sample letter from the insurance company requesting additional information on a claim sent by Dr. Lee's office, and abstracting information from Jimmy Miarecki's treatment notes, create a response letter that provides the information requested by the insurance company.

Valley Health Insurance Company
327 Maple Street
Belmont, CT 03219

December 15, 2008

Dear Dr. Lee,

We received your claims for services provided to Jimmy Miarecki on October 28, 2008 and October 30, 2008. The claim states the following services were rendered:

10/28/2008 – office visit
10/28/2008 – diagnostic testing
10/28/2008 – therapeutic treatment
10/30/2008 – office visit
10/30/2008 – diagnostic testing

In order to process these claims, we need additional information, including treatment notes on the patient and clinical diagnosis.

Please supply this information by November 30, 2008 or the claim will be denied.

Sincerely,

Janet G. Veloz

Janet G. Veloz
Director of Claims

PROCEDURE 13-1 – RESPONDING TO WRITTEN COMMUNICATIONS

Name _____   Date _____   Score _____

                                          Instructor _____

Task
Respond to a written communication.

Conditions
Correspondence from an outside party
Patient chart
Paper
Computer

Time: _____

Standard
In the time specified and within scoring parameters determined by the instructor, the student will success-fully respond to written correspondence by creating a response letter.

Points assigned reflect importance of step to meeting the task

Important = 1 pt.
Essential = 5 pts.
Critical = 15 pts.

Automatic failure results if any of the **CRITICAL TASKS** are omitted or performed incorrectly.

(To use a pass/fail system, instructors can record "P" or "F" in the "points earned (pass/fail)" column.)

PERFORMANCE STANDARDS	PTS	PTS EARNED (Pass/Fail)	COMMENTS
1. Read the correspondence received by the office from an outside party.	5	_____	_____
2. Chose the appropriate letter style for the required response.	5	_____	_____
3. Constructed a response letter. Used information from the patient's chart as well as appropriate language, grammar, and spelling.	15	_____	_____
4. Proofread the letter.	15	_____	_____
5. Placed the letter on the physician's (instructor's) desk for her review and signature.	5	_____	_____

PERFORMANCE STANDARDS (cont.)	PTS	PTS EARNED (Pass/Fail)	COMMENTS
6. Photocopied the signed letter and put a copy in the patient's chart.	1	_____	_____ _____
7. Using the computer and printer, addressed the envelope and indicated on the envelope the amount of postage that you would affix in the correct area for postage.	5	_____	_____ _____ _____ _____

TOTAL POINTS	51		

DOCUMENTATION

COMMENTS

_____

_____

_____

_____

Instructions for Procedure 13-2

Create a thank-you letter to be sent to Dr. Giordano for referring E. J. Bruschi to the Baybridge Orthopedic Group.

PROCEDURE 13-2 – INITIATING WRITTEN COMMUNICATIONS

Name _____   Date _____   Score _____

Instructor _____

Task

Initiate a written letter thanking a physician for a patient referral.

Conditions

Patient chart
Paper
Computer

Time: _____

Standard

In the time specified and within the scoring parameters determined by the instructor, the student will successfully initiate written correspondence relating to patient care.

Points assigned reflect importance of step to meeting the task

Important = 1 pt.
Essential = 5 pts.
Critical = 15 pts.

Automatic failure results if any of the **CRITICAL TASKS** are omitted or performed incorrectly.

(To use a pass/fail system, instructors can record "P" or "F" in the "points earned (pass/fail)" column.)

PERFORMANCE STANDARDS	PTS	PTS EARNED (Pass/Fail)	COMMENTS
1. Referred to the patient's chart, as needed.	5	_____	_____ _____
2. Chose the appropriate letter style for the required correspondence.	1	_____	_____ _____
3. Constructed a letter thanking a physician for a patient referral, using appropriate language, grammar, and spelling.	15	_____	_____ _____ _____
4. Proofread the letter.	15	_____	_____
5. Placed the letter on the physician's (instructor's) desk for her review and signature.	5	_____	_____ _____

TOTAL POINTS	41		

DOCUMENTATION

COMMENTS

Medical Records Management

Key Term Review   *Define the following key terms:*

1. **tickler file** _____

2. **consecutive filing** filing system that uses sequential numbers to order medical records.

3. **unit** Each part of a patients name or i.d. number used in a filing system.

4. **terminal digit filing** System that uses the last digits of an id. number as the primary indexing unit.

5. **middle digit filing** Numeric system that uses the middle digits of the i.d. number as the primary indexing unit.

6. **purging** permanent removal of medical records that are no longer in use.

7. **accession record** record of numbers assigned to each new patient record.

8. **cross reference** guide placed where a medical record could be misfiled to indicate the correct location of the file.

9. **out guide** Marker used to indicate that a medical record has been taken from the filing system.

10. **archives** Storage place for records that are no longer in use but are kept for legal purposes.

Review Questions

1. List and discuss the equipment and supplies necessary for a filing system.

   Fasteners are used to secure papers.
   Tabs are a small section of the folder that projects beyond the other
   side of the folder. Units are any portion of a persons name,
   accession number, or other numerical filing designation used to order
   and identify the medical record.

2. A well-organized, easy-to-use record-management system includes rules for:

   _____

   _____

   _____

   _____

3. Discuss the four basic forms of filing.

   _____

   _____

   _____

   _____

4. Using the color key on page 177 in your textbook, list the color tabs that would be used for the following list of patients:

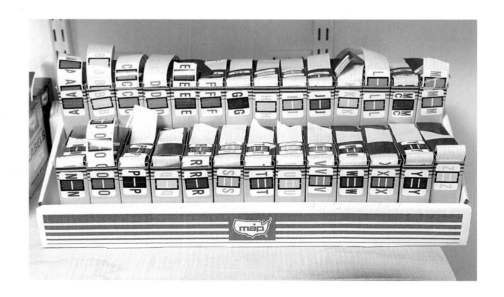

2. Numeric filing: File the following numbers in consecutive, middle digit, and terminal digit order.

	Consecutive Filing Order	Middle Digit Order	Terminal Digit Order
72 37 02			
70 37 10			
71 36 10			
70 36 09			
71 35 08			
71 37 11			
71 35 18			
72 34 18			
72 37 08			
70 35 07			

Teamwork Exercise

1. Divide into groups of three or four students. Read and discuss the following scenario, and then as a group answer the questions regarding the scenario. Finally, come together as a class, and discuss each group's answers.

    You've noticed that the newly hired CMA, Janice, has been misfiling patient charts. The rest of the staff has noticed as well and begin to complain about Janice. Your office manager asks you to help Janice with the proper procedures for filing.

Questions regarding the scenario:

    How you would go about this?
    What teamwork skills would you use?

2. Divide into groups of two or three. Your instructor will provide each group with supplies to make patient charts. Discuss as a group how to organize and establish a patient chart. Each student in the group will make a file on him- or herself. Once all charts have been created for each group, make the charts accessible for all students to practice their filing techniques.

PROCEDURE 14-1 – CREATING AND FILING A MEDICAL RECORD

Name _____   Date _____   Score _____

                                           Instructor _____

Task
Create a medical record and file it using alphabetical filing rules.

Conditions
File folder
Colored letter labels
Patient intake form
Signed HIPAA statement
Pen
Other stickers (provided by the instructor, such as allergy indicators)

Time: _____

Standards
In the time specified by the instructor, create a medical record and file it in an alphabetical file with classmates' medical records.

Points assigned reflect importance of step to meeting the task

Important = 1 pt.
Essential = 5 pts.
Critical = 15 pts.

Automatic failure results if any of the **CRITICAL TASKS** are omitted or performed incorrectly.

(To use a pass/fail system, instructors can record "P" or "F" in the "points earned (pass/fail)" column.)

PERFORMANCE STANDARDS	PTS	PTS EARNED (Pass/Fail)	COMMENTS
1. Filled out the patient intake form.	1	_____	_____
2. Explained the HIPAA information to a patient and had the patient sign a signature on the HIPAA form to indicate that the patient had received, read, and understood the document.	5	_____	_____
3. Inserted the patient intake form into the medical record by using the fastener to attach it to the right inside of the medical record.	1	_____	_____
4. Placed the correct colored letter labels on the outside right edge of the folder, folding the sticker over the edge.	1	_____	_____

PERFORMANCE STANDARDS *(cont.)*	PTS	PTS EARNED (Pass/Fail)	COMMENTS
5. Placed the allergy alert, insurance, or physician labels on the outside of the folder as indicated by your instructor.	1	_____	_____ _____ _____
6. Accurately filed patient file in filing cabinet.	15	_____	_____ _____

TOTAL POINTS	24		

DOCUMENTATION

COMMENTS

_____

_____

_____

_____

Office Management

CHAPTER 15

Key Term Review *Define the following key terms:*

1. policies and procedures manual

2. job description

3. agenda

4. internal marketing

5. external marketing

6. brainstorming

7. cross-training

8. constructive criticism

Review Questions

1. List six responsibilities of an office manager:

   _____

   _____

   _____

   _____

2. Compare and contrast the roles of an office manager with those of a human resource director.

   _____

   _____

   _____

   _____

3. What are some qualities of a good office manager?

   _____

   _____

   _____

   _____

4. What are some pertinent questions to ask a prospective employee during an interview?

   _____

   _____

   _____

   _____

5. What are some questions you are not allowed to ask a job applicant during an interview?

   _____

   _____

   _____

   _____

6. Compare and contrast an office policy with an office procedure.

_____

_____

_____

_____

7. What is the purpose of conducting routine staff meetings in the medical office?

_____

_____

_____

_____

8. Discuss the importance of working as a team. What makes a team work well together?

_____

_____

_____

_____

Critical Thinking

1. As the office manager for your facility, you are responsible for interviewing and hiring new staff. You just interviewed Peg Brunell for a clinical medical assisting position. You are about to call the office manager at her last place of employment, whom Peg has given you as a reference. What kind of questions will you ask?

_____

_____

_____

_____

2. Develop a job description for the following medical office positions:

   a. clinical medical assistant

_____

_____

_____

_____

b. administrative medical assistant

_____

_____

_____

_____

c. billing clerk

_____

_____

_____

_____

d. privacy compliance officer

_____

_____

_____

_____

Teamwork Exercises

1. Emily Mazar is due for her 6-month employee evaluation. She was hired upon graduating with her medical assisting degree. You have seen an improvement in her skills but observed that she still has difficulty with working efficiently. With a classmate, role-play the employee evaluation.

2. With a classmate, role-play interview techniques/questions for the following positions:

   - clinical medical assistant
   - billing coordinator

PROCEDURE 15-1 – TRAINING NEW PERSONNEL USING THE POLICIES AND PROCEDURES MANUAL

Name _____ Date _____ Score _____

Instructor _____

Task
Orient new personnel to the information contained in the policies and procedures manual.

Conditions
Policies and procedures manual
New employee personnel file

Time: _____

Standard
In the time specified and within the scoring parameters determined by the instructor, the student will successfully train new personnel using the policies and procedures manual.

Points assigned reflect importance of step to meeting the task

Important = 1 pt.
Essential = 5 pts.
Critical = 15 pts.

Automatic failure results if any of the **CRITICAL TASKS** are omitted or performed incorrectly.

(To use a pass/fail system, instructors can record "P" or "F" in the "points earned (pass/fail)" column.)

PERFORMANCE STANDARDS	PTS	PTS EARNED (Pass/Fail)	COMMENTS
1. Role-played the supervisor and then the new employee with a classmate. The new employee read a section of the policies and procedures manual. The supervisor then answered questions posed by the new employee. The supervisor ensured that the new employee understood the policies and procedures by asking questions.	15	_____	
2. Asked the new employee to read a section of the policies and procedures manual (as directed by the instructor).	15	_____	
3. Asked the new employee to relate the policy and procedure outlined and give a rationale for the item.	5	_____	

PERFORMANCE STANDARDS (cont.)	PTS	PTS EARNED (Pass/Fail)	COMMENTS
4. Gave the new employee an opportunity to ask questions.	5	_____	_____ _____
5. Answered the employee's questions and was sure to ask if the explanation was clear.	5	_____	_____ _____ _____
6. Asked the new employee to sign a statement in her personnel file to indicate that she had read and understood the policies and procedures manual (or designated section).	15	_____	_____ _____ _____ _____

TOTAL POINTS	60		

DOCUMENTATION

COMMENTS

PROCEDURE 15-2 – TAKING AND REORDERING INVENTORY, PERFORMING MAINTENANCE, AND CHECKING SAFETY

Name _____   Date _____   Score _____

Instructor _____

Tasks
Take an inventory of equipment and supplies and reorder supplies, perform routine equipment maintenance, and check laboratory safety.

Conditions
Various equipment and supplies in the classroom and laboratory
Inventory log
Reorder form
Equipment safety and maintenance instructions (provided by the manufacturer)
Equipment quality-control log
Pen

Time: _____

Standards
In the time specified and within the scoring parameters determined by the instructor, the student will successfully perform an inventory of equipment and supplies in the classroom and laboratory, fill out the reorder form, perform routine maintenance on equipment as directed by the instructor, check the condition of the laboratory and classroom for safety violations, and correct any violations.

Points assigned reflect importance of step to meeting the task

Important = 1 pt.
Essential = 5 pts.
Critical = 15 pts.

Automatic failure results if any of the **CRITICAL TASKS** are omitted or performed incorrectly.

(To use a pass/fail system, instructors can record "P" or "F" in the "points earned (pass/fail)" column.)

PERFORMANCE STANDARDS	PTS	PTS EARNED (Pass/Fail)	COMMENTS
1. Using the inventory log and reorder form, counted supplies and equipment and noted items that need to be reordered. Was sure to check the contents of open packages.	15	_____	_____
2. Inspected the equipment for missing or broken parts, frayed electrical cords, or other safety hazards.	1	_____	_____
3. Reported the condition of the equipment, noting the serial number on each item. Equipment to examine included: **a.** autoclave	15	_____	_____

PERFORMANCE STANDARDS (cont.)	PTS	PTS EARNED (Pass/Fail)	COMMENTS
b. ECG machine			_____
c. computers			_____
d. height and weight scale			_____
e. wall-mounted sphygmo-manometer (blood pressure cuff)			_____
f. wall-mounted ophthalmoscope/otoscope unit			_____
g. glucometer			_____
h. cholesterol meter			_____
4. Ran a quality-control check on a machine (as directed by your instructor). Filled out the results in the quality-control log. Dated and initialed your work.	15	_____	_____ _____ _____
5. Cleaned the autoclave as directed by the manufacturer's instruction manual.	15	_____	_____ _____
6. Checked the entire laboratory for safety hazards and marked the laboratory safety inspection sheet. Was sure to inspect:	15	_____	_____ _____
a. electrical cords for fraying or malfunctioning			_____
b. electrical outlets for loose covers or damage			_____
c. computer keyboards, monitors, towers, other components, and wiring			_____
d. light sources and rechargeable batteries			_____
e. ECG leads and wires			_____
f. other equipment (as directed by the instructor)			_____
7. Initiated repairs to the equipment (as directed by the instructor).	15	_____	_____ _____

TOTAL POINTS	91		

DOCUMENTATION

COMMENTS

PROCEDURE 15-3 – PREPARING PHYSICIAN TRAVEL

Name _____   Date _____   Score _____

Instructor _____

Task

Prepare the physician's itinerary for travel arrangements, hotel and rental car reservations, and seminar registration.

Conditions

Computer with access to the Internet
Physician or company credit card

Time: _____

Standard

In the time specified and within the scoring parameters determined by the instructor, the student will successfully arrange travel plans for the physician, including travel arrangements, hotel and rental car reservations, and seminar registration.

Points assigned reflect importance of step to meeting the task

Important = 1 pt.
Essential = 5 pts.
Critical = 15 pts.

Automatic failure results if any of the **CRITICAL TASKS** are omitted or performed incorrectly

(To use a pass/fail system, Instructors can record "P" or "F" in the "points earned (pass/fail)" column.)

PERFORMANCE STANDARDS	PTS	PTS EARNED (Pass/Fail)	COMMENTS
1. Discussed with the physician what city she needs to fly to, the dates of the flight, and her preference for rental car, plane seating, and hotel accommodations.	15	_____	_____ _____ _____
2. Researched flights from your local airport to the destination.	15	_____	_____ _____
3. Researched hotels that are near the seminar and that meet the physician's criteria.	15	_____	_____ _____
4. Found a rental car at the destination airport that meets the physician's criteria.	15	_____	_____ _____

PERFORMANCE STANDARDS *(cont.)*	PTS	PTS EARNED (Pass/Fail)	COMMENTS
5. Printed the travel information and confirmed it with the physician.	15	_____	_____ _____
6. Created a confirmation notification for the physician that confirms travel reservations.	5	_____	_____ _____

TOTAL POINTS	80		

DOCUMENTATION

COMMENTS

_____
_____
_____
_____

Key Term Review   *Define the following key terms:*

1. capitation

2. demographics

3. write-off

4. modifier

5. PPO

6. *Current Procedural Terminology,* 4th edition

7. referral

8. beneficiary

9. superbill

10. coordination of benefits

11. benefit year

Key Term Review *cont.*

12. utilization review _____

_____

13. premium _____

_____

14. copayment _____

_____

15. upcode _____

_____

16. policyholder _____

_____

17. registration _____

_____

18. fee for service _____

_____

19. verification _____

_____

20. birthday rule _____

_____

Review Questions

1. What is the medical assistant's role in accurate claims filing?

_____

_____

_____

_____

2. What is the purpose of the CMS-1500 form?

_____

_____

_____

_____

3. Discuss the purpose of the CPT-4 coding system.

_____

_____

_____

_____

4. List the six sections of category I codes in the CPT manual.

_____

_____

_____

_____

5. Which CPT codes are used to describe physician services?

_____

_____

_____

_____

6. What is the purpose of Category II codes?

_____

_____

_____

_____

7. What is the purpose of Category III codes?

_____

_____

_____

_____

8. Explain the use of CPT modifiers.

_____

_____

_____

_____

9. In what types of situation are HCPCS codes used?

_____

_____

_____

_____

10. Which system is used to code diagnoses?

_____

_____

_____

_____

11. Explain why it is important that diagnosis codes support the procedural codes when filing a patient claim.

_____

_____

_____

_____

12. List the various volumes associated with the ICD9-CM code book and describe what is included in each volume.

_____

_____

_____

_____

13. Explain the purpose of V codes and provide an example of when a V code would be used.

_____

_____

_____

_____

14. Explain the purpose of E codes and provide an example of when an E code would be used.

_____

_____

_____

_____

15. How should a medical assistant code multiple diagnoses on a CMS-1500 form?

_____

_____

_____

_____

16. Discuss the changes that will occur when the ICD-9-CM system converts to the ICD-10 system.

_____

_____

_____

_____

17. What is the importance of the superbill, and how is it used in a medical office?

_____

_____

_____

_____

18. Explain what methods managed care utilizes to provide health insurance while controlling costs.

_____

_____

_____

_____

19. Discuss the importance of utilization review procedures.

_____

_____

_____

_____

20. Describe how an HMO works.

_____

_____

_____

_____

21. List the three types of managed care health plan models.

_____

_____

_____

_____

22. How does traditional insurance differ from managed care plans?

_____

_____

_____

_____

23. How does a consumer-driven health plan work?

_____

_____

_____

_____

24. Compare and contrast HSAs with HRAs.

_____

_____

_____

_____

25. Discuss the specifics of the Medicare program.

_____

_____

_____

_____

26. List 10 services Medicaid must cover.

_____

_____

_____

_____

27. Compare and contrast CHAMPUS with CHAMPVA.

_____

_____

_____

_____

28. How does Worker's Compensation operate?

_____

_____

_____

_____

29. Explain the procedure for billing a patient who has multiple coverage.

_____

_____

_____

_____

30. What is the purpose of the Consolidated Omnibus Budget Reconciliation Act of 1986?

_____

_____

_____

_____

Coding Review

Match the modifier with its corresponding service:

Modifier

1. 21 _____
2. 22 _____
3. 23 _____
4. 26 _____
5. 32 _____
6. 47 _____
7. 50 _____
8. 52 _____
9. 53 _____
10. 55 _____
11. 57 _____
12. 76 _____
13. 80 _____
14. 91 _____
15. 99 _____

Service/Procedure

a. mandated services

b. repeat clinical diagnostic laboratory test

c. anesthesia by surgeon

d. repeat procedure by same physician

e. unusual anesthesia

f. reduced services

g. prolonged EM services

h. professional component

i. assistant surgeon

j. decision for surgery

k. bilateral procedure

l. d/c procedure

m. unusual procedural services

n. post-op management only

o. multiple modifiers

ICD-9-CM Coding Exercise

Using an ICD-9-CM coding book, code the following conditions:

1. pesticide dust inhalation _____

2. acute cholecystitis _____

3. routine Pap exam _____

4. well baby check _____

5. fatigue _____

6. nausea/vomiting, unknown cause _____

7. senile dementia _____

8. symptomatic HIV _____

9. iron deficiency anemia due
   to blood loss _____

10. acute alcoholic hepatitis _____

11. benign essential hypertension _____

12. history of thrombophlebitis _____

13. deviated septum _____

14. flat feet _____

15. ACL tear with medial meniscus
    of left knee _____

16. ingrown toenail _____

17. acne vulgaris _____

18. MMR vaccination _____

19. renal insufficiency _____

20. family history of mental
    retardation _____

CPT Coding Exercise

Using a CPT-4 coding book, code the following procedures:

1. established outpatient visit _____

2. fitting of contact lenses with medical supervision _____

3. ova and parasite study on stool _____

4. blood typing for paternity testing _____

5. transvaginal ultrasound _____

6. ACL reconstruction with allograft _____

7. entire spine survey, AP and lateral _____

8. otoplasty _____

9. neurofibromatosis with glaucoma _____

10. ventriculoperitoneal shunt _____

11. excision of brain tumor, temporal lobe _____

12. abdominal hysterectomy _____

13. postpartum care _____

14. subtotal suprapubic prostatectomy _____

15. tonsillectomy 8-year-old girl _____

16. comprehensive history, detailed exam, moderate medical decision making _____

17. rapid streptococcal test for strep throat _____

18. nasal septum button _____

19. MRI left knee _____

20. closed reduction and 11/2 hip spica cast application _____

Critical Thinking

1. As the billing and coding coordinator of your facility, you've noticed one employee who consistently upcodes procedures. When you bring it to her attention, she states, "This is how we did it an my former office." How do you respond to her? What training would you provide this employee?

   _____

   _____

   _____

   _____

2. Mrs. Szantyr calls your office, her primary care provider, complaining about a bill she received from her consult with an orthopedic surgeon. When you retrieve her file, you notice that Dr. Greer did not refer her to an orthopedic office and instead prescribed physical therapy for the patient. Explain to Mrs. Szantyr how the referral process works with her insurance company and why she received a bill.

   _____

   _____

   _____

   _____

Teamwork Exercises

1. Divide into groups of two or threee. Work together on the following CPT and ICD-9 coding exercises. Talk through each code to see which one best fits the scenario. Compare your group's results with the rest of the class.

2. Divide into groups of two or three. Your instructor will assign each group one of the following types of health insurance. Each group will develop a fact sheet on its assigned insurance. Information on the fact sheet should include type of coverage, covered services, copayment (if any), specific procedures not covered, preexisting conditions not covered (if any), medication benefits, inpatient benefits, and outpatient benefits.

   a. Medicare

   b. Medicaid

c. COBRA

d. CHAMPUS

e. CHAMPVA

f. Blue Cross/Blue Shield of your state

g. Local HMO

PROCEDURE 16-1 – CODING PROCEDURES AND DIAGNOSES

Name _____   Date _____   Score _____

                                                  Instructor _____

Task
Using a superbill and CPT-4 and ICD-9-CM coding manuals, choose the correct procedural and diagnostic codes for a patient visit and correctly fill out the appropriate fields on the CMS-1500 form.

Conditions
Pen
Superbill
CMS-1500 form (obtained from instructor)
CPT-4 and ICD-9-CM coding manuals

Time: _____

Standards
In the time specified and within the scoring parameters determined by the instructor, the student will accurately choose codes for a patient visit and correctly fill out the appropriate fields on the CMS-1500 form.

Points assigned reflect importance of step to meeting the task

Important = 1 pt.
Essential = 5 pts.
Critical = 15 pts.

Automatic failure results if any of the **CRITICAL TASKS** are omitted or performed incorrectly.

(To use a pass/fail system, instructors can record "P" or "F" in the "points earned (pass/fail)" column.)

PERFORMANCE STANDARDS	PTS	PTS EARNED (Pass/Fail)	COMMENTS
1. Referred to the patient superbill and noted the procedures and diagnosis written by the physician.	5	_____	_____ _____
2. Using the CPT-4 coding manual, assigned the appropriate office visit code, laboratory code, and office surgical procedure code.	15	_____	_____ _____ _____ _____
3. Using the ICD-9-CM coding manual, assigned the appropriate diagnosis codes for the patient. Wrote the procedure and diagnostic codes on the superbill.	15	_____	_____ _____ _____ _____
4. Filled out the appropriate fields on the CMS-1500 form, being sure to link the diagnosis and procedure codes.	15	_____	_____ _____ _____ _____

PERFORMANCE STANDARDS (cont.)	PTS	PTS EARNED (Pass/Fail)	COMMENTS
5. Rechecked the CPT-4 and ICD-9-CM codes against each coding manual.	5	_____	_____ _____

TOTAL POINTS	55		

DOCUMENTATION

COMMENTS

PROCEDURE 16-2 – SUBMITTING A CMS-1500 FORM TO A THIRD-PARTY PAYOR

Name _____   Date _____   Score _____

                                                  Instructor _____

Task

Submit a CMS-1500 form to a third-party payor in electronic or hard-copy format.

Conditions

Patient medical record
Superbill
CMS-1500 forms in printer (for mailed claims)
Computer with CMS-1500 software

Time: _____

Standard

In the time specified and within the scoring parameters determined by the instructor, the student will accurately submit a claim for payment using CMS-1500 compatible software or by referring to the patient's medical record.

Points assigned reflect importance of step to meeting the task

Important = 1 pt.
Essential = 5 pts.
Critical = 15 pts.

Automatic failure results if any of the **CRITICAL TASKS** are omitted or performed incorrectly.

(To use a pass/fail system, instructors can record "P" or "F" in the "points earned (pass/fail)" column.)

PERFORMANCE STANDARDS	PTS	PTS EARNED (Pass/Fail)	COMMENTS
1. Referred to the patient's medical record (containing the patient registration form and photocopy of the patient's insurance card) or the patient database to insert the name, address, telephone number, and insurance information into the CMS form (lines 1 through 13).	15	_____	_____ _____ _____ _____ _____
2. Rechecked all information for accuracy.	5	_____	_____ _____
3. Referred to the superbill to fill out the following lines of the CMS form: **a.** #14—illness (first symptom) OR injury (accident) **b.** #15—date patient has had same or similar illness (if applicable)	15	_____	_____ _____ _____ _____ _____

PERFORMANCE STANDARDS (cont.)	PTS	PTS EARNED (Pass/Fail)	COMMENTS

c. #16—dates unable to work (if applicable) _____

d. #17—referring provider and that providers national provider identification number (NPI) (if applicable) _____

e. #18—dates of hospitalization (if applicable) _____

f. #21—diagnosis code(s), using the ICD-9-CM codes from the superbill (entered the codes in spaces 1, 2, 3, and 4) _____

g. #24 A—date of service _____

h. #24 B—place of service code (The physician's office code is 11.) _____

i. #24 D—CPT codes from the superbill with modifiers (if applicable) _____

j. #24 F—charge for the procedure listed _____

k. #24G—"1" in the days/units column _____

l. #25—federal tax identification number or physician Social Security number (as determined by office policy) _____

m. #26—patient's account number (as designated by the practice) _____

n. #27—check box to accept (yes) or reject (no) assignment, as designated by office policy _____

o. #28—total charges for the procedures entered _____

p. #29—amount paid by the patient (if any) _____

q. #30—balance due _____

r. #31—indication of physician's signature on file _____

s. #33—billing provider name, address, and phone number _____

t. #33 a—physician's NPI _____

4. Saved and printed the claim form.   5   _____   _____

PERFORMANCE STANDARDS (cont.)	PTS	PTS EARNED (Pass/Fail)	COMMENTS
5. Made a copy of the completed form for the patient's medical record.	5	_____	_____
6. If filing the claim electronically, saved the claim and sent it via electronic claims submission protocols. (The password-protected software encrypts the data for secure transmission.) If filing by mail, addressed the envelope to the claims department, enclosed the CMS-1500 form, and sealed the envelope.	15	_____	_____
7. Documented the date of submission of the claim.	1	_____	_____
8. Backed up the data onto a separate data-storage device, such as a USB drive.	1	_____	_____

TOTAL POINTS	62		

DOCUMENTATION

COMMENTS

_____

PROCEDURE 16-3 – COMMUNICATING WITH A THIRD-PARTY PAYOR

Name _____   Date _____   Score _____

Instructor _____

Task
Write a letter to a third-party payor requesting an appeal for a denied claim.

Conditions
Patient medical record
CMS-1500 claim form sent to third-party payor
    for payment
Denial notification from third-party payor
Office letterhead
Computer

Time: _____

Standard
In the time specified and within the scoring parameters determined by the instructor, the student will successfully write a letter of appeal for payment of a denied claim.

Points assigned reflect importance of step to meeting the task

Important = 1 pt.
Essential = 5 pts.
Critical = 15 pts.

Automatic failure results if any of the **CRITICAL TASKS** are omitted or performed incorrectly.

(To use a pass/fail system, instructors can record "P" or "F" in the "points earned (pass/fail)" column.)

PERFORMANCE STANDARDS	PTS	PTS EARNED (Pass/Fail)	COMMENTS
1. Read information from the patient's medical record.	15	_____	_____
2. Reread the CMS-1500 form originally submitted.	15	_____	_____
3. Read the denial notification on the explanation of benefits.	15	_____	_____
4. Composed a letter requesting payment of the claim based on medical necessity as proven by the patient's medical record. Was sure to refute the reasons given for denial of the claim.	15	_____	_____
5. Reprinted the CMS-1500 form.	5	_____	_____

PERFORMANCE STANDARDS (cont.)	PTS	PTS EARNED (Pass/Fail)	COMMENTS
6. Signed the letter and submitted it to the insurance company (your instructor).	5	_____	_____ _____

TOTAL POINTS	70		

DOCUMENTATION

COMMENTS

_____

_____

_____

_____

_____

Billing and Collections

Key Term Review *Define the following key terms:*

1.   monthly billing _____

_____

2.   aging accounts _____

_____

3.   cycle billing _____

_____

4.   cash flow _____

_____

5.   copayments _____

_____

6.   collection agency _____

_____

Review Questions

1. Explain the importance of timely billing and collections in the physician's office.

2. Discuss the medical assistant's role in office billing.

3. Discuss the proper procedure for explaining office fees to patients.

4. List eight items that should be included on a patient's bill.

5. Compare and contrast cycle billing and monthly billing.

6. Discuss the process of aging accounts.

7. Discuss the medical assistant's role in credit and collections.

_____

_____

_____

_____

8. Describe the various options for collecting overdue accounts.

_____

_____

_____

_____

9. What is the proper procedure for telephone collections?

_____

_____

_____

_____

10. Describe the purpose of using a collection agency to collect overdue payments.

_____

_____

_____

_____

Critical Thinking

1. You are the business manager for a newly operating medical clinic. Devise a collections and credit policy for your new office.

_____

_____

_____

_____

2. Come up with some situations in which a medical practice may use a small-claims court to obtain money that is owed.

_____

_____

_____

_____

Teamwork Exercises

1. Divide into groups of three or four. Your instructor will assign one of the following special collection situations for each group to research and report on to the rest of the class.

   a. Patient has died and has an estate.

   b. Patent has filed for bankruptcy.

   c. The statute of limitations for a patient's bill is up.

   d. The patient has moved and has not left a forwarding address.

PROCEDURE 17-1 – EXPLAINING OFFICE FINANCIAL POLICIES TO A PATIENT

Name _____   Date _____   Score _____

Instructor _____

Task
Explain the office financial policies to a new patient.

Conditions
Office brochure
Financial policies document
Patient's medical record

Time: _____

Standard
In the time specified and within the scoring parameters determined by the instructor, the student will successfully explain the financial policies of the office to the patient as outlined in the financial policies document.

Points assigned reflect importance of step to meeting the task

Important = 1 pt.
Essential = 5 pts.
Critical = 15 pts.

Automatic failure results if any of the **CRITICAL TASKS** are omitted or performed incorrectly.

(To use a pass/fail system, instructors can record "P" or "F" in the "points earned (pass/fail)" column.)

PERFORMANCE STANDARDS	PTS	PTS EARNED (Pass/Fail)	COMMENTS
1. Introduced yourself to the patient and asked her to read the office financial policies brochure.	5	_____	_____ _____
2. Asked the patient if she had any questions regarding the office policies listed in the brochure.	5	_____	_____ _____
3. Asked the patient to sign the financial policies document.	15	_____	_____ _____
4. Placed the signed financial policies document in the patient's medical record.	5	_____	_____ _____

TOTAL POINTS	30		

DOCUMENTATION

COMMENTS

© copyright 2009 F.A. Davis Company

PROCEDURE 17-2 – CREATING A COLLECTION LETTER

Name _____   Date _____   Score _____

                                            Instructor _____

Task
Create a collection letter for a past-due account.

Conditions
Record of patient's account
Computer
Office letterhead

Time: _____

Standard
In the time specified and within the scoring parameters determined by the instructor, the student will successfully create a letter to a patient regarding his past-due account.

Points assigned reflect importance of step to meeting the task

Important = 1 pt.
Essential = 5 pts.
Critical = 15 pts.

Automatic failure results if any of the **CRITICAL TASKS** are omitted or performed incorrectly.

(To use a pass/fail system, instructors can record "P" or "F" in the "points earned (pass/fail)" column.)

PERFORMANCE STANDARDS	PTS	PTS EARNED (Pass/Fail)	COMMENTS
1. Referred to the patient's financial account.	5	_____	
2. Determined the appropriate collection agency to use (as provided by your instructor or using your local telephone book).	5	_____	
3. Composed a letter to the patient, explaining that his account will be sent to the collection agency (using name in letter) if it remains unpaid.	15	_____	
4. Made a copy of the letter and placed it in the patient's medical record.	5	_____	

TOTAL POINTS	30		

DOCUMENTATION

COMMENTS

Accounting and Banking

Key Term Review   *Define the following key terms:*

1. financial accounting _____

2. accounts payable _____

_____

3. managerial accounting _____

4. liability _____

_____

5. accounts receivable _____

6. collection ratio _____

_____

7. variable costs _____

_____

8. cost ratio _____

_____

9. fixed costs _____

_____

10. balance sheet _____

_____

Review Questions

1. Explain the two main categories of accounting practices.

_____

_____

_____

_____

2. Does a fixed cost vary by the number of patients being seen in the practice? Explain your answer.

_____

_____

_____

_____

3. Give some examples of fixed costs in the medical office.

_____

_____

_____

_____

4. Compare and contrast fixed costs with variable costs.

_____

_____

_____

_____

5. Describe what happens when the fixed costs per patient declines.

_____

_____

_____

_____

6. Explain what the analysis of finances provides.

_____

_____

_____

_____

7. What can a manager predict from cost analysis?

_____
_____
_____
_____

8. Explain what a balance sheet does.

_____
_____
_____
_____

9. How are insurance reimbursement procedures started?

_____
_____
_____
_____

10. Why should an employee check the items received against the packing slip?

_____
_____
_____
_____

11. List the items to record when writing a check.

_____
_____
_____
_____

12. Explain what the W-4 shows.

_____
_____
_____
_____

13. Explain when and how all federal and state taxes should be paid.

_____

_____

_____

_____

14. Describe the steps to record and deposit money and checks into the practice's checking account.

_____

_____

_____

_____

15. Explain what petty cash is used for.

_____

_____

_____

_____

Critical Thinking Questions

1. Seth Coulter works 40 hours a week, with an hourly rate of $16.40. How much will his gross salary be? One week, Seth works 5 hours of overtime. Calculate his gross salary for this week.

_____

_____

_____

_____

2. As the office manager, the physicians in your group practice want you to research if it is cost effective for the office to provide in-office phlebotomy services to their patients. What are the things you must take into consideration when developing your proposal?

_____

_____

_____

_____

3. Tracey is a medical assisting student externing in your office. She is trying to manually balance a day sheet, and it will not balance out correctly. What suggestions can you give her?

_____

_____

_____

_____

Teamwork Exercises

1. First, as a class, come up with a list of the available medical office software programs currently on the market. Feel free to contact local medical offices to see which software program they are currently employing. Next, divide the class into groups of three to four students and assign each group one of the brands of medical software from the list. Each group will research the software, including its applications, cost, training provided, etc. If from your research there is a local medical office using a group's software, contact them for their input on the user-friendliness and functionality of the software.

2. Two medical offices have a plan to merge into one larger health facility. One office uses manual bookkeeping procedures while the other office uses computerized bookkeeping software. Divide the class into two groups, one being the manual users and the other being the software users. Each group will come up with a proposal as to why their current system of bookkeeping is better and should be used by the new health facility. Both groups will give an oral presentation to the office manager (your instructor).

PROCEDURE 18-1 – POSTING CHARGES, ADJUSTMENTS, AND PAYMENTS AND BALANCING A DAY SHEET

Name _____   Date _____   Score _____

Instructor _____

Tasks

Post charges, adjustments, and payments from an insurance company, patients, and a collection agency to a day sheet, and balance the day sheet.

Conditions

Computer and printer or manual day sheet
Checks (from insurance companies and patients)
Collection agency payment
Pen

Time: _____

Standards

In the time specified and within the scoring parameters determined by the instructor, the student will success-fully post charges, adjustments, and payments and balance a day sheet.

Points assigned reflect importance of step to meeting the task

Important = 1 pt.
Essential = 5 pts.
Critical = 15 pts.

Automatic failure results if any of the **CRITICAL TASKS** are omitted or performed incorrectly.

(To use a pass/fail system, Instructors can record "P" or "F" in the "points earned (pass/fail)" column.)

PERFORMANCE STANDARDS	PTS	PTS EARNED (Pass/Fail)	COMMENTS
1. Posted charges and payments to the ledger cards for these patients, who visited the office on April 22, 2008:	15	_____	
a. Andrew Stevenson came in for an office visit ($40 charge) and paid a $10 copayment in cash.			
b. Jenna Collins came in for an office visit and urinalysis (combined charge of $75) and paid a $15 copayment by check (#534).			
c. Barry Chen came in for an x-ray ($75 charge) and paid a $25 copayment in cash.			
d. John Rivera came in for an office visit and urinalysis and paid a $10 copayment by check (#1766).			
e. Hannah Martin came in for an ECG (charge $105).			

PERFORMANCE STANDARDS (cont.)	PTS	PTS EARNED (Pass/Fail)	COMMENTS
2. Created a computerized day sheet or used a manual day sheet (provided by your instructor).	15	_____	
3. Posted entries on the day sheet according to the activities listed above.	15	_____	
4. Posted the insurance payment from United Health Systems to the day sheet and applied payments to the patient accounts on the ledger cards.	15	_____	
5. Applied the amount allowed from the insurance company's explanation of benefits, adjusting the patient balances to reflect only the amount allowed.	15	_____	
6. Posted the collection agency payment from ACME Collections, Inc., on the patient ledger card and day sheet.	15	_____	
7. Included the following adjustments to the day sheet and the appropriate patient's ledger card: **a.** Hannah Martin—Medicare adjustment $15 **b.** John Rivera—HMO adjustment $15 **c.** Barry Chen—HMO adjustment $47	15	_____	
8. Balanced the day sheet.	15	_____	

TOTAL POINTS	120		

DOCUMENTATION

COMMENTS

Please use the materials below to complete Procedure 18-1.

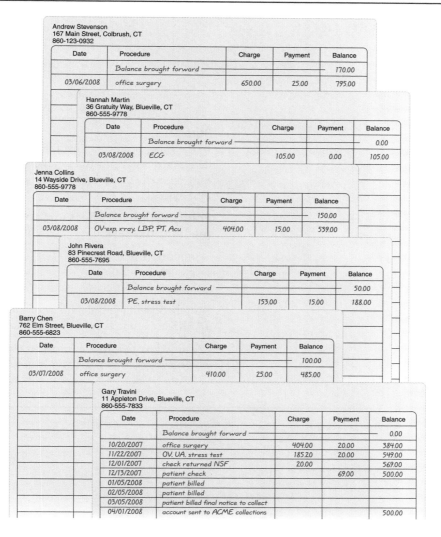

Andrew Stevenson
167 Main Street, Colbrush, CT
860-123-0932

Date	Procedure	Charge	Payment	Balance
	Balance brought forward			170.00
03/06/2008	office surgery	650.00	25.00	795.00

Hannah Martin
36 Gratuity Way, Blueville, CT
860-555-9778

Date	Procedure	Charge	Payment	Balance
	Balance brought forward			0.00
03/08/2008	ECG	105.00	0.00	105.00

Jenna Collins
14 Wayside Drive, Blueville, CT
860-555-9778

Date	Procedure	Charge	Payment	Balance
	Balance brought forward			150.00
03/08/2008	OV-exp. xray. LBP. PT. Acu	404.00	15.00	539.00

John Rivera
83 Pinecrest Road, Blueville, CT
860-555-7695

Date	Procedure	Charge	Payment	Balance
	Balance brought forward			50.00
03/08/2008	PE. stress test	153.00	15.00	188.00

Barry Chen
762 Elm Street, Blueville, CT
860-555-6823

Date	Procedure	Charge	Payment	Balance
	Balance brought forward			100.00
03/07/2008	office surgery	410.00	25.00	485.00

Gary Travini
11 Appleton Drive, Blueville, CT
860-555-7833

Date	Procedure	Charge	Payment	Balance
	Balance brought forward			0.00
10/20/2007	office surgery	404.00	20.00	384.00
11/22/2007	OV. UA. stress test	185.20	20.00	549.00
12/01/2007	check returned NSF	20.00		569.00
12/13/2007	patient check		69.00	500.00
01/05/2008	patient billed			
02/05/2008	patient billed			
03/05/2008	patient billed final notice to collect			
04/01/2008	account sent to ACME collections			500.00

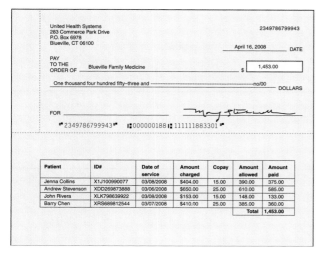

United Health Systems
283 Commerce Park Drive
P.O. Box 6978
Blueville, CT 06100

2349786799943

April 16, 2008   DATE

PAY TO THE ORDER OF   Blueville Family Medicine $ 1,453.00

One thousand four hundred fifty-three and ------------------------------no/00   DOLLARS

FOR

⑈2349786799943⑈ ⑆000000188⑆ 111111883301⑈

Patient	ID#	Date of service	Amount charged	Copay	Amount allowed	Amount paid
Jenna Collins	X1J100990077	03/08/2008	$404.00	15.00	390.00	375.00
Andrew Stevenson	XDD269873888	03/06/2008	$650.00	25.00	610.00	585.00
John Rivera	XLK798639922	03/08/2008	$153.00	15.00	148.00	133.00
Barry Chen	XRS689812544	03/07/2008	$410.00	25.00	385.00	360.00
					Total	1,453.00

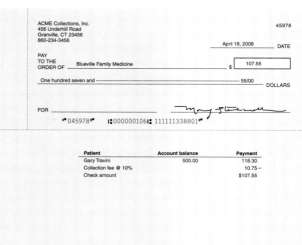

ACME Collections, Inc.
456 Underhill Road
Granville, CT 23456
860-234-3456

45978

April 18, 2008   DATE

PAY TO THE ORDER OF   Blueville Family Medicine $ 107.55

One hundred seven and -- 55/00   DOLLARS

FOR

⑈045978⑈ ⑆000000106⑆ 111111338801⑈

Patient	Account balance	Payment
Gary Travini	500.00	118.30
Collection fee @ 10%		10.75 −
Check amount		$107.55

PROCEDURE 18-2 – PROCESSING A CREDIT BALANCE AND REFUND AND POSTING AN NSF CHECK

Name _____ Date _____ Score _____

Instructor _____

Tasks
Process a credit balance, process a refund, and post a not sufficient funds (NSF) check.

Conditions
Day sheet
Checks (insurance and patient checks)
Collection agency payment
Pen

Time: _____

Standards
In the time specified and within the scoring parameters determined by the instructor, the student will successfully process a credit balance and a refund and post an NSF check.

Points assigned reflect importance of step to meeting the task

Important = 1 pt.
Essential = 5 pts.
Critical = 15 pts.

Automatic failure results if any of the **CRITICAL TASKS** are omitted or performed incorrectly.

(To use a pass/fail system, Instructors can record "P" or "F" in the "points earned (pass/fail)" column.)

PERFORMANCE STANDARDS	PTS	PTS EARNED (Pass/Fail)	COMMENTS
1. Posted the insurance check for Irina Sharapova to her ledger card.	15	_____	_____
2. Wrote a refund check to Mrs. Sharapova and recorded her balance as zero.	15	_____	_____
3. Posted the returned check from Ariana Klieger on the day sheet and on the patient's ledger card.	15	_____	_____
TOTAL POINTS	45		

DOCUMENTATION

_____ | _____
_____ | _____
_____ | _____
_____ | _____

COMMENTS

_____

_____

_____

_____

Please use the materials below to complete Procedure 18-2.

Universal HMO
1 Vista Boulevard
Regionville, NY 04321
800-888-8765

0088678721

April 20, 2008   DATE

PAY
TO THE
ORDER OF ___ Blueville Family Medicine ___ $ 30.00

Thirty and _____ 00/100 ___ DOLLARS

FOR _____

⑆0088678721⑆ ⑈000000886⑈ 771117354301⑈

Name	Procedure	Amount charged	Allowed	Copay	Paid
Irina Sharapova	99204	85.00	70.00	40.00	30.00

Irina Sharapova
211 Elm Street, Blueville, CT
860-555-1129

Date	Procedure	Charge	Payment	Balance
	Balance brought forward			0.00
03/07/2008	OV exp	85.00	15.00 (writeoff)	70.00
03/07/2008	Payment, personal check #859		50.00	20.00

BLUEVILLE FAMILY MEDICINE
15 MAIN STREET
BLUEVILLE, CT 06000
860-555-3212

11432

_____ DATE

PAY
TO THE
ORDER OF _____ $ [   ]

_____ DOLLARS

BLUEVILLE SAVINGS BANK

FOR _____

⑆011432⑆ ⑈000000105⑈ 111111333301⑆

Arianna Klieger
769 Elm Street
Blueville, CT 06000

772

April 7, 2008   DATE

PAY
TO THE
ORDER OF ___ Blueville Family Medicine ___ $ 45.00

Forty-five and _____ no/100 ___ DOLLARS

NSF

PRESLEY SAVINGS AND LOAN

MEMO _____   Arianna Klieger

⑈0440088804⑈ 960130629721⑆ 1000

Arianna Klieger
769 Elm Street, Blueville, CT
860-555-9733

Date	Procedure	Charge	Payment	Balance
	Balance brought forward			0.00
04/07/2008	office surgery	410.00	45.00	365.00

PROCEDURE 18-3 – RECONCILING A BANK STATEMENT

Name _____   Date _____   Score _____

Instructor _____

Task
Reconcile the monthly deposit and withdrawal report with a bank statement.

Conditions
Office check register
Bank statement
Adding machine
Pen

Time: _____

Standard
In the time specified and within the scoring parameters determined by the instructor, the student will successfully reconcile the deposit and withdrawal report with a bank statement.

Points assigned reflect importance of step to meeting the task

Important = 1 pt.
Essential = 5 pts.
Critical = 15 pts.

Automatic failure results if any of the **CRITICAL TASKS** are omitted or performed incorrectly.

(To use a pass/fail system, Instructors can record "P" or "F" in the "points earned (pass/fail)" column.)

PERFORMANCE STANDARDS	PTS	PTS EARNED (Pass/Fail)	COMMENTS
1. Using the bank statement dated April 1, 2008, and the deposit and withdrawal report for that same period, compared the totals and noted the difference in the amounts, if any.	15	_____	_____ _____ _____ _____
2. Compared each withdrawal and deposit on the bank statement to the report.	5	_____	_____ _____
3. In comparing each item, was sure to determine if the amount on the statement and the report matched.	15	_____	_____ _____
4. For each matching item, made a check mark next to the item on the report and the corresponding item on the bank statement.	5	_____	_____ _____ _____

PERFORMANCE STANDARDS (cont.)	PTS	PTS EARNED (Pass/Fail)	COMMENTS
5. Drew a circle around any item on the report that was not also included on the bank statement as well as any item on the statement that was not on the report.	5	_____	_____ _____ _____
6. Using the adding machine, added all circled withdrawals. Then added all circled deposits on the report.	15	_____	_____ _____ _____
7. Subtracted the total outstanding withdrawals from the bank statement ending balance.	15	_____	_____ _____ _____
8. Added the total outstanding deposits to the bank statement ending balance.	15	_____	_____ _____ _____
9. Confirmed that the resulting amount matched the balance of the deposit and withdrawal report.	5	_____	_____ _____ _____

TOTAL POINTS	85		

DOCUMENTATION

_____	_____
_____	_____
_____	_____

COMMENTS

_____

_____

_____

_____

Please use the materials below to complete Procedure 18-3.

Blueville Savings Bank
122 Main Street
Blueville, CT 06000

860-555-1298
www.bluevillesavings.com

Statement Account s#6869750033
Blueville Family Medicine
15 Main Street
Blueville, CT
860-555-3212

Bank Statement April 1, 2008
Beginning balance $59,008.31
Ending balance $57,778.19

Average balance $55,715.89

Check #	Date of Transaction	Withdrawal	Deposit Date	Deposit Amount
11733	03/08/08	$458.25	03/14/08	$8,231.44
11734	03/09/08	$611.90		
11735	03/09/08	$734.47	03/21/08	$11,772.11
11736	03/09/08	$1248.22		
11737	03/09/08	$3019.39		
11738	03/09/08	$2033.22		
11739	03/09/08	$1338.33		
11740		missing in sequence		
11741	03/09/08	$324.11		
	03/09/08	$250.00		
11742	03/09/08	$475.88		
11743	03/09/08	$294.11		
11744	03/09/08	$1585.55		
11745		missing in sequence		
11746	03/21/08	$6400.00		
Totals	**checks and withdrawals**	**$18,773.43**	**deposits and interest**	**$20,003.55**

Deposit and Withdrawal Report – March 2008

Number	Date	Description of Transaction	C	Debit (-)	Credit (+)	Balance
		Previous balance				$59,008.31
11733	03/07/08	Payroll- Kelly Manera, CMA		$458.25		$58,550.06
11734	03/07/08	Payroll- Cindy Smith, CMA		$611.90		$57,938.16
11735	03/07/08	Payroll- Sharon Piecek, APRN		$734.47		$57,203.69
11736	03/07/08	Payroll- Henry Lee, MD		$1248.22		$55,955.47
11737	03/07/08	Payroll- Robert Greer, MD		$3019.39		$52,936.08
11738	03/07/08	Payroll- Hector Rodriguez, MD		$2033.22		$50,902.86
11739	03/07/08	Payroll- Ann Wilson, MD		$1338.33		$49,564.53
11740	03/07/08	Payroll- Shelly Gonzalez, CMA		$356.08		$49,208.45
11741	03/07/08	Payroll- Jennifer Morgan, CMA		$324.11		$48,884.34
11742	03/07/08	Payroll- Wendy Jones		$475.88		$48,408.46
11743	03/07/08	Payroll- Carol Chapin		$294.11		$48,114.35
11744	03/07/08	Payroll taxes		$1585.55		$46,528.80
	03/09/08	Cash withdrawal for office party supplies		$250.00		$46,278.80
	03/11/08					
11745		Patterson Office Supply		$136.12		$46,142.68
	03/14/08	Deposit insurance & personal cks			$8,231.44	$54,374.12
11746	03/16/08	Henderson Realty- Office rent for April 2008		$6400.00		$47,974.12
	03/21/08	Deposit insurance & personal cks			$11,772.11	$59,746.23
	03/31/08	Deposit insurance & personal cks			$9,763.07	$69,509.30

PROCEDURE 18-4 – PREPARING A BANK DEPOSIT

Name _____   Date _____   Score _____

                                            Instructor _____

Task
Prepare a bank deposit.

Conditions
Bank deposit form
Checks (insurance and patient checks)
Cash received
Office checkbook register
Pen

Time: _____

Standard
In the time specified and within the scoring parameters determined by the instructor, the student will successfully prepare a bank deposit and record the deposit in the office checkbook register.

Points assigned reflect importance of step to meeting the task

Important = 1 pt.
Essential = 5 pts.
Critical = 15 pts.

Automatic failure results if any of the **CRITICAL TASKS** are omitted or performed incorrectly.

(To use a pass/fail system, Instructors can record "P" or "F" in the "points earned (pass/fail)" column.)

PERFORMANCE STANDARDS	PTS	PTS EARNED (Pass/Fail)	COMMENTS
1. Using the personal checks from patients, the United Health Systems check, and the bank deposit form, entered the check numbers and amounts of all checks on the deposit slip.	15	_____	_____ _____ _____ _____
2. Totaled the cash received from the day sheet in Procedure 18-1 and entered the amount on the deposit slip in the appropriate section.	15	_____	_____ _____ _____ _____
3. Totaled the amount of the checks and cash using an adding machine. Rechecked your total.	15	_____	_____ _____ _____
4. Wrote the total amount of the deposit in the Total column.	5	_____	_____ _____ _____

PERFORMANCE STANDARDS (cont.)	PTS	PTS EARNED (Pass/Fail)	COMMENTS
5. Wrote the amount of the deposit in the office checkbook register (below) and added it to the previous balance.	5	_____	_____ _____ _____
6. Rechecked your math before writing the new balance in the register.	5	_____	_____ _____

TOTAL POINTS	60		

DOCUMENTATION

COMMENTS

_____

_____

_____

_____

Please use the materials below to complete Procedure 18-4.

Brenda Capshaw
1 Circle Drive
Redtown, CT 06111

457

April 19, 2008 DATE

PAY TO THE ORDER OF Blueville Family Medicine $ 15.00

Fifteen and   no/100 DOLLARS

Blueville Trust
Blueville, CT

Brenda Capshaw

Michael McGuinniss
7125 Main Street
Blueville, CT 06101

3239

April 19, 2008 DATE

PAY TO THE ORDER OF Blueville Family Medicine $ 20.00

Twenty and   no/100 DOLLARS

Blueville First Bank
Blueville, CT

FOR

Michael McGuinniss

⑆123456780⑆ 0301 123 456⑈ 7⑈

Charles Ayers
1719 Lake Avenue
Green Lake, CT 06088

466

April 19, 2008 DATE

PAY TO THE ORDER OF Blueville Family Medicine $ 15.00

Fifteen and   no/100 DOLLARS

1st Green Lake Bank
Green Lake, CT

Charles Ayers

Alicia Carter
43 East End Avenue
Redtown, CT 06111

337

April 19, 2008 DATE

PAY TO THE ORDER OF Blueville Family Medicine $ 20.00

Twenty and   no/100 DOLLARS

1st Green Lake Bank
Green Lake, CT

FOR

Alicia Carter

⑆123456780⑆ 0301 123 456⑈ 7⑈

Kirsten Tremblay
231 Purple Place
Blueville, CT 06000

199

April 19, 2008 DATE

PAY TO THE ORDER OF Blueville Family Medicine $ 15.00

Fifteen and   no/100 DOLLARS

Blueville National Bank
Blueville, CT

FOR

Kirsten Tremblay

⑆123456780⑆ 0301 123 456⑈ 7⑈

10549

Date _4/16/08_

To _____

_____

Amount _____

Deposit _____ $66,387.45

10550

Date _4/16/08_

To _Clinic One Supply_

_____

Amount _$136.12_ $66,251.33

Deposit _$22,766.21_ $89,017.54

10551

Date _4/22/08_

To _Henderson Realty_

Office rent May 2008

Amount _$6,400.00_

Deposit _____ $82,617.54

10552

Date _4/22/08_

To _Yellow Page.com –_

advertising

Amount _$1,250.00_

Deposit _____ $81,367.54

10553

Date _____

To _____

_____

Amount _____

Deposit _____

BLUEVILLE FAMILY MEDICINE
15 MAIN STREET
BLUEVILLE, CT 06100
860-555-3212

10553

_____ DATE

PAY
TO THE
ORDER OF _____ $ [   ]

_____ DOLLARS

BLUEVILLE SAVINGS BANK

FOR _____ _____

⑈010553⑈ ⑆ 000000105⑆111111333301⑈

Date	Profit description	Amount
10/01/08	Carpenters Local 896 check	2,477.08
10/03/08	Allied Health Services check	17,344.99
10/03/08	Medicare check	7,990.44
10/03/08	Aetna Life check	4,337.01
10/03/08	Guardian Life check	8,907.45
10/15/08	Carpenters Local 896 check	3,551.98
10/16/08	Allied Health Services check	11,445.07
10/16/08	Medicare ceck	3,221.08
10/16/08	Aetna Life check	6,997.07
10/16/08	Guardian Life check	2,407.09
10/16/08	Mutual of Omaha check	1,104.56
10/17/08	Casino Workers Local 445 check	874.22
10/21/08	ABC Collection Corporation	1,456.02
10/01-10/31	Front desk cash/check copayments	8,800.00
10/01-10/31	Patient balances paid by personal checks	1,759.30
		82,673.36

Date	Expense description	Amount
10/01/08	Henderson Realty office rent	6,400.00
10/01/08	Office supplies	435.00
10/01/08	Clinical supplies	1,550.00
10/21/08	Telephone bill and advertising in Yellow Pages	683.44
10/21/08	Payroll taxes	16,433.07
10/21/08	Total payroll for October	45,488.58
		70,989.58

Total income for October 2008 $82,673.36
Total expenses for October 2008 $70,989.58
Net profit for October 2008 $11,683.78

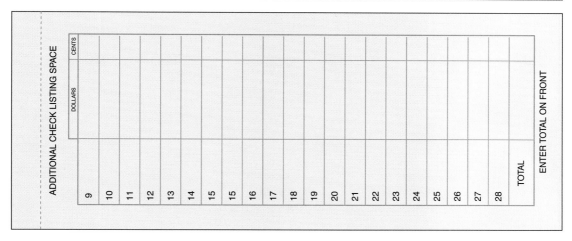

DEPOSIT TICKET

Blueville Family Medicine
15 Main Street
Blueville, CT
860-555-3212

Date _____

Blueville Savings Bank
122 Main Street
Blueville, CT 06000
860-555-1298
www.bluevillesavings.com

PLEASE ENTER TOTAL

PLEASE BE SURE ALL ITEMS ARE PROPERLY ENDORSED

$

⑆001001⑆ ⑈6869750033⑇ 12345678⑆

200033

LIST CHECKS INDIVIDUALLY		DOLLARS	CENTS
COIN			
CURRENCY			
1			
2			
3			
4			
5			
6			
7			
8			
Total from other side			
TOTAL			

ADDITIONAL CHECK LISTING SPACE

	DOLLARS	CENTS
9		
10		
11		
12		
13		
14		
15		
15		
16		
17		
18		
19		
20		
21		
22		
23		
24		
25		
26		
27		
28		
TOTAL		

ENTER TOTAL ON FRONT

UNIT III

Clinical

Infection Control and Medical Asepsis

Key Term Review *Define the following key terms:*

1.   phagocytosis _____

   _____

2.   virulence _____

   _____

3.   aerobe _____

   _____

4.   fomite _____

   _____

5.   purulent _____

   _____

6.   leukocytes _____

   _____

7.   pathogen _____

   _____

8.   microorganisms _____

   _____

9.   spores _____

   _____

10.   antibody _____

   _____

11.   anaerobe _____

   _____

Key Term Review *cont.*

12. histamine _____

13. vectors _____

14. normal flora _____

15. lymphocytes _____

16. prodrome _____

17. antigen _____

18. symptomatic _____

19. host _____

20. fungi _____

Review Questions

1. What is the medical assistant's role in infection control?

    _____

    _____

    _____

    _____

2. Are all microorganisms harmful? Explain.

    _____

    _____

    _____

3. What is normal flora?

_____

_____

_____

_____

4. Describe five categories of pathogenic microorganisms. Provide at least one disease each type can cause.

_____

_____

_____

_____

5. Describe the five stages of disease.

_____

_____

_____

_____

6. What is the body's first line of defense when coming into contact with a pathogen?

_____

_____

_____

_____

7. How does the inflammatory response work?

_____

_____

_____

_____

8. How do lymphocytes aid in the body's defense?

_____

_____

_____

_____

9. Describe active and passive immunity.

_____

_____

_____

_____

10. What is a fomite? How can it be involved in disease transmission?

_____

_____

_____

_____

11. What is a vector? Give three examples of vectors.

_____

_____

_____

_____

12. Discuss the differences between bacteria and viruses.

_____

_____

_____

_____

13. List six times throughout the day when a medical assistant should wash his or her hands.

_____

_____

_____

_____

14. What is OSHA? What is its function?

_____

_____

_____

_____

15. List five types of PPEs.

_____

_____

_____

_____

16. Describe some workplace practices an employer must provide.

_____

_____

_____

_____

17. List some office safety tips as they apply to standard precautions (on infection control).

_____

_____

_____

_____

18. List five body fluids that are considered Other Potentially Infectious Material (OPIM).

_____

_____

_____

_____

19. Compare and contrast medical asepsis with surgical asepsis.

_____

_____

_____

_____

20. Differentiate between sanitization, disinfection, and sterilization.

_____

_____

_____

_____

21. Explain the proper steps in sterilizing surgical packs using an autoclave.

_____

_____

_____

_____

Critical Thinking

1. The facility you work for asks you to develop a pamphlet for patients. The pamphlet is to inform patients about commonsense, everyday measures they can use to prevent disease transmission to keep healthy during cold and flu season. What data will you include?

_____

_____

_____

_____

2. You are currently working as a medical assistant in patient care. As part of your duties you disinfect the examination areas and all other patient contact surfaces in the back office every night before leaving. The front office medical assistant observes you doing this and asks why you have to do this every day. She states that she only bothers cleaning the front desk if something has spilled on it. What is your response to her?

_____

_____

_____

_____

3. Does a person get sick every time he or she is exposed to a pathogen? Explain your answer.

_____

_____

_____

_____

4. Using the chain of infection diagram as a guide, explain how the influenza virus could get into a person, cause the flu, and be transmitted to someone else.

_____

_____

_____

_____

Teamwork Exercises

1. Divide into groups of three or four students. Each group is to simulate a biohazard spill and then follow the procedure for cleaning up and documenting the cleanup.

2. Divide into groups of three or four students. Form work stations for hand washing, equipment sterilization and/or disinfection, wrapping articles for sterilization, and using the autoclave. Have each group of students rotate through each station, with students in each group teaching each other how to do the procedure for that station.

PROCEDURE 19-1 – WASHING HANDS WITH SOAP AND WATER

Name _____   Date _____   Score _____

Instructor _____

Task
Perform hand washing.

Conditions
Sink
Soap
Timer
Nail stick or brush
Paper towels
Waste container

Time: _____

Standard
In the time specified and within the scoring parameters determined by the instructor, the student will successfully perform hand washing with soap and water.

Points assigned reflect importance of step to meeting the task

Important = 1 pt.
Essential = 5 pts.
Critical = 15 pts.

Automatic failure results if any of the **CRITICAL TASKS** are omitted or performed incorrectly.

(To use a pass/fail system, Instructors can record "P" or "F" in the "points earned (pass/fail)" column.)

PERFORMANCE STANDARDS	PTS	PTS EARNED (Pass/Fail)	COMMENTS
1. Removed all rings and jewelry and pushed your watchband up to expose your wrists.	1	_____	_____ _____
2. Stood in front of the sink without touching the sink edge or counter top.	1	_____	_____ _____
3. Turned on the water to a comfortable temperature.	1	_____	_____ _____
4. Applied soap to your hands (approximately 5 ml or 1 tsp) and worked it into a lather, being sure to cover all parts of your hands and wrists. Using friction, continued to wash hands and wrists for 15 seconds.	15	_____	_____ _____ _____ _____ _____
5. Using an orange stick or a fingernail, cleaned under the edges of all of your fingernails.	5	_____	_____ _____ _____

PERFORMANCE STANDARDS (cont.)	PTS	PTS EARNED (Pass/Fail)	COMMENTS
6. Pointing your hands and fingers down, rinsed your hands under the running water.	5	_____	_____ _____
7. Dried your hands with a disposable towel, then discarded the used towel in a waste container.	5	_____	_____ _____
8. Used a dry, disposable towel to turn off the water.	15	_____	_____ _____
9. Disposed of the towel in a waste container.	1	_____	_____ _____

TOTAL POINTS	49		

DOCUMENTATION

COMMENTS

_____

_____

_____

_____

PROCEDURE 19-2 – SANITIZING HANDS WITH AN ALCOHOL-BASED HAND SANITIZER

Name _____   Date _____   Score _____

                                           Instructor _____

Task
Sanitize hands using an alcohol-based hand sanitizer.

Conditions
Alcohol-based hand sanitizer

Time: _____

Standard
In the time specified and within the scoring parameters determined by the instructor, the student will success-fully perform hand sanitization using an alcohol-based hand sanitizer.

Points assigned reflect importance of step to meeting the task

Important = 1 pt.
Essential = 5 pts.
Critical = 15 pts.

Automatic failure results if any of the **CRITICAL TASKS** are omitted or performed incorrectly.

(To use a pass/fail system, Instructors can record "P" or "F" in the "points earned (pass/fail)" column.)

PERFORMANCE STANDARDS	PTS	PTS EARNED (Pass/Fail)	COMMENTS
1. Removed all rings and jewelry and pushed your watchband up to expose your wrists.	1	_____	
2. Read the label of the alcohol-based hand sanitizer and verified that it contains 60% to 95% alcohol.	1	_____	
3. Applied enough sanitizer to cover all the surfaces of your hands and wrists.	15	_____	
4. Rubbed the sanitizer over the surfaces of your hands, fingers, fingernails, and wrists.	15	_____	

PERFORMANCE STANDARDS (cont.)	PTS	PTS EARNED (Pass/Fail)	COMMENTS
5. Allowed your hands to air-dry.	5	_____	_____

TOTAL POINTS	37	

DOCUMENTATION

COMMENTS

_____
_____
_____
_____

PROCEDURE 19-3 – SANITIZING EQUIPMENT

Name _____   Date _____   Score _____

Instructor _____

Task
Perform sanitization of equipment.

Conditions
Sink
Brush with stiff bristles
Low-sudsing, chemical disinfectant soap
Gown or apron with a plastic, leakproof backing
Utility gloves
Goggles
Towels
Soap

Time: _____

Standard
In the time specified and within the scoring parameters determined by the instructor, the student will successfully sanitize equipment for reuse.

Points assigned reflect importance of step to meeting the task

Important = 1 pt.
Essential = 5 pts.
Critical = 15 pts.

Automatic failure results if any of the **CRITICAL TASKS** are omitted or performed incorrectly.

(To use a pass/fail system, Instructors can record "P" or "F" in the "points earned (pass/fail)" column.)

PERFORMANCE STANDARDS	PTS	PTS EARNED (Pass/Fail)	COMMENTS
1. Washed or sanitized your hands and assembled supplies.	5	_____	_____ _____
2. Using soap, scrubbed all instruments with a bristle brush under running water.	15	_____	_____ _____ _____
3. Cleaned all surfaces of the instruments and opened any hinges.	5	_____	_____ _____
4. Rinsed the instruments thoroughly with hot water.	5	_____	_____ _____
5. Placed the instruments on a towel for drying.	1	_____	_____ _____

PERFORMANCE STANDARDS (cont.)	PTS	PTS EARNED (Pass/Fail)	COMMENTS
6. Removed your gloves and washed your hands	1	_____	_____ _____

TOTAL POINTS	32		

DOCUMENTATION

COMMENTS

_____

_____

_____

_____

PROCEDURE 19-4 – DISINFECTING EQUIPMENT

Name _____   Date _____   Score _____

Instructor _____

Task
Perform equipment disinfection.

Conditions
Sink
Disinfectant chemical solution
Container for instruments
Timer
Water

Time: _____

Standard
In the time specified and within the scoring parameters determined by the instructor, the student will successfully disinfect equipment.

Points assigned reflect importance of step to meeting the task

Important = 1 pt.
Essential = 5 pts.
Critical = 15 pts.

Automatic failure results if any of the **CRITICAL TASKS** are omitted or performed incorrectly.

(To use a pass/fail system, Instructors can record "P" or "F" in the "points earned (pass/fail)" column.)

PERFORMANCE STANDARDS	PTS	PTS EARNED (Pass/Fail)	COMMENTS
1. Washed or sanitized your hands and assembled supplies.	5	_____	_____
2. Put on utility gloves.	1	_____	_____
3. Sanitized all instruments prior to disinfecting.	1	_____	_____
4. Read the manufacturer's instructions on the label of the disinfectant solution.	5	_____	_____
5. Prepared the disinfectant as directed.	15	_____	_____
6. Placed the sanitized instruments into a container.	15	_____	_____
7. Applied the disinfectant to the instruments.	5	_____	_____

PERFORMANCE STANDARDS (cont.)	PTS	PTS EARNED (Pass/Fail)	COMMENTS
8. Soaked the instruments for the required time, according to the manufacturer's instructions.	15	_____	_____ _____
9. Dried the instruments with towels.	1	_____	_____
10. Stored the instruments appropriately for future use.	1	_____	_____ _____
11. Removed your gloves and wash your hands.	1	_____	_____ _____

TOTAL POINTS	65		

DOCUMENTATION

COMMENTS

_____

_____

_____

_____

PROCEDURE 19-5 – WRAPPING A PACK FOR AUTOCLAVING

Name _____   Date _____   Score _____

                                          Instructor _____

Task
Wrap a pack for autoclaving.

Conditions
Disinfectant chemical solution
Container for instruments
Timer
Water
Sanitized instruments to be sterilized
Wrapping towels (2)
Sterile indicator strips and tape for securing contents
Marker pen

Time: _____

Standard
In the time specified and within the scoring parameters determined by the instructor, the student will successfully wrap a pack for sterilization.

Points assigned reflect importance of step to meeting the task

Important = 1 pt.
Essential = 5 pts.
Critical = 15 pts.

Automatic failure results if any of the **CRITICAL TASKS** are omitted or performed incorrectly.

(To use a pass/fail system, Instructors can record "P" or "F" in the "points earned (pass/fail)" column.)

PERFORMANCE STANDARDS	PTS	PTS EARNED (Pass/Fail)	COMMENTS
1. Washed or sanitized your hands.	5	_____	_____
2. Identified the type of pack to be used. Gathered the instruments and other equipment.	5	_____	_____ _____
3. Laid the towels flat in a diamond configuration and placed the instruments in the center.	5	_____	_____ _____
4. Opened all hinged instruments. If the hinged instruments could touch, separated them with a 2 × 2 gauze pad.	15	_____	_____ _____
5. Placed the sterile indicator strip at the top of the contents.	15	_____	_____ _____
6. Brought the bottom of the diamond up to cover the contents and folded the tip of the corner.	1	_____	_____ _____

PERFORMANCE STANDARDS (cont.)	PTS	PTS EARNED (Pass/Fail)	COMMENTS
7. Brought one side of the wrap over to cover the contents and folded up the tip of the corner.	1	_____	_____ _____
8. Brought the other side of the wrap over to cover the contents and folded up the tip of the corner.	1	_____	_____ _____
9. Folded the bottom of the wrap over, including the instruments, to align with the top edges of the side folds.	1	_____	_____ _____ _____
10. For packages that must be double wrapped, placed the package in the center of a second sheet of wrapping material and repeated steps 6–9.	5	_____	_____ _____ _____
11. Brought the top of the wrap down and sealed the top flap with sterile indicator tape.	15	_____	_____ _____
12. Labeled the tape with the contents, the date, and your initials.	15	_____	_____ _____

TOTAL POINTS	84		

DOCUMENTATION

COMMENTS

The Patient Interview

Key Term Review

Define the following key terms:

1. rapport _____

2. medical jargon _____
_____

3. acronym _____
_____

4. redirecting _____
_____

5. summarizing _____
_____

6. active listening _____
_____

7. open-ended question _____
_____

8. layperson _____
_____

9. reflecting _____
_____

10. restating _____
_____

11. closed question _____
_____

Key Term Review *cont.*

12. problem-oriented
medical record _____
_____

13. silence _____
_____

14. directive
statements _____
_____

15. source-oriented
medical record _____
_____

Review Questions

1. Describe the purpose of the three main parts of the patient interview process.

_____
_____
_____
_____

2. List the nine interviewing techniques and the purpose of each.

_____
_____
_____
_____

3. Describe how you would handle a talkative patient during an interview.

_____
_____
_____
_____

4. List five obstacles to effective interviewing and give an effective alternative strategy for each.

_____

_____

_____

_____

_____

5. How can a medical assistant help patients feel comfortable when asking sensitive questions?

_____

_____

_____

_____

6. Give four different interview techniques that can be used when working with children.

_____

_____

_____

_____

7. What are some methods that can be used when interviewing elderly patients?

_____

_____

_____

_____

8. What are the benefits of having a patient complete a self-assessment questionnaire?

_____

_____

_____

_____

9. What are three purposes the patient's medical chart serves?

_____

_____

_____

_____

10. List the various components of a medical history.

_____

_____

_____

_____

11. Describe some charting dos and don'ts.

_____

_____

_____

_____

12. Compare and contrast the source-oriented medical record with the problem-oriented medical record.

_____

_____

_____

_____

13. Give three examples of an objective symptom.

_____

_____

_____

_____

14. Give three examples of a subjective symptom.

_____

_____

_____

_____

Critical Thinking

1. Jake Ellis is a 44-year-old patient who is in for a long-overdue physical exam. Develop five open-ended interview questions you will ask him during the initial patient interview.

   _____

   _____

   _____

   _____

2. Shannon Murphy is a 5-year-old girl who is a new patient to your practice. When you call her and her mother into the exam room, you observe that she seems very apprehensive. What techniques can you use to put Shannon at ease and obtain a full medical history?

   _____

   _____

   _____

   _____

3. For each patient symptom, identify whether it is a subjective (S) or objective (O) symptom:

   a. Feeling of nausea _____

   b. Lightheaded and dizzy _____

   c. Flush skin _____

   d. Left leg limp _____

   e. BP 154/92 _____

   f. Muscle aches in both arms _____

   g. Petechiae rash on trunk of body _____

   h. Sore throat _____

   i. Surgical scar with purulent discharge _____

4. For the following statements, tell whether they are an open-ended questions (OE), a closed question (C), or a directive statement (D).

   a. "Does your arm hurt when you raise it above your head?" _____

   b. "Tell me what you were doing when the pain first began." _____

c. "How would you describe the pain?" _____

d. "When was your last physical exam?" _____

e. "Tell me why you are here today." _____

f. "What medications are you taking?" _____

g. "How are you feeling right before you take your insulin?" _____

h. "Did you take anything for your pain?" _____

i. "What type of over-the-counter medicines do you take?" _____

j. "Do you exercise?" _____

Teamwork Exercises

1. Group students in pairs. Using the blank patient history form, role-play taking a patient history. Students playing the patient should come up with different chief complaints and pretend to be of various age groups. Students should also document appropriately.

2. In groups of two, role-play the following scenarios. As the medical assistant, ask open-ended and closed questions along with directive statements.

   a. 17-year-old Alysha Payne is in with a sore knee.

   b. 35-year-old Jim Ring has been experiencing heartburn the past few weeks.

   c. 51-year-old Thom Patrick has had trouble sleeping.

   d. 22-year-old Cammy DeLisle has been experiencing frequent burning sensation.

PROCEDURE 20-1 – OBTAINING A MEDICAL HISTORY

Name _____   Date _____   Score _____

Instructor _____

Task
Interview a patient to obtain a medical history.

Conditions
Patient history form
Black and red ink pens
Clipboard
Private area to conduct the interview

Time: _____

Standard
In the time specified and within the scoring parameters determined by the instructor, the student will successfully conduct a patient interview to obtain the patient's health history.

Points assigned reflect importance of step to meeting the task

Important = 1 pt.
Essential = 5 pts.
Critical = 15 pts.

Automatic failure results if any of the **CRITICAL TASKS** are omitted or performed incorrectly.

(To use a pass/fail system, Instructors can record "P" or "F" in the "points earned (pass/fail)" column.)

PERFORMANCE STANDARDS	PTS	PTS EARNED (Pass/Fail)	COMMENTS
1. Washed or sanitized your hands and assembled supplies.	5	_____	_____
2. Greeted and identified the patient by his last name. Used a pleasant, professional manner and introduced yourself.	5	_____	_____
3. Guided the patient to a private, quiet, comfortable area. Explained the purpose and nature of the interview.	5	_____	_____
4. Gathered medical information using therapeutic communication techniques.	15	_____	_____
5. Reviewed the self-history section if one was completed.	15	_____	_____

PERFORMANCE STANDARDS (cont.)	PTS	PTS EARNED (Pass/Fail)	COMMENTS
6. Throughout the interview, explained or translated any medical terms the patient did not understand.	15	_____	_____
7. Allowed the patient adequate time to answer each question.	5	_____	_____
8. Recorded the patient's allergies in red ink.	5	_____	_____
9. Spoke in a pleasant, unhurried manner using adequate volume and enunciation.	5	_____	_____
10. Used culturally appropriate body language.	5	_____	_____
11. Repeated the patient's answers as needed for clarification or confirmation.	5	_____	_____
12. Wrote legibly in black ink.	5	_____	_____
13. Documented all data accurately and objectively in measurable terms.	15	_____	_____
14. If more explanation was needed than the space on the form allows, marked it with an asterisk (*) and wrote an explanation in the "comments" section.	5	_____	_____
15. Thanked the patient and explained the next step in the examination.	1	_____	_____
16. Invited the patient to use the restroom (and collected a specimen if appropriate) before the examination.	5	_____	_____

TOTAL POINTS	116		

DOCUMENTATION

COMMENTS

Vital Signs

Key Term Review *Define the following key terms:*

1. diurnal rhythm

2. tachypnea

3. febrile

4. arrhythmia

5. diastolic pressure

6. pulse deficit

7. ausculatory gap

8. pyrexia

9. systolic pressure

10. hypertension

11. apnea

12. Korotkoff
     sounds

13. orthostatic
     hypotension

14. bradypnea

15. diaphoresis

Review Questions

1. Describe how body temperature is regulated.

2. What is the diurnal rhythm?

3. Describe some symptoms that occur when a patient has a fever.

4. Discuss the differences between the following types of fevers:

a. remittent:

_____

_____

_____

_____

b. continuous:

_____

_____

_____

_____

c. intermittent:

_____

_____

_____

_____

5. What are some considerations that must be taken into account when choosing the right thermometer?

_____

_____

_____

_____

6. Discuss the pros and cons of using the following thermometers:

a. glass:

_____

_____

_____

_____

b. digital:

_____

_____

_____

_____

c. tympanic:

_____

_____

_____

_____

d. chemical:

_____

_____

_____

_____

e. temporal:

_____

_____

_____

_____

7. Describe the proper means of disinfecting the various types of thermometers.

_____

_____

_____

8. List some factors that affect a pulse rate, rhythm, and strength.

_____

_____

_____

_____

9. Discuss the importance of taking an apical pulse.

_____

_____

_____

_____

10. Discuss the processes of inspiration and expiration.

_____

_____

_____

_____

11. Explain the proper procedure of a medical assistant to take a patient's respiration without his or her knowledge.

_____

_____

_____

_____

12. Differentiate between internal and external respiration.

_____

_____

_____

_____

13. List some factors that affect the respiratory rate.

_____

_____

_____

_____

14. Why is it important to also determine a patient's rhythm and depth of respiration?

_____

_____

_____

_____

15. What does a blood pressure represent?

_____

_____

_____

_____

16. Differentiate between systolic and diastolic blood pressure.

_____

_____

_____

_____

17. Discuss some non-modifiable risk factors for hypertension.

_____

_____

_____

_____

18. What are some factors that affect a patient's blood pressure?

_____

_____

_____

_____

19. Discuss some tips a medical assistant should know when taking a patient's blood pressure.

_____

_____

_____

_____

20. Describe the five types of sounds commonly heard when obtaining a blood pressure.

_____

_____

_____

_____

21. Explain how a pulse oximeter measures blood oxygen levels.

_____

_____

_____

_____

22. List the normal adult ranges for each vital sign.

_____

_____

_____

_____

Critical Thinking

1. Insert pulse site illustration (see Figure 22-1 in chapter) and have students identify each pulse site (temporal, carotid, brachial, radial, apical, femoral, popliteal, dorsal pedis, posterior tibialis).

_____

_____

_____

_____

2. For the following factors that could interfere with an oxygen saturation measurement, provide some corrective action:

a. The LED reading is of questionable accuracy:

_____

_____

_____

_____

b. The motion of a patient's hand or finger is interfering with the reading:

_____

_____

_____

_____

c. The patient's hands and fingers are edematous:

_____

_____

_____

_____

d. There is interference from an outside light source:

_____

_____

_____

_____

e. The patient's hands and fingers are pale and cool:

_____

_____

_____

_____

f. The probe is too tight on the patient's finger:

_____

_____

_____

_____

g. Carbon monoxide caused by smoke inhalation or poisoning artificially elevates the SpO_2 reading:

_____

_____

_____

_____

h. A patient who is jaundiced:

_____

_____

_____

_____

Teamwork Exercises

1. Using a partner, practice taking vital signs on each other. Use the following chart to document your readings.

Vital Sign	Reading 1	Reading 2	Reading 3	Reading 4	Reading 5
Temperature					
Pulse					
Respiration					
Blood pressure					

2. Using a partner, take turns locating each of the different pulse sites.

PROCEDURE 21-1: MEASURING ORAL TEMPERATURE USING A DIGITAL THERMOMETER

Name _____   Date _____   Score _____

Instructor _____

Task
Measure oral body temperature using a digital thermometer.

Conditions
Digital thermometer
Oral probe
Probe cover
Waste container
Pen
Patient's medical record

Time: _____

Standard
In the time specified and within the scoring parameters determined by the instructor, the student will successfully measure and record a patient's oral temperature using a digital thermometer.

Points assigned reflect importance of step to meeting the task

Important = 1 pt.
Essential = 5 pts.
Critical = 15 pts.

Automatic failure results if any of the **CRITICAL TASKS** are omitted or performed incorrectly.

(To use a pass/fail system, instructors can record "P" or "F" in the "points earned (pass/fail)" column.)

PERFORMANCE STANDARDS	PTS	PTS EARNED (Pass/Fail)	COMMENTS
1. Washed or sanitized your hands and assembled supplies.	5	_____	_____
2. Prepared the oral probe for use according to the manufacturer's directions.	5	_____	_____
3. Greeted and identified your patient and introduced yourself. Explained the procedure and asked if the patient had smoked, exercised, or had anything to eat or drink within the past 30 minutes.	5	_____	_____
4. Applied the disposable probe cover, making sure it locked into place.	1	_____	_____
5. Placed the probe under patient's tongue in the pocket on either side of the frenulum linguae.	5	_____	_____

PERFORMANCE STANDARDS (cont.)	PTS	PTS EARNED (Pass/Fail)	COMMENTS
6. Instructed the patient to close his mouth. Continued holding the end of the probe.	1	_____	_____
7. Removed the probe after the thermometer beeped and read the number on the digital display screen. Ejected the probe cover into the waste container by pressing the ejection button and without touching the probe cover.	15	_____	_____
8. Returned the probe to its storage position in the thermometer unit and returned the thermometer to its base.	1	_____	_____
9. Washed or sanitized your hands and disinfected equipment if indicated.	5	_____	_____
10. Recorded the patient's temperature in the medical record, including the date and time.	15	_____	_____

TOTAL POINTS	58		

DOCUMENTATION

COMMENTS

PROCEDURE 21-2 – MEASURING AXILLARY TEMPERATURE USING A DIGITAL THERMOMETER

Name _____   Date _____   Score _____

Instructor _____

Task
Measure axillary body temperature using a digital thermometer.

Conditions
Digital thermometer
Oral probe
Probe cover
Waste container
Pen
Patient's medical record

Time: _____

Standard
In the time specified and within the scoring parameters determined by the instructor, the student will successfully measure and record an individual's axillary temperature using a digital thermometer.

Points assigned reflect importance of step to meeting the task

Important = 1 pt.
Essential = 5 pts.
Critical = 15 pts.

Automatic failure results if any of the **CRITICAL TASKS** are omitted or performed incorrectly.

(To use a pass/fail system, instructors can record "P" or "F" in the "points earned (pass/fail)" column.)

PERFORMANCE STANDARDS	PTS	PTS EARNED (Pass/Fail)	COMMENTS
1. Washed or sanitized your hands and assembled supplies.	5	_____	_____
2. Greeted and identified your patient, introduced yourself, and explained the procedure.	5	_____	_____
3. Prepared the oral probe for use according to the manufacturer's directions.	1	_____	_____
4. Assisted the patient in removing or loosening clothing around the shoulder and arm as needed.	1	_____	_____
5. Patted the axilla dry if needed.	1	_____	_____
6. Applied a disposable probe cover, making sure it locked into place.	1	_____	_____

PERFORMANCE STANDARDS (cont.)	PTS	PTS EARNED (Pass/Fail)	COMMENTS
7. Inserted the probe into the center of the axilla pointing toward the upper chest. Told the patient to hold his upper arm snugly against the side of his ribcage and assisted him as necessary. Held the probe in place until you heard the beep sound that indicated the reading was complete.	15	_____	_____
8. Removed the probe and read the number on the digital display screen. Ejected the probe cover into the waste container by pressing the ejection button without touching the probe cover.	15	_____	_____
9. Returned the probe to its storage position in the thermometer unit and returned the thermometer to its base.	1	_____	_____
10. Washed or sanitized your hands and disinfected equipment if indicated.	5	_____	_____
11. Recorded the patient's temperature in the medical record, including the method of measurement (in this case, axillary), the date, and the time.	15	_____	_____

TOTAL POINTS	60		

DOCUMENTATION

COMMENTS

PROCEDURE 21-3: MEASURING RECTAL TEMPERATURE USING A DIGITAL THERMOMETER

Name _____   Date _____   Score _____

Instructor _____

Task
Measure rectal body temperature.

Conditions
Digital rectal thermometer
Rectal probe
Probe cover
Lubricant
Tissues
Nonsterile examination gloves
Waste container
Pen
Patient's medical record

Time: _____

Standard
In the time specified and within the scoring parameters determined by the instructor, the student will successfully measure and record the patient's rectal temperature.

Points assigned reflect importance of step to meeting the task

Important = 1 pt.
Essential = 5 pts.
Critical = 15 pts.

Automatic failure results if any of the **CRITICAL TASKS** are omitted or performed incorrectly.

(To use a pass/fail system, instructors can record "P" or "F" in the "points earned (pass/fail)" column.)

PERFORMANCE STANDARDS	PTS	PTS EARNED (Pass/Fail)	COMMENTS
1. Washed or sanitized your hands and assembled supplies.	5	_____	_____
2. Greeted and identified the patient and introduced yourself.	5	_____	_____
3. Prepared the rectal probe for use, according to the manufacturer's instructions. Applied a disposable probe cover, making sure it locked into place.	1	_____	_____
4. Applied nonsterile examination gloves.	1	_____	_____

PERFORMANCE STANDARDS (cont.)	PTS	PTS EARNED (Pass/Fail)	COMMENTS
5. Assisted the patient in removing clothing below the waist. Assisted the adult or child patient into a Sims or side-lying position. Draped the patient as completely as possible, exposing only the anal area. Positioned the infant patient on his abdomen.	1	_____	_____
6. Applied lubricant to the tip of the thermometer. Inserted the thermometer into the rectum past the external sphincter. For an infant or small child, took care to insert it no more than $1/2$ inch and no more than 1 inch for an older child or adult. Continued holding the probe end.	15	_____	_____
7. Removed the probe after the beeping sound. Ejected the probe cover into the waste container without touching the probe cover and disposed of examination gloves.	5	_____	_____
8. Read the number on the digital display screen.	15	_____	_____
9. Offered tissues to the adult or child patient. Wiped excess lubricant from the infant.	1	_____	_____
10. Returned the probe to its storage position in the thermometer unit and returned the thermometer to its base.	1	_____	_____
11. Washed or sanitized your hands and disinfected equipment if indicated.	1	_____	_____
12. Assisted the patient with positioning and dressing as needed.	1	_____	_____

PERFORMANCE STANDARDS (cont.)	PTS	PTS EARNED (Pass/Fail)	COMMENTS
13. Recorded the patient's temperature in the medical record, including the method of measurement (in this case, rectal), the date, and the time.	15	_____	_____ _____ _____

TOTAL POINTS	67		

DOCUMENTATION

COMMENTS

PROCEDURE 21-4 – MEASURING TEMPERATURE USING A TYMPANIC THERMOMETER

Name _____ Date _____ Score _____

Instructor _____

Task
Measure body temperature using a tympanic thermometer.

Conditions
Tympanic thermometer
Probe cover
Waste container
Pen
Patient's medical record

Time: _____

Standard
In the time specified and within the scoring parameters determined by the instructor, the student will successfully measure and record a patient's body temperature using a tympanic thermometer.

Points assigned reflect importance of step to meeting the task

Important = 1 pt.
Essential = 5 pts.
Critical = 15 pts.

Automatic failure results if any of the **CRITICAL TASKS** are omitted or performed incorrectly.

(To use a pass/fail system, instructors can record "P" or "F" in the "points earned (pass/fail)" column.)

PERFORMANCE STANDARDS	PTS	PTS EARNED (Pass/Fail)	COMMENTS
1. Washed or sanitized your hands and assembled supplies.	5	_____	_____
2. Greeted and identified your patient, introduced yourself, and explained the procedure.	5	_____	_____
3. Prepared the tympanic thermometer for use, according to the manufacturer's directions, making sure that probe lens was clean and the display screen was adjusted for the patient's age.	1	_____	_____
4. Applied the disposable probe cover, making sure that it snapped into place.	1	_____	_____

PERFORMANCE STANDARDS (cont.)	PTS	PTS EARNED (Pass/Fail)	COMMENTS
5. When the thermometer display read ready, straightened the patient's ear canal with your other hand by gently pulling the auricle up and backward for patients over age 3 or by gently pulling the pinna down and backward for younger patients.	15	_____	_____ _____ _____ _____ _____ _____
6. Inserted the probe into the patient's ear canal just far enough to seal the opening but without applying pressure.	15	_____	_____ _____ _____ _____
7. Pressed the button and held it down briefly, as indicated in the manufacturer's instructions. Checked the temperature reading that appeared on the display screen.	15	_____	_____ _____ _____ _____
8. Removed the probe and ejected the probe cover into a waste receptacle without touching it.	5	_____	_____ _____ _____
9. Recorded the patient's temperature in the medical record, including the method of measurement (in this case, tympanic) along with the ear in which it was measured, the date, and the time.	15	_____	_____ _____ _____ _____ _____ _____

TOTAL POINTS	77		

DOCUMENTATION

COMMENTS

PROCEDURE 21-5 – MEASURING TEMPERATURE USING A TEMPORAL THERMOMETER

Name _____   Date _____   Score _____

                                            Instructor _____

Task
Measure body temperature using a temporal thermometer.

Conditions
Temporal thermometer
Probe cover or disinfectant wipe
Waste container
Pen
Patient's medical record

Time: _____

Standard
In the time specified and within the scoring parameters determined by the instructor, the student will accurately measure and record a patient's temporal temperature.

Points assigned reflect importance of step to meeting the task

Important = 1 pt.
Essential = 5 pts.
Critical = 15 pts.

Automatic failure results if any of the **CRITICAL TASKS** are omitted or performed incorrectly.

(To use a pass/fail system, instructors can record "P" or "F" in the "points earned (pass/fail)" column.)

PERFORMANCE STANDARDS	PTS	PTS EARNED (Pass/Fail)	COMMENTS
1. Washed or sanitized your hands and assembled supplies.	5	_____	_____
2. Greeted and identified the patient, introduced yourself, and explained the procedure.	5	_____	_____
3. Applied a disposable probe cover, as necessary.	1	_____	_____
4. Scanned the probe across the patient's forehead over the temporal artery, as indicated in the manufacturer's instructions.	15	_____	_____
5. Read the temperature on the digital display screen.	15	_____	_____

PERFORMANCE STANDARDS (cont.)	PTS	PTS EARNED (Pass/Fail)	COMMENTS
6. Ejected the probe cover into the waste container without touching the probe cover or cleaned the probe with a disinfectant wipe.	5	_____	_____ _____ _____
7. Washed or sanitized your hands.	1	_____	_____
8. Recorded the patient's temperature in the medical record, including the method of measurement (in this case, temporal), the date, and the time.	15	_____	_____ _____ _____

TOTAL POINTS	62		

DOCUMENTATION

COMMENTS

PROCEDURE 21-6 – MEASURING RADIAL PULSE AND RESPIRATIONS

Name _____   Date _____   Score _____

Instructor _____

Task
Measure and record radial pulse and respirations.

Conditions
Clock or watch
Pen
Patient's medical record

Time: _____

Standard
In the time specified and within the scoring parameters determined by the instructor, the student will accurately measure and record radial pulse and respirations.

Points assigned reflect importance of step to meeting the task

Important = 1 pt.
Essential = 5 pts.
Critical = 15 pts.

Automatic failure results if any of the **CRITICAL TASKS** are omitted or performed incorrectly.

(To use a pass/fail system, instructors can record "P" or "F" in the "points earned (pass/fail)" column.)

PERFORMANCE STANDARDS	PTS	PTS EARNED (Pass/Fail)	COMMENTS
1. Washed or sanitized your hands and assembled supplies.	5	_____	_____ _____
2. Greeted and identified the patient, introduced yourself, and explained the procedure.	5	_____	_____ _____
3. Assisted the patient into a comfortable sitting position with his arm relaxed and slightly flexed.	1	_____	_____ _____
4. Grasped the patient's wrist with the pads of your middle three fingers placed over the radial site and applied just enough pressure to distinctly palpate the pulse. Did not palpate with the thumb.	15	_____	_____ _____ _____ _____
5. Counted the pulse for 30 seconds as measured with your watch and multiplied by two.	15	_____	_____ _____

PERFORMANCE STANDARDS (cont.)	PTS	PTS EARNED (Pass/Fail)	COMMENTS
6. To count respirations, continued holding the patient's wrist while looking at your watch. Counted the patient's respirations for 30 seconds, then multiplied by two. Was sure to note the character of the respirations, including depth and rhythm.	15	_____	_____
7. Recorded the patient's pulse and respirations in the medical record, including date and time.	15	_____	_____
8. Washed or sanitized your hands.	1	_____	_____

TOTAL POINTS	72		

DOCUMENTATION

COMMENTS

PROCEDURE 21-7 – MEASURING APICAL HEART RATE

Name _____ Date _____ Score _____

Instructor _____

Task
Measure and record a patient's apical heart rate.

Conditions
Watch with a second hand
Stethoscope
Patient examination gown
Antiseptic wipe
Pen
Patient's medical record

Time: _____

Standard
In the time specified and within the scoring parameters determined by the instructor, the student will accurately measure and record the apical heart rate.

Points assigned reflect importance of step to meeting the task

Important = 1 pt.
Essential = 5 pts.
Critical = 15 pts.

Automatic failure results if any of the **CRITICAL TASKS** are omitted or performed incorrectly.

(To use a pass/fail system, instructors can record "P" or "F" in the "points earned (pass/fail)" column.)

PERFORMANCE STANDARDS	PTS	PTS EARNED (Pass/Fail)	COMMENTS
1. Washed or sanitized your hands and assembled supplies.	5	_____	
2. Greeted and identified the patient, introduced yourself, and explained the procedure.	5	_____	
3. Cleaned the earpieces and chest piece of the stethoscope with an antiseptic wipe.	1	_____	
4. Assisted the patient in undressing from the waist up and putting on examination gown, if preferred, with the opening in the front. Placed patient in a sitting or reclining position.	5	_____	
5. Placed the bell of the stethoscope over the apical area, applying just enough pressure to ensure full contact with the skin.	5	_____	

PERFORMANCE STANDARDS *(cont.)*	PTS	PTS EARNED (Pass/Fail)	COMMENTS
6. Counted the heart beat for a full minute as measured with your watch.	15	_____	_____ _____
7. Washed or sanitized your hands and sanitized the earpieces and chest piece of the stethoscope.	5	_____	_____
8. Recorded the patient's apical heart rate and rhythm in the medical record, including the date and time.	15	_____	_____ _____

TOTAL POINTS	56		

DOCUMENTATION

COMMENTS

PROCEDURE 21-8 – MEASURING BLOOD PRESSURE

Name _____ Date _____ Score _____

Instructor _____

Task	**Standard**
Measure and record blood pressure.	In the time specified and within the scoring parameters determined by the instructor, the student will accurately measure and record the patient's blood pressure.
Conditions	
Sphygmomanometer (blood pressure cuff) Antiseptic wipes Stethoscope Waste container	**Points assigned reflect importance of step to meeting the task**
Time: _____	Important = 1 pt. Essential = 5 pts. Critical = 15 pts.
	Automatic failure results if any of the **CRITICAL TASKS** are omitted or performed incorrectly.
	(To use a pass/fail system, instructors can record "P" or "F" in the "points earned (pass/fail)" column.)

PERFORMANCE STANDARDS	PTS	PTS EARNED (Pass/Fail)	COMMENTS
1. Seated the patient in a quiet room for several minutes prior to checking her blood pressure.	1	_____	_____
2. Washed or sanitized your hands and assembled supplies.	5	_____	_____
3. Greeted and identified the patient, introduced yourself, and explained the procedure.	5	_____	_____
4. Minimized room noise by turning off music (if playing) and asking the patient to refrain from talking.	1	_____	_____
5. Rolled up the patient's sleeve about 5 inches above the elbow or assisted the patient in removing her arm from clothing.	5	_____	_____

PERFORMANCE STANDARDS *(cont.)*	PTS	PTS EARNED (Pass/Fail)	COMMENTS
6. Selected the proper size cuff for each patient. The cuff bladder was long enough to wrap around 80% of the patient's arm and wide enough to cover two-thirds of the upper arm.	15	_____	_____ _____ _____
7. Applied the deflated cuff to the patient's upper arm with the arrow over the brachial artery and the lower cuff edge at least 1 inch above the bend of the elbow.	15	_____	_____ _____ _____
8. Positioned the gauge so you could easily read it.	5	_____	_____ _____
9. Palpated the brachial pulse with one hand and tightened the valve on the inflation bulb with the other hand. Then inflated the cuff and noted the reading on the gauge when you were no longer able to palpate the pulse.	5	_____	_____ _____ _____ _____
10. Applied the stethoscope to the area of the brachial pulse, making sure the earpieces fit snugly and comfortably in your ears and were pointed forward and downward.	5	_____	_____ _____ _____ _____
11. Placed the stethoscope diaphragm directly on the patients' skin over the site of the brachial artery.	15	_____	_____ _____
12. Made sure the patients' arm is relaxed at heart level. With the patient's arm fully extended, held the stethoscope over the brachial pulse with your thumb, while pressing the back of the elbow with your index and middle finger.	5	_____	_____ _____ _____ _____ _____
13. Positioned the stethoscope tubing so that it hung freely without rubbing on anything.	1	_____	_____ _____
14. Quickly inflated the bulb until the gauge measured approximately 30 mm Hg higher than the palpated reading.	15	_____	_____ _____ _____

PERFORMANCE STANDARDS (cont.)	PTS	PTS EARNED (Pass/Fail)	COMMENTS
15. Released the pressure at a steady rate of 2–3 mm Hg per second.	15	_____	
16. Noted when the first sounds were heard (phase I) and recorded this measurement as the systolic pressure even if the sounds disappeared and then returned again (auscultatory gap). Was sure to note the auscultatory gap in the patient's medical record because, depending on the patient, it could be an abnormal finding.	15	_____	
17. Noted when the sounds completely disappeared and recorded this as the diastolic pressure.	15	_____	
18. Measured and recorded blood pressure in both arms during an initial patient assessment and any time the reading was in doubt.	15	_____	
19. Waited at least 1 minute between measurements if a repeat blood pressure measurement was required.	5	_____	
20. Recorded blood pressure in even numbers as a fraction (such as 132/72).	15	_____	
21. Removed the cuff from the patient's arm and returned it to the appropriate place. Cleaned the stethoscope earpieces with alcohol or another antiseptic solution as dictated by office policy and returned it to its appropriate place.	5	_____	
22. Washed or sanitized your hands.	1	_____	
23. Recorded the patient's blood pressure measurement in the medical record, including the date and time.	15	_____	

TOTAL POINTS	199		

DOCUMENTATION

COMMENTS

Student Activity Manual to Accompany The Professional Medical Assistant

PROCEDURE 21-9 – MEASURING OXYGEN SATURATION USING A PULSE OXIMETER

Name _____   Date _____   Score _____

Instructor _____

Task

Measure and record arterial oxygen saturation using a pulse oximeter.

Conditions

Pulse oximeter with probe
Acetone or nail polish remover
Antiseptic wipe
Pen
Patient's medical record

Time: _____

Standard

In the time specified and within the scoring parameters determined by the instructor, the student will successfully measure the patients oxygen saturation with a pulse oximeter.

Points assigned reflect importance of step to meeting the task

Important = 1 pt.
Essential = 5 pts.
Critical = 15 pts.

Automatic failure results if any of the **CRITICAL TASKS** are omitted or performed incorrectly.

(To use a pass/fail system, instructors can record "P" or "F" in the "points earned (pass/fail)" column.)

PERFORMANCE STANDARDS	PTS	PTS EARNED (Pass/Fail)	COMMENTS
1. Washed or sanitized your hands and assembled supplies.	5	_____	_____
2. Greeted and identified your patient and introduced yourself.	5	_____	_____
3. Explained the procedure and reassured the patient that it would not hurt.	1	_____	_____
4. Cleaned the probe with an antiseptic wipe.	1	_____	_____
5. Identified the patient's baseline reading, if available in the medical record.	5	_____	_____
6. Identified the most appropriate site for the sensor probe and selected the appropriate probe.	1	_____	_____

PERFORMANCE STANDARDS *(cont.)*	PTS	PTS EARNED (Pass/Fail)	COMMENTS
7. Positioned the patient comfortably and instructed him to breathe normally.	1	_____	_____
8. If a digital sensor was used on the finger, removed any nail polish and supported the patient's lower arm.	5	_____	_____
9. Applied the probe and activated the oximeter. Waited several seconds and observed the pulse waveform and audible beep. Noted the LED reading when it reached a constant value. If necessary, checked the radial pulse.	15	_____	_____
10. Removed the probe and cleaned it with a disinfectant wipe.	1	_____	_____
11. Returned the oximeter to its correct location.	1	_____	_____
12. Washed or sanitized your hands.	1	_____	_____
13. Recorded the SpO_2 level in the patient's medical record, including the date and time. Included data regarding oxygen use and the presence of fever.	15	_____	_____

TOTAL POINTS	57		

DOCUMENTATION

COMMENTS

Physical Examination

Key Term Review   *Define the following key terms:*

1. manipulation
2. semi-Fowler position
3. dorsal recumbent position
4. lithotomy position
5. skin turgor
6. auscultation
7. knee-chest position
8. percussion
9. supine position
10. mensuration
11. inspection
12. Sims position

Key Term Review *cont.*

13. Fowler position _____

    _____

14. palpation _____

    _____

15. Trendelenburg _____

    position _____

16. jack-knife _____

    position _____

Review Questions

1. What is the purpose of the physical examination?

   _____

   _____

   _____

   _____

2. Discuss some considerations to take into account when scheduling a patient for a physical exam.

   _____

   _____

   _____

   _____

3. List and describe six examination techniques commonly used by the physician during a physical exam. Provide an example of each type of technique.

   _____

   _____

   _____

   _____

4. List at least 10 components of the physical exam.

General apperance, skin, head,neck, arms, hands, head, neck, eyes, ears, nose, mouth and pharynx, chest/lungs, cardiovascular function, breasts, abdomen, genitalia/rectum, legs and feet, mental status.

5. List some terms used to describe abnormal findings of the skin during a physical exam.

6. When assessing a patient's general appearance, what are some things to look for?

color, affect, gate, speech, hair, physical activity, hearing, responsiveness, smell.

7. What are some common abnormal findings when examining the eyes?

8. What are some common abnormal findings when examining the chest and lungs?

Weezing, crackling, irregular respirations, squeeks,

9. What sort of conditions would the physician observe to assess the mental status of a patient?

Affect, personal hygiene, nutritional status, cooperation, attitude, mental exam.

10. List and describe supplies and equipment most commonly used in the physical exam, and describe the purpose of each item.

Thermometer to take temperature, Stethoscope to take BP listen to lungs. Sphgmomanometer to take BP. Pen light for eyes. Reflex hammer for reflexes. Opthalmoscope and otoscope to look in ears and mouth. Vaginal speculum for papsmear, scale for weight/height tongue depressors, lubricating jelly for pap, cotton swabs, alcohol pads,

11. Discuss the medical assistant's role in preparing the examination room. Gauze pads, gloves urine sample cup, stool sampler card, developer. Broom, pap developer jelly.

_____

_____

_____

12. Describe the medical assistant's role in preparing a patient for a physical exam.

_____

_____

_____

_____

13. Provide at least two reasons or examination procedures that would require the patient to be in the above positions.

If your pregnant, If you have swelling, Medications. diuretic, diabetic, weight loss/gain.

_____

_____

14. Explain how the medical assistant helps the physician and patient during the physical exam.

_____

_____

_____

15. Provide at least three reasons why a patient's weight is measured during each office visit.

_____

_____

_____

_____

16. Discuss the differences when measuring the height of an adult and the height of an infant or child.

_____

_____

_____

_____

Position Identification

Identify the name of each position shown in Figures 22–1 through 22–10.

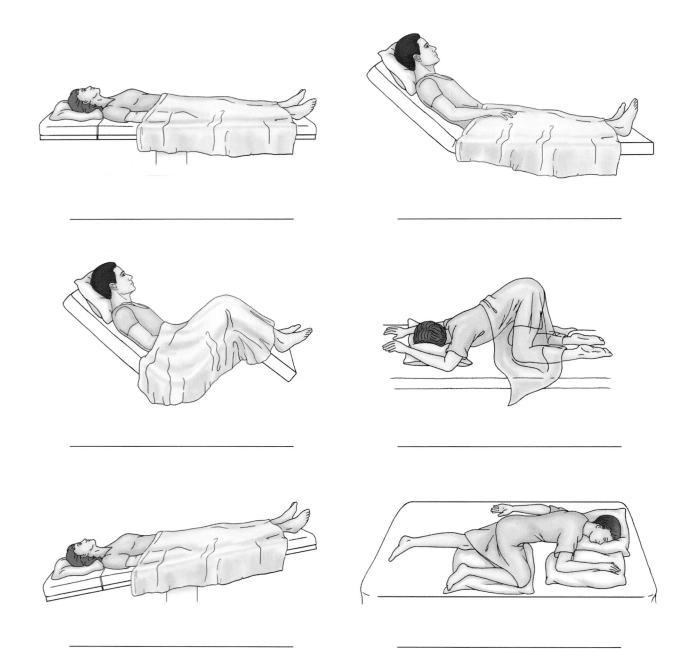

_____

_____

_____

_____

_____

_____

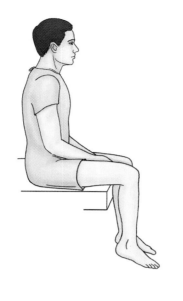

_____

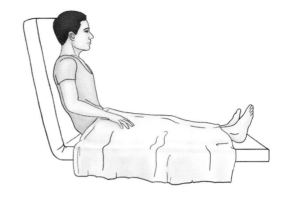

_____

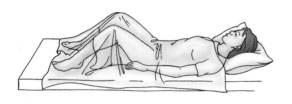

_____

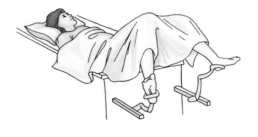

_____

Critical Thinking

1. Julian Vhooris, age 44, is in for his annual physical exam. Upon taking his initial medical history, you notice he appears confused and is having difficulty answering your questions. What would you do?

    _____

    _____

    _____

    _____

2. You are the site supervisor for Ming, a medical assisting student who is externing in your office. You are showing her how to set up Dr. Hite's examination room for a physical exam when she asks, "Why does Dr. Hite need all these supplies and equipment for a simple physical exam?" How would you respond to Ming?

    _____

    _____

    _____

    _____

Teamwork Exercises

1. In groups of two, practice putting each other in the various patient examination positions. Once in each position, drape the patient in the proper manner. As the students are putting each other in the various positions, they should also be explaining the uses for that position.

2. In groups of two or three, practice taking each other's height and weight. Each student can also practice his or her documentation techniques by properly recording their results.

PROCEDURE 22-1 – ASSISTING WITH THE PHYSICAL EXAMINATION

Name _____   Date _____   Score _____

Instructor _____

Task
Assist the physician with a physical examination.

Conditions
Examination table
Specific supplies and equipment for the type of
  examination being performed
Drape
Patient examination gown

Time: _____

Standard
In the time specified and within the scoring parameters determined by the instructor, the student will successfully assist the physician with the physical examination of a patient.

Points assigned reflect importance of step to meeting the task

Important = 1 pt.
Essential = 5 pts.
Critical = 15 pts.

Automatic failure results if any of the **CRITICAL TASKS** are omitted or performed incorrectly.

(To use a pass/fail system, instructors can record "P" or "F" in the "points earned (pass/fail)" column.)

PERFORMANCE STANDARDS	PTS	PTS EARNED (Pass/Fail)	COMMENTS
1. Prepared the examination room, ensuring adequate room temperature and lighting.	1	_____	_____ _____
2. Washed or sanitized your hands.	5	_____	_____
3. Assembled supplies and equipment in the order in which they would be used.	5	_____	_____ _____
4. Obtained the patient's medical record, greeted and identified the patient, and introduced yourself.	5	_____	_____ _____
5. Obtained the patient's weight and height if needed and escorted her to the examination room.	15	_____	_____ _____

PERFORMANCE STANDARDS (cont.)	PTS	PTS EARNED (Pass/Fail)	COMMENTS
6. Reviewed the record with the patient, making sure that the medication list and allergy information were current.	5	_____	_____ _____ _____
7. Inquired about the purpose of the visit. Recorded the patient's complaint and symptoms to the degree of detail preferred by the physician.	15	_____	_____ _____ _____ _____
8. Obtained the patient's vital signs.	15	_____	_____
9. Drew blood if needed for laboratory tests. Performed an ECG if ordered.	15	_____	_____ _____
10. Invited the patient to empty her bladder. If a urine specimen was needed, provided instructions and a specimen container.	5	_____	_____ _____ _____
11. Provided the patient with an examination gown and drape. Instructed her to remove all clothing, pointing out where she may hang or lay her clothing. Explained that the gown should be worn with the opening in the front and how the drape should be used.	5	_____	_____ _____ _____ _____ _____ _____ _____
12. Explained that the patient should sit on the end of the examination table and that the physician would be with her soon.	5	_____	_____ _____ _____ _____
13. Left the room so the patient may change in privacy. However, if she was elderly, weak, frail, or had any symptoms of dizziness, remained in the room to assist her. Helped her sit in a regular chair to wait for the physician.	1	_____	_____ _____ _____ _____ _____ _____
14. Placed the medical record in the designated place for the physician to retrieve and let him know that the patient was ready.	1	_____	_____ _____ _____ _____

PERFORMANCE STANDARDS (cont.)	PTS	PTS EARNED (Pass/Fail)	COMMENTS
15. Returned to the room when directed by the physician.	1	_____	_____
16. Assisted the physician with a general body system examination, including:	15	_____	_____

a. Assisted the patient into a sitting position on the end of the table if she was not already there. Arranged the drape over her lap.

b. As the physician examined the patient's upper body (eyes, ears, nose, mouth, throat, and chest), was prepared to hand her items as needed, such as the otoscope, ophthalmoscope, penlight, and tongue depressor.

c. Dimmed the lights if directed when the physician examined the patient's eyes.

d. Throughout the remainder of the examination, continued to hand needed items to the physician and assisted the patient in assuming the positions directed by the physician.

e. Followed standard precautions and took care to handle potentially contaminated items from the physician (such as a tongue depressor, a speculum, and swabs) in a manner that prevented exposure to you.

f. Disposed of all waste in appropriate containers.

g. Placed specimens in appropriately labelled containers.

| **17.** Upon completion of the examination, assisted the patient down from the table and instructed her to get dressed. Left the room for a few minutes so the patient could change in privacy unless she required your assistance. | 5 | _____ | _____ |

PERFORMANCE STANDARDS _(cont.)_	PTS	PTS EARNED (Pass/Fail)	COMMENTS
18. Provided the patient with educational information or instructions as directed by the physician and answered questions she may have had. Consulted the physician or nurse if you were unsure of the answer to a patient's question.	5	_____	_____ _____ _____ _____ _____
19. Scheduled ordered follow-up tests or appointments.	5	_____	_____ _____
20. Directed the patient back to the reception area. Assisted her if needed.	1	_____	_____ _____
21. Documented patient education, instructions, or scheduled tests in the medical record.	5	_____	_____ _____
22. Cleaned, sanitized, and restocked the examination room as needed.	1	_____	_____ _____

TOTAL POINTS		

DOCUMENTATION

_____	_____
_____	_____
_____	_____
_____	_____

COMMENTS

_____

_____

_____

_____

PROCEDURE 22-2 – ASSISTING THE PATIENT VARIOUS EXAMINATION POSITIONS

Name _____   Date _____   Score _____

Instructor _____

Task
Assist the patient into the sitting position.

Conditions
Examination table
Table paper
Examination gown
Disposable drape or sheet

Time: _____

Standard
In the time specified and within the scoring parameters determined by the instructor, the student will successfully assist the patient into the sitting position.

Points assigned reflect importance of step to meeting the task

Important = 1 pt.
Essential = 5 pts.
Critical = 15 pts.

Automatic failure results if any of the **CRITICAL TASKS** are omitted or performed incorrectly.

(To use a pass/fail system, instructors can record "P" or "F" in the "points earned (pass/fail)" column.)

PERFORMANCE STANDARDS	PTS	PTS EARNED (Pass/Fail)	COMMENTS
1. Greeted and identified the patient, introduced yourself, and explained the procedure.	5	_____	_____ _____
2. Washed or sanitized your hands.	5	_____	_____
3. Provided the patient with an examination gown. Described how fully the patient should undress. Pointed out where the patient may hang or lay his clothing. Explained that the gown should be worn with the opening in the front.	5	_____	_____ _____ _____ _____ _____ _____

Assisting the patient into the sitting position

4. Pulled out the footrest of the examination table and explained that he should sit securely on the end of the table with the drape over his lap.	15	_____	_____ _____ _____

PERFORMANCE STANDARDS (cont.)	PTS	PTS EARNED (Pass/Fail)	COMMENTS
5. Left the room for a few minutes so the patient could change in privacy unless he required your assistance.	1	_____	_____ _____
6. Assisted the physician as needed with the examination.	5	_____	_____ _____

Assisting the patient into the supine and dorsal recumbent positions

7. Instructed the patient to lay back and rest his head on the pillow. As he did so, pulled out the table extension.	15	_____	_____ _____
8. Ensured that he was lying flat and the drape was positioned properly over his abdomen and legs.	1	_____	_____ _____
9. To assist the patient into the dorsal recumbent position, instructed him to place the soles of both feet flat on the table with his knees flexed.	5	_____	_____ _____ _____

Assisting the patient into the Sims position

10. Assisted the patient into a sitting position. Then instructed him to lay back and rest his head on the pillow. As he did this, pulled out the table extension.	15	_____	_____ _____ _____ _____
11. Instructed the patient to turn onto his left side. Provided support as needed.	1	_____	_____ _____
12. Positioned him with his left arm behind his body and his right arm forward with his elbow bent. Instructed him to flex his left leg slightly and his right leg sharply. Placed a pillow between his knees.	15	_____	_____ _____ _____ _____ _____
13. Ensured that the drape was positioned.	5	_____	_____ _____

PERFORMANCE STANDARDS (cont.)	PTS	PTS EARNED (Pass/Fail)	COMMENTS

Assisting the patient into the lithotomy position

14. Assisted the patient into a sitting position. Then instructed her to lay back and rest her head on the pillow. As she did this, pulled out the table extension. Next, pulled out the stirrups and adjusted their position for the patient's size. Instructed her to slide down to the bottom of the table and guided her feet into the stirrups.   **15**   _____   _____

15. Adjusted the drape so that it lay in a diamond formation with one corner draped between the patient's legs.   **5**   _____   _____

Assisting the patient into the semi-Fowler and Fowler positions

16. Assisted the patient into a sitting position. Then assisted him into the semi-Fowler position by raising the head of the examination table to a 45-degree angle.   **15**   _____   _____

17. To assist the patient into the Fowler position, raised the head of the examination table to 90 degrees.   **15**   _____   _____

18. Then instructed the patient to lay back and rest his head on the pillow. As he did this, pulled out the table extension.   **1**   _____   _____

19. Ensured that the drape was positioned properly.   **5**   _____   _____

Assisting the patient into the Trendelenburg position

20. Adjusted the table so that the head of the table was tilted downward. Ensured that the drape is positioned properly. Alternatively, the footrest may be tilted downward so that the knees bend.   **15**   _____   _____

PERFORMANCE STANDARDS (cont.)	PTS	PTS EARNED (Pass/Fail)	COMMENTS

Assisting the patient into the knee-chest position

21. Assisted the patient to a sitting position. Then asked him to move back on the table as you pulled out the table extension. Assisted him into the supine position and then into the prone position by turning onto his side and then onto his stomach. Was sure that he rolled toward you rather than away from you. — **15**

22. Placed a drape over him diagonally with one corner draped over his buttocks and another one over his back. — **5**

23. Instructed patient to bend his elbows and rest his arms along side of his head, then to raise his buttocks and chest off the table. — **5**

24. Placed a pillow beneath his chest for support and instructed him to lower his chest while keeping his buttocks elevated and his back straight. — **1**

25. Instructed him to separate his knees and lower legs approximately 12 inches. — **1**

26. Upon completion of the examination, assisted the patient down from the table and instructed him to get dressed. Returned the table footrest to the normal position. Left the room for a few minutes so the patient could change in privacy unless he required your assistance. — **5**

27. Cleaned, sanitized, and restocked the examination room as needed. — **1**

TOTAL POINTS		

DOCUMENTATION

COMMENTS

PROCEDURE 22-3 – MEASURING WEIGHT AND HEIGHT

Name _____   Date _____   Score _____

                                              Instructor _____

Task
Measure the patient's weight and height.

Conditions
Upright balance scale or digital stand-up scale
Pen
Patient's medical record

Time: _____

Standard
In the time specified and within the scoring parameters determined by the instructor, the student will success-fully measure the patient's weight and height.

Points assigned reflect importance of step to meeting the task

Important = 1 pt.
Essential = 5 pts.
Critical = 15 pts.

Automatic failure results if any of the **CRITICAL TASKS** are omitted or performed incorrectly.

(To use a pass/fail system, instructors can record "P" or "F" in the "points earned (pass/fail)" column.)

PERFORMANCE STANDARDS	PTS	PTS EARNED (Pass/Fail)	COMMENTS
1. Checked the scale to be sure that the pointer floats in the center of the balance frame when all weights are on zero. If the scale is digital, checked to make sure it was properly zeroed.	5	_____	_____ _____ _____ _____
2. Greeted and identified the patient, introduced yourself, and explained the procedure.	5	_____	_____ _____ _____
3. Washed or sanitized your hands.	5	_____	_____
4. Instructed the patient to remove her coat or sweater, shoes, and purse. Placed a paper towel on the scale and instructed the patient to step onto the scale. Provided assistance as needed.	1	_____	_____ _____ _____ _____ _____

PERFORMANCE STANDARDS _(cont.)_	PTS	PTS EARNED (Pass/Fail)	COMMENTS
5. Instructed the patient to stay still.	1	_____	_____
6. Slid the large lower weight to the right to the furthest notched groove that did not cause the pointer to drop to the bottom of the balance frame. Made sure that the weight was securely seated in the groove.	15	_____	_____
7. Slid the smaller upper weight to the right until the pointer was balanced in the center of the balance frame.	15	_____	_____
8. Added the numbers from the bottom and top together to arrive at the patient's weight to the nearest $\frac{1}{4}$ lb. If the scale was digital, noted the reading when patient was standing still on the scale.	15	_____	_____
9. Assisted the patient off the scale.	1	_____	_____
10. Slid the calibration rod up above the patient's approximate height and opened the height bar.	5	_____	_____
11. Assisted the patient back onto the scale with her back to it and instructed her to look straight forward.	5	_____	_____
12. Adjusted the height bar so that it just touched the top of the patient's head.	15	_____	_____
13. Instructed the patient to step off the scale while ensuring that the height bar did not move.	15	_____	_____
14. Read the measurement where the stationary calibration rod and moveable calibration rods met to the nearest $\frac{1}{4}$ inch.	15	_____	_____

PERFORMANCE STANDARDS (cont.)	PTS	PTS EARNED (Pass/Fail)	COMMENTS
15. Charted the patient's height and weight in the medical record. Recorded the weight in pounds or kilograms, depending on office policy	5	_____	_____ _____ _____

TOTAL POINTS		

DOCUMENTATION

COMMENTS

Essentials of Medical Terminology

Key Term Review

Define the following key terms:

1. pathological term

   _____

2. combining vowel

   _____

3. directional term

   _____

4. prefix

   _____

5. combining form

   _____

6. suffix

   _____

7. word root

   _____

Review Questions

1. List the five main categories of word elements, and give an example of each.

   _____

   _____

   _____

   _____

2. Write the plural forms for the following words:

   a. streptococcus:

   _____

   _____

   _____

   _____

   b. ovary:

   _____

   _____

   _____

   _____

   c. pleura:

   _____

   _____

   _____

   _____

   d. diagnosis:

   _____

   _____

   _____

   _____

e. appendix:

_____

_____

_____

f. bacterium:

_____

_____

_____

g. bronchus:

_____

_____

_____

Directional Term Review

Match the meaning with the proper term.

Directional term

1. distal _____

2. anterior _____

3. posterior _____

4. proximal _____

5. medial _____

6. superior _____

7. lateral _____

8. inferior _____

Definition

a. nearer to the origin or point

b. toward the midline

c. above or near to the head

d. toward or nearer to the front

e. farther from the origin or point of attachment

f. away from the midline toward the side

g. beneath or nearer to the feet

h. toward or nearer to the back

9. adduction _____

10. dorsal _____

11. ventral _____

12. deep _____

13. abduction _____

14. superficial _____

i. front

j. farther into the body

k. movement away from the body

l. back

m. nearer the surface of the body

n. movement toward the body

Prefix Review

Given the meaning, provide the proper prefix.

1. large: _____

2. before, forward: _____

3. within, inner: _____

4. one: _____

5. between: _____

6. poison: _____

7. without, absence of: _____

8. after, following: _____

9. against: _____

10. four: _____

11. above, upon: _____

12. away from: _____

13. good, normal: _____

14. in, within: _____

15. slow: _____

16. around: _____

17. through, across: _____

18. double, twin: _____

19. two: _____

20. rapid: _____

21. painful, difficult: _____

22. away from, external: _____

23. excessive, above: _____

24. below, beneath: _____

25. half: _____

Suffix Review

Given the meaning, provide the proper suffix.

1. instrument used for measuring: _____

2. abnormal condition: _____

3. deficiency: _____

4. nourishment or growth: _____

5. pain: _____

6. hernia: _____

7. cell: _____

8. excision, surgical removal: _____

9. condition of the blood: _____

10. creating, producing: _____

11. sensation: _____

12. bursting forth: _____

13. vision: _____

14. kill: _____

15. disease: _____

16. resembling: _____

17. cessation, stopping: _____

18. crushing: _____

19. pertaining to: _____

20. surgical puncture: _____

21. swelling: _____

22. record: _____

23. condition: _____

24. slight or partial paralysis: _____

25. inflammation: _____

26. formation or growth: _____

27. before, in front of: _____

28. vomiting: _____

29. drooping or prolapse: _____

30. tumor: _____

31. weakness, debility: _____

32. binding, fixation: _____

33. skin: _____

34. movement: _____

35. stone: _____

36. appetite: _____

37. softening: _____

38. pregnancy: _____

39. enlargement: _____

40. narrowing, stricture: _____

41. digestion: _____

42. speech: _____

43. surgical repair: _____

44. suture: _____

45. childbirth, labor: _____

46. urine: _____

47. head: _____

48. thirst: _____

49. fear: _____

50. contraction, tension: _____

Abbreviation Review

Provide the meaning for the following abbreviations.

1. RR   _____

2. BM   _____

3. qh   _____

4. Tx   _____

5. bid   _____

6. NPO   _____

7. Kg   _____

8. Ca   _____

9. Mg   _____

10. qhs   _____

11. stat _____

12. Rx   _____

13. INR   _____

14. c/o   _____

15. Dx   _____

16. IV   _____

17. FH   _____

18. 1PE   _____

19. PO   _____

20. Sx   _____

21. N&V   _____

22.	PMH	_____
23.	Hx	_____
24.	K	_____
25.	NG	_____

Medical Term Review

Define the following medical terms:

1.	antenatal:	_____
2.	circumoral:	_____
3.	parahepatic:	_____
4.	diploid:	_____
5.	epicardia:	_____
6.	hemigastrectomy:	_____
7.	dermal:	_____
8.	osteoblast:	_____
9.	pleurodesis:	_____
10.	exotropia:	_____
11.	syndesis:	_____
12.	toxemia:	_____
13.	rectocele:	_____
14.	polydipsia:	_____
15.	euthyroid:	_____
16.	cyanoderma:	_____

17. gastric: _____

18. electrocardiogram: _____

19. cholelithiasis: _____

20. hyperkinesis: _____

21. vaginosis: _____

22. hysteroptosis: _____

23. arteriospasm: _____

24. mastopexy: _____

25. dyspepsia: _____

26. vasorrhaphy: _____

27. atrophy: _____

28. hematuria: _____

29. craniotome: _____

30. dystocia: _____

Critical Thinking Activities

1. Using the textbook as well as a medical dictionary, put the following charting entries into layman's terms:

   a. Patient's father had a history of COPD and a myocardial infarction at age 57. Mother died from a severe staphylococcal infection due to complications of a mastectomy. Two siblings died from CVD due to hypertension and hyperlipidemia.

   _____

   _____

   _____

   _____

b. Patient referred to orthopedic surgeon for excision of anterior lateral lipoma on left arm.

_____

_____

_____

_____

c. Patient appeared cyanotic and showed signs of dyspnea. Extremities appeared edematous. Patient complained of orthopnea the last three nights. The physician ordered spirometry testing.

_____

_____

_____

_____

d. Patient complained of lower abdominal pain and dysuria. Recent medical history indicated multiple bouts of cystitis. Pelvic examination revealed purulent discharge, which was collected and sent for STD analysis.

_____

_____

_____

_____

2. Access the Web site www.lcsc.edu/healthocc/enable02/java/termbot2.htm. Click on "click here for new term" and a medical term will appear at the top of the screen. Try to define the term, based on your knowledge of prefixes, suffixes, and word roots.

_____

_____

_____

Teamwork Exercises

1. Divide the class into teams of three or four students. Have each team come up with a list of 10 medical terms. Collect all terms and use them in a medical terminology guessing game. Using a whiteboard or flip chart, draw lines to represent the exact number of letters in the word being used. Starting with one team, allow them to provide you with a letter they think is in the word. If the letter appears in the word, write that letter in the proper space. Allow that team to continue until the letter they select is not in the word. Then it is the next team's turn to choose a letter. The first team to correctly identify the word wins.

2. Divide into groups of two or three. Each group will make a medical terminology word search. The word search can be made by hand or done on the computer. Each group will make copies of their word search and hand one out to the rest of the students in the class to practice their medical terminology.

3. Group the class into pairs. Have each pair create flashcards of the terms found in chapter 23. Take turns quizzing each other with the flashcards. Even if this activity is not done in class, it makes for a great out-of-class group studying activity.

Office Project: Medical Terminology in Different Languages

Based on the languages spoken by the students at your school or in the community, develop as a class a list of medical terms or common medical phrases (such as "Where does it hurt?" or "Are you in pain?") in those various languages. Contact the local hospital to see if they have a medical interpreter who may be able to assist the class or even come speak to the class.

Surgical Asepsis and Assisting With Minor Surgery

Key Term Review *Define the following key terms:*

1. swag _____

_____

2. electrosurgery _____

_____

3. anesthesia _____

_____

4. sterile technique _____

_____

5. bandages _____

_____

6. approximation _____

_____

7. suture _____

_____

8. microsurgery _____

_____

9. dressings _____

_____

10. cryosurgery _____

_____

11. endoscopy _____

_____

12.   laser surgery   _____

_____

13.   sterile toss   _____

_____

14.   surgical asepsis   _____

_____

Review Questions

1. Describe the categories and common features of surgical instruments used in the medical office.

_____

_____

_____

_____

2. Discuss three types of scissors and their purpose.

_____

_____

_____

_____

3. Discuss three types of grasping and clamping instruments and their purpose.

_____

_____

_____

_____

4. Discuss three types of probing and dilating instruments and their purpose.

_____

_____

_____

_____

5. What is the purpose of the ratchet on certain instruments?

_____

_____

_____

_____

6. Why do some instruments have serrations, or teeth, on them?

_____

_____

_____

_____

7. How are suture needles categorized? What are some of the types of needles used?

_____

_____

_____

_____

8. Explain how suture materials are sized.

_____

_____

_____

_____

9. Explain the different types of suture materials that are available. How does a physician select which suture size and material to use?

_____

_____

_____

_____

10. What are the benefits of using surgical staples?

_____

_____

_____

_____

11. What is the purpose of a surgical wick?

_____

_____

_____

_____

12. Describe the difference between a bandage and a dressing.

_____

_____

_____

_____

13. What types of anesthetics are commonly used in the medical office?

_____

_____

_____

_____

14. For the following solutions used to clean a wound, discuss the pro's and con's of using each:

a. sterile saline:

_____

_____

_____

_____

b. Betadine:

_____

_____

_____

_____

   c. Hibiclens:

_____

_____

_____

_____

   d. isopropyl alcohol:

_____

_____

_____

_____

   e. hydrogen peroxide:

_____

_____

_____

_____

15. List three types of specialty instruments and reasons for their use.

_____

_____

_____

_____

16. What is a biopsy? What type of specimen is collected for a biopsy?

_____

_____

_____

_____

17. What are some ways a biopsy is obtained?

_____

_____

_____

_____

18. Describe seven principles of sterile technique that a medical assistant should follow.

_____

_____

_____

_____

19. Describe the medical assistant's role in minor office surgery.

_____

_____

_____

_____

20. Compare and contrast medical asepsis with surgical asepsis.

_____

_____

_____

_____

21. Compare and contrast the surgical hand scrub to the typical handwashing procedure.

_____

_____

_____

_____

22. For each of the listed surgical procedures, provide the following information:

- Purpose of the specific type

- Uses for

- Any special patient preparation

a. endoscopy:

_____

_____

_____

_____

b. cryosurgery:

_____

_____

_____

c. laser surgery:

_____

_____

_____

_____

d. microsurgery:

_____

_____

_____

_____

e. electrosurgery:

_____

_____

_____

_____

23. Discuss some preoperative instructions that the medical assistant may give to the patient.

_____

_____

_____

_____

24. List six general postoperative guidelines a medical assistant would provide to a patient.

_____

_____

_____

_____

25. What are some postoperative warning signs a patient needs to be aware of?

_____

_____

_____

_____

Critical Thinking

1. Identify the following surgical instruments and provide one reason for its use:

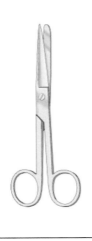

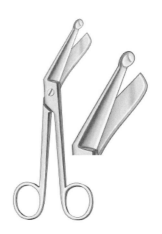

_____   _____

_____   _____

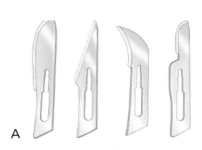

A

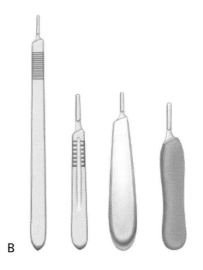

B

_____

_____

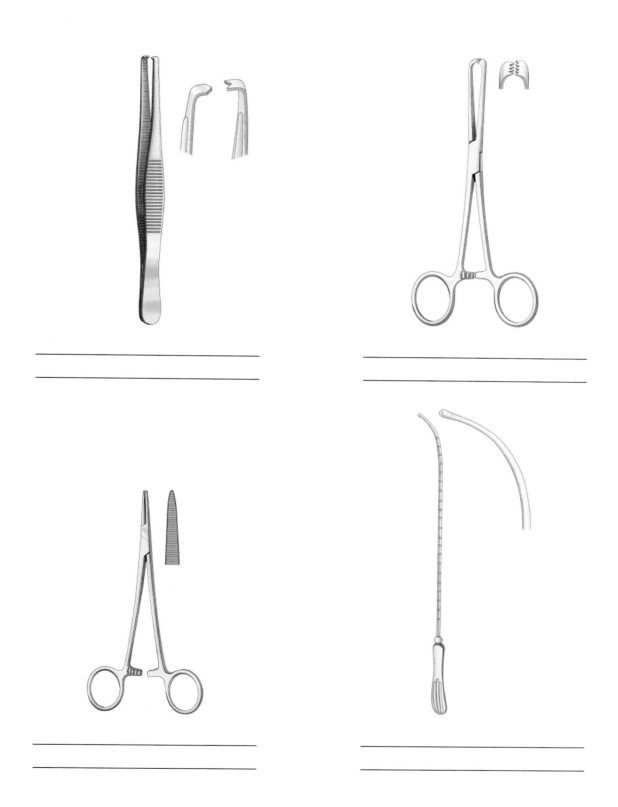

_____

_____

_____

_____

_____

_____

_____

_____

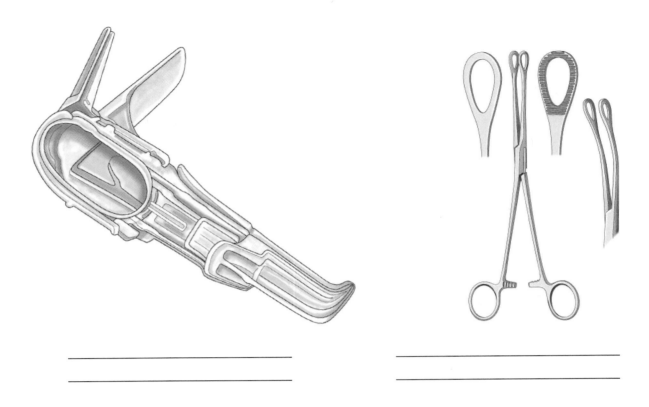

_____   _____

_____   _____

2. Heather Szmyc is at the office today for the removal of 15 staples from her shoulder surgery to remove a lipoma.

   a. What supplies and equipment will you need to gather for this procedure?

   _____

   _____

   _____

   _____

   b. Upon removing the dressing, you notice the skin is red around the incision site and there is greenish-yellow discharge at some of the staple sites. What do you think is going on? What should you do? Please explain.

   _____

   _____

   _____

   _____

Teamwork Exercises

1. Divide into teams of three or four. Select one of the following scenarios and create a role-playing skit to present to the rest of the class:

   a. Pre-operative teaching for a patient scheduled to undergo a laparoscopic tubal ligation

   b. Post-operative teaching for a patient who has undergone reattachment of a severed thumb

   c. Post-operative teaching for a patient who has undergone arthroscopic surgery on his knee

   d. Post-operative teaching regarding wound care for a patient who underwent surgical repair and suturing related to a laceration in his leg from a chain saw

   e. Post-operative teaching for a patient who had the surgical removal of an ingrown toenail

2. Divide into teams of three or four. Each student will take turns practicing putting on sterile gloves and setting up a sterile field. The other students in the group will watch the student perform the procedures and then provide comments/suggestions/questions regarding the student's performance.

PROCEDURE 24-1 – PERFORMING A SURGICAL SCRUB

Name _____   Date _____   Score _____

Instructor _____

Task
Perform a surgical scrub.

Conditions
Deep sink or a surgical sink with foot, knee, or arm
  controls (if available)
Surgical soap
Nail file or fingernail stick
Surgical scrub brush
Clean or sterile towels

Time: _____

Standard
In the time specified and within the scoring parameters
determined by the instructor, the student will successfully perform a surgical scrub.

**Points assigned reflect importance of step to
meeting the task**

Important = 1 pt.
Essential = 5 pts.
Critical = 15 pts.

Automatic failure results if any of the **CRITICAL
TASKS** are omitted or performed incorrectly.

*(To use a pass/fail system, instructors can record "P" or "F"
in the "points earned (pass/fail)" column.)*

PERFORMANCE STANDARDS	PTS	PTS EARNED (Pass/Fail)	COMMENTS
1. Removed all jewelry on hands and arms.	1	_____	_____
2. Rolled long sleeves up above the elbows.	1	_____	_____
3. Examined hands and fingernails for breaks or rough areas.	1	_____	_____
4. Turned on the water to a warm temperature. Avoided touching the body to the sink's edge.	15	_____	_____
5. Wet hands under the water while holding them upright above waist level.	5	_____	_____
6. Cleaned under all fingernails with a nail file, fingernail stick, or the nail attachment of the scrub brush, if provided.	15	_____	_____

PERFORMANCE STANDARDS *(cont.)*	PTS	PTS EARNED (Pass/Fail)	COMMENTS
7. Discarded the file or stick without lowering the hands.			
8. Rinsed nails by continuing to hold the hands upright, allowing water to run over the hands from nails downward and off of the elbows.	15	_____	
9. Applied surgical soap or used a disposable brush impregnated with surgical soap and scrubbed the palms of the hands in a circular motion.	15	_____	
10. While continuing to hold the hands and fingers upward, followed a set pattern for scrubbing the thumbs and each finger, taking care to scrub the base, along each side, and across the nails.	15	_____	
11. Scrubbed the back of each hand in a circular motion. Total scrub time for each hand should be a minimum of 5 minutes.	15	_____	
12. Scrubbed the wrists and the forearms from the distal to the proximal side.	15	_____	
13. Rinsed each arm separately by continuing to hold hands upright, allowing the water to run downward and off of the elbows.	15	_____	
14. Discarded the scrub brush.	1	_____	
15. Turned off the water using a clean paper towel (or the foot or knee lever on a surgical sink).	15	_____	
16. Continued to hold the hands upright and dried one hand and arm with a towel, moving from the distal to the proximal side. If sterile gowning and closed gloving are required, was sure to use a sterile towel for drying.	15	_____	

PERFORMANCE STANDARDS (cont.)	PTS	PTS EARNED (Pass/Fail)	COMMENTS
17. Using the other end of the towel, repeated the drying process on the other hand and arm.	15	_____	

TOTAL POINTS	174		

DOCUMENTATION

COMMENTS

PROCEDURE 24-2 – SETTING UP A STERILE FIELD

Name _____   Date _____   Score _____

                                                          Instructor _____

Task
Set up a sterile field.

Conditions
Mayo stand or other small table on wheels
Sterile drape
Waste receptacle
Other supplies, as needed for the procedure, such
  as (used in this example):

  Sterile solution, such as saline or povidone-iodine
    (Betadine)
  Sterile transfer forceps
  Small sterile cup or basin
  Two sterile, wrapped 4 × 4 sponges

Time: _____

Standards
In the time specified and within the scoring parameters determined by the instructor, the student will successfully set up a sterile field, add items to the field by sterile toss, use sterile transfer forceps to add an item to the field, and pour a sterile solution.

Points assigned reflect importance of step to meeting the task

  Important = 1 pt.
  Essential = 5 pts.
  Critical = 15 pts.

Automatic failure results if any of the **CRITICAL TASKS** are omitted or performed incorrectly.

(To use a pass/fail system, instructors can record "P" or "F" in the "points earned (pass/fail)" column.)

PERFORMANCE STANDARDS	PTS	PTS EARNED (Pass/Fail)	COMMENTS
1. Selected a clean, dry surface above waist level, such as a Mayo stand.	1	_____	_____
2. Assembled the necessary supplies and checked the expiration dates on the packages. Checked the label on each.	5	_____	_____
3. Placed the waste receptacle within easy reach of the work area.	1	_____	_____
4. Washed or sanitized hands.	5	_____	_____
5. Laid a sterile wrapped drape on the surface in front of self with the top flap pointing toward body.	1	_____	_____
6. Grasped and removed the sterilization seal or tape.	1	_____	_____

PERFORMANCE STANDARDS (cont.)	PTS	PTS EARNED (Pass/Fail)	COMMENTS
7. Grasped the top flap of the wrap by the outer surface near the tip. Lifted and opened it away from self.	1	_____	_____
8. Grasped the side flap by the outer surface near the tip, the lifted and opened it to the side.	1	_____	_____
9. Grasped the other side flap by the outer surface near the tip. Lifted and opened it to the side, taking care not to touch any of the sterile contents with fingers.	1	_____	_____
10. Carefully picked up top edge of remaining corner of the folded drape.	1	_____	_____
11. Lifted the drape and let it unfold itself by gravity, rather than shaking it, and made sure that it did not touch anything	5	_____	_____
12. Holding the drape by the outer top corners, laid it over the work surface.	1	_____	_____
13. If sterile 4 × 4 gauze pads were used, took a wrapped pad and grasped each flap of the wrapper between the thumbs and fingers and opened the package outward, taking care not to touch the inner contents with nonsterile fingers.	15	_____	_____
14. Upon opening the package approximately three-quarters of the way, moved over the sterile field and gently tossed or dropped the item onto the field, and took care not to touch any nonsterile item to the field.	15	_____	_____
15. Disposed of the outer wrap in the waste receptacle.	1	_____	_____
16. Repeated steps 12 to 14 to add any other needed items to the field.	15	_____	_____

PERFORMANCE STANDARDS *(cont.)*	PTS	PTS EARNED (Pass/Fail)	COMMENTS
17. Opened the package containing the sterile basin; left the basin on its sterile wrapper.	15	_____	_____ _____ _____
Using sterile transfer forceps			
18. Opened the package containing the sterile transfer forceps and grasped them by the handles only.	1	_____	_____ _____
19. Using sterile forceps, grasped the sterile basin and placed it in the sterile field where desired.	15	_____	_____ _____ _____
Pouring a sterile solution onto the sterile field			
20. Grasped the sterile container, removed the seal, and then removed the cap. Held the cap with the open side downward in your nondominant hand or placed it nearby (but not on the sterile field) with the open side up	15	_____	_____ _____ _____ _____ _____
21. Carefully poured in the required amount of solution, holding the bottle between 1 and 4 inches above the basin.	15	_____	_____ _____ _____
22. Recapped the sterile bottle and set it aside but not on the sterile field.	1	_____	_____ _____

TOTAL POINTS	132		

DOCUMENTATION

COMMENTS

PROCEDURE 24-3 – APPLYING STERILE GLOVES

Name _____   Date _____   Score _____

                                                  Instructor _____

Task
Apply sterile gloves.

Conditions
Package of sterile gloves in the appropriate size
Clean, dry surface such as the top of a Mayo stand

Time: _____

Standard
In the time specified and within the scoring parameters determined by the instructor, the student will successfully apply sterile gloves.

Points assigned reflect importance of step to meeting the task

Important = 1 pt.
Essential = 5 pts.
Critical = 15 pts.

Automatic failure results if any of the **CRITICAL TASKS** are omitted or performed incorrectly.

(To use a pass/fail system, instructors can record "P" or "F" in the "points earned (pass/fail)" column.)

PERFORMANCE STANDARDS	PTS	PTS EARNED (Pass/Fail)	COMMENTS
1. Washed hands with warm water and soap. Dried thoroughly.	5	_____	_____ _____
2. Opened the outer wrapper, removed the inner pack, and laid the inner pack on the table, slightly above waist level.	5	_____	_____ _____ _____ _____
3. Grasped paper fold in each hand and opened outward without disturbing the gloves inside.	1	_____	_____ _____
4. Identified the right and left glove.	1	_____	_____ _____
5. With the first two fingers and thumb of the nondominant hand, grasped the cuff of the dominant hand glove by touching only the inside surface.	5	_____	_____ _____ _____ _____ _____

PERFORMANCE STANDARDS (cont.)	PTS	PTS EARNED (Pass/Fail)	COMMENTS
6. Inserted dominant hand into the glove while carefully pulling it on with the nondominant hand.	5	_____	_____ _____
7. With sterile-gloved, dominant hand, slipped fingers under the cuff of the other glove, touching only the sterile side, and lifted it off the table.	5	_____	_____ _____ _____ _____ _____
8. Inserted nondominant hand into the glove and carefully pulled glove on by pulling upward and outward under its cuff with the fingers of the other hand. Used caution not to touch sterile-gloved fingers or thumb to any nonsterile surface. Kept gloved thumb abducted.	5	_____	_____ _____ _____ _____ _____ _____ _____ _____
9. If long sleeves are worn, continued pulling the cuff upward in the manner describe above until the cuff encircled sleeve cuff.	1	_____	_____ _____ _____ _____
10. After applying the second glove, interlocked hands and adjusted the fingers of the gloves if necessary.	1	_____	_____ _____
Removing gloves			
11. Grasped the outer cuff of one glove with the other hand. Did not touch wrist with the fingers of the contaminated glove	5	_____	_____ _____ _____
12. Pulled the glove off, turned it inside out, and wadded it up in the other gloved hand.	5	_____	_____ _____
13. Placed the fingers of ungloved hand under the cuff of the gloved hand (next to the skin) and pulled the glove off, turning it inside out while enclosing the other glove in the process.	5	_____	_____ _____ _____ _____

PERFORMANCE STANDARDS (cont.)	PTS	PTS EARNED (Pass/Fail)	COMMENTS
14. Discarded in waste receptacle.	1	_____	_____ _____

TOTAL POINTS	**50**		

DOCUMENTATION

COMMENTS

PROCEDURE 24-4 – ASSISTING WITH MINOR SURGERY

Name _____   Date _____   Score _____

Instructor _____

Task
Prepare patient for and assist physician with minor surgery, including application of sterile gloves, setup of the sterile field, and surgical skin preparation.

Conditions
Mayo stand
Needles and syringes for anesthesia
Betadine solution and preparation bowls or cups (at least 2)
Sterile saline solution
Sterile gauze sponges
Scalpel and blade
Operating scissors
Fenestrated drape
Hemostats, curved and blunt
Thumb dressing forceps
Thumb tissue forceps
Needle holder
Suture pack
Transfer forceps

Side table
Package of sterile gloves
Labeled biopsy containers (with formalin)
Laboratory requisition
Anesthesia vial
Alcohol wipes
Dressing materials, including tape, bandages, and 4 × 4 gauze pads
Biohazard container
Betadine solution

Time: _____

Standard
In the time specified and within the scoring parameters determined by the instructor, the student will successfully assist with a minor surgical procedure.

Points assigned reflect importance of step to meeting the task

Important = 1 pt.
Essential = 5 pts.
Critical = 15 pts.

Automatic failure results if any of the **CRITICAL TASKS** are omitted or performed incorrectly.

(To use a pass/fail system, instructors can record "P" or "F" in the "points earned (pass/fail)" column.)

PERFORMANCE STANDARDS	PTS	PTS EARNED (Pass/Fail)	COMMENTS
1. Selected a clean, dry surface above waist level, such as a Mayo stand.	1	_____	_____ _____
2. Checked the room for cleanliness.	1	_____	_____
3. Assembled the supplies for the procedure, inspecting each item for expiration date or contamination.	5	_____	_____ _____
4. Washed hands.	5	_____	_____
5. Set up a side table with nonsterile items.	1	_____	_____ _____
6. Set up a sterile field on a clean, dry surface.	15	_____	_____ _____
7. Added sterile items to the sterile field as needed.	15	_____	_____ _____
8. Applied sterile gloves.	5	_____	_____
9. Arranged the sterile instruments according to order of use.	1	_____	_____ _____
10. Covered the sterile field with a sterile towel if not used immediately.	15	_____	_____ _____
11. Identified the patient and explained the procedure.	5	_____	_____ _____
Surgical skin preparation			
12. Prepared the patient's skin according to office procedure or following these steps:	15	_____	_____ _____
a. Applied clean examination gloves.	1	_____	_____
b. Removed hair from the operative site by carefully shaving, holding the skin taut and shaving in the direction of hair growth or by clipping hair short.	5	_____	_____ _____ _____
c. Rinsed the area with sterile saline solution and patted it dry.	1	_____	_____

PERFORMANCE STANDARDS (cont.)	PTS	PTS EARNED (Pass/Fail)	COMMENTS
d. Cleansed the areas with an antiseptic solution and a surgical scrub brush by scrubbing gently in a circular motion moving from inward to outward. Did not retrace over the previously scrubbed area.	15	_____	_____
e. Rinsed the area with sterile saline saturated gauze pads and blotted it dry.	1	_____	_____
f. Cleaned the area with antiseptic povidone-iodine (Betadine) or alcohol swabs.	15	_____	_____
g. Allowed the area to air dry.	1	_____	_____
h. Removed gloves.	1	_____	
i. Sanitized hands.	5	_____	
13. Removed the sterile towel from the sterile field as the physician applied sterile gloves.	5	_____	_____
14. Assisted the physician with the procedure, according to her requests.	15	_____	_____
15. Throughout the procedure:			_____
a. Ensured that the physician had the necessary equipment and supplies.	1	_____	_____
b. Ensured that the lighting was adequate for the physician to view the surgical field.	1	_____	_____
c. Comforted the patient (if awake) during the procedure.	1	_____	_____
d. Handed instruments to the physician as requested.	1	_____	_____
e. Held the biopsy container for the physician to place the tissue specimen into, if necessary.	1	_____	_____
f. Ensured the biopsy containers or other specimens are properly labeled, tightly covered, and sent to the laboratory with an appropriately completed laboratory requisition form.	15	_____	_____

PERFORMANCE STANDARDS (cont.)	PTS	PTS EARNED (Pass/Fail)	COMMENTS
16. Upon completion of the procedure, assisted the physician as needed with the application of a dressing.	5	_____	
17. Disposed of contaminated supplies and sharps in an appropriate biohazard sharps container.	5	_____	
18. Rinsed used surgical instruments and soaked, sanitized, and sterilized them for reuse.	5	_____	
19. Removed and appropriately disposed of gloves, gown, and other PPE and washed hands.	5	_____	
20. Applied clean gloves and other PPE as needed.	5	_____	
21. Disinfected the treatment area per office protocol.	5	_____	
22. Washed hands.	5	_____	
23. Provided the patient's medical record to the physician.	5	_____	

TOTAL POINTS	109		

DOCUMENTATION

COMMENTS

PROCEDURE 24-5 – PERFORMING SUTURE REMOVAL

Name _____

Date _____   Score _____

Instructor _____

Task
Perform removal of skin sutures.

Conditions
Gauze sponges
Bandage scissors
Biohazard waste container
Tape
Sponge forceps
Suture scissors or staple remover
Thumb forceps
4 × 4 gauze pads
Sterile gloves
Betadine solution or wash

Time: _____

Standard
In the time specified and within the scoring parameters determined by the instructor, the student will successfully remove sutures from a wound.

Points assigned reflect importance of step to meeting the task

Important = 1 pt.
Essential = 5 pts.
Critical = 15 pts.

Automatic failure results if any of the **CRITICAL TASKS** are omitted or performed incorrectly.

(To use a pass/fail system, instructors can record "P" or "F" in the "points earned (pass/fail)" column.)

PERFORMANCE STANDARDS	PTS	PTS EARNED (Pass/Fail)	COMMENTS
1. Washed or sanitized hands.	5	_____	_____
2. Identified the patient and explained the procedure.	5	_____	_____ _____
3. Opened the suture-removal kit.	1	_____	_____
4. Applied sterile gloves.	5	_____	_____
5. Using thumb forceps, gently picked up one knot of a suture.	15	_____	_____ _____
6. Gently pulled upward toward the suture line.	5	_____	_____ _____
7. Inserted the curved notch of the suture-removal scissors beneath the suture and cut one side of the suture as close to the skin as possible.	15	_____	_____ _____ _____

PERFORMANCE STANDARDS (cont.)	PTS	PTS EARNED (Pass/Fail)	COMMENTS
8. Pulled the suture through the skin, being careful to avoid contaminating the wound with the suture tip.	15	_____	_____ _____
9. Removed all sutures in the same manner.	15	_____	_____ _____
10. Placed each suture on a sterile gauze sponge.	5	_____	_____ _____
11. Examined the wound to be sure that you had removed all of the sutures.	5	_____	_____ _____
12. Applied povidone-iodine solution to the area, unless the patient is allergic to iodine.	5	_____	_____ _____
13. Applied a sterile dressing if directed.	1	_____	_____
14. Removed gloves and disposed of them in a biohazardous waste container.	5	_____	_____ _____
15. Disposed of all used items per OSHA regulations.	5	_____	_____ _____
16. Washed hands.	5	_____	_____
17. Explained wound care to the patient, providing written and verbal instructions.	5	_____	_____ _____
18. Documented the procedure.	5	_____	_____ _____

TOTAL POINTS	122		

DOCUMENTATION

COMMENTS

PROCEDURE 24-6 – REMOVING A DRESSING AND APPLYING A NEW STERILE DRESSING

Name _____ Date _____ Score _____

Instructor _____

Task

Demonstrate the removal and application of a sterile dressing.

Conditions

Sterile gloves
Sterile gauze dressings as needed
Examination gloves
Tape
Biohazard waste container
Sterile saline solution
Tape, roller gauze, or elastic net as desired

Time: _____

Standard

In the time specified and within the scoring parameters determined by the instructor, the student will successfully remove an old dressing and apply a new, dry, sterile dressing.

Points assigned reflect importance of step to meeting the task

Important = 1 pt.
Essential = 5 pts.
Critical = 15 pts.

Automatic failure results if any of the **CRITICAL TASKS** are omitted or performed incorrectly.

(To use a pass/fail system, instructors can record "P" or "F" in the "points earned (pass/fail)" column.)

PERFORMANCE STANDARDS	PTS	PTS EARNED (Pass/Fail)	COMMENTS
1. Washed or sanitized your hands.	5	_____	_____
2. Introduced yourself to the patient and explained the procedure.	5	_____	_____
3. Noted the location, size, and depth of the wound as well as the current dressing material used.	5	_____	_____
4. Reviewed the physician's order for wound care and dressing change.	15	_____	_____
5. Gathered the needed supplies.	1	_____	_____
6. Evaluated the patient's current degree of discomfort and whether pain medication was needed.	1	_____	_____
7. Took measures to ensure privacy for the patient.	1	_____	_____

PERFORMANCE STANDARDS (cont.)	PTS	PTS EARNED (Pass/Fail)	COMMENTS

8. Positioned the patient on the examination table in a manner that maximized patient comfort and provided optimal access to the wound.   **5**   _____

9. Washed or sanitized your hands.   **5**   _____

10. Set up a sterile field and needed supplies.   **15**   _____

Removing the old dressing

11. Applied clean examination gloves and removed the old dressing by following these steps: **15**   _____

   a. Stabilized the old dressing with one hand while carefully pulling the tape off toward the wound.   **5**   _____

   b. Gently removed the dressing in layers.   **5**   _____

   c. Before disposing of the dressing, noted the amount and character of drainage on the dressing material.   **5**   _____

   d. Removed your contaminated gloves and disposed of them in the biohazard waste container.   **5**   _____

12. Washed or sanitized your hands.   **5**   _____

Applying the new dressing

13. Applied sterile gloves.   **5**   _____

14. Noted the wound's appearance, including size, depth, and any signs of infection.   **5**   _____

15. Cleaned the wound, as ordered. Used sterile saline moistened gauze to clean from the most to least contaminated area (from wound outward) and from wound margins outward. Alternatively, irrigated the wound with sterile saline, flushing in one direction.   **5**   _____

PERFORMANCE STANDARDS (cont.)	PTS	PTS EARNED (Pass/Fail)	COMMENTS
16. Patted the area dry with dry sterile gauze.	1	_____	_____
17. Applied a sterile dry dressing material as needed over the wound.	15	_____	_____
18. Secured the dressing in place with tape or another bandage material, such as roller gauze or elastic net.	5	_____	_____
19. Documented the procedure and any patient education about wound care or signs of infection	5	_____	_____

TOTAL POINTS	139		

DOCUMENTATION

COMMENTS

Dermatology

Key Term Review

Define the following key terms:

1. dermabrasion _____

_____

2. pruritus _____

_____

3. benign _____

_____

4. edema _____

_____

5. intradermal _____

_____

6. teratogenic _____

_____

7. malignant _____

_____

8. allergen _____

_____

9. verruca vulgaris _____

_____

10. metastasize _____

_____

11. dermatitis _____

_____

12. comedo _____

_____

Key Term Review *cont.*

13. aerobic _____

_____

14. laceration _____

_____

15. biopsy _____

_____

16. tinea _____

_____

17. wheal _____

_____

18. dysplasia _____

_____

19. neoplasm _____

_____

20. erythema _____

_____

Review Questions

1. Describe the three layers of skin and provide the function of each layer.

_____

_____

_____

_____

2. List the important functions the skin serves.

_____

_____

_____

_____

3. Discuss seven warning signs of skin cancer.

_____

_____

_____

4. Identify the characteristics of a malignant melanoma.

_____

_____

_____

5. List and describe four types of allergy testing.

_____

_____

_____

6. Explain why it is important to perform a culture and sensitivity test prior to treating an infection.

_____

_____

_____

7. List and describe five types of image enhancement procedures.

_____

_____

_____

8. List six accessory structures of the skin.

_____

_____

_____

9. Compare and contrast HSV-1 with HSV-2.

_____

_____

_____

_____

10. What is pediculosis? Describe how it is diagnosed and treated.

_____

_____

_____

_____

Medical Terminology Review

Give the proper medical term for the definition provided:

1. a tumor composed of fat: _____

2. pertaining to the skin: _____

3. an abnormal condition of hardening: _____

4. disease of the hair: _____

5. the study of cells: _____

6. an abnormal condition of fungus: _____

7. surgical repair of the skin: _____

8. fear of hair: _____

9. softening of the nail: _____

10. dry skin: _____

Disease/Condition Review

Match the disease/condition with its definition:

Disease/condition

1. psoriasis _____

2. cellulites _____

3. tinea pedis _____

4. shingles _____

5. eczema _____

6. pediculosis _____

7. scabies _____

8. acne _____

9. folliculitis _____

10. warts _____

11. impetigo _____

12. basal cell carcinoma _____

13. nevus _____

14. alopecia _____

15. squamous cell carcinoma _____

Definition

a. hyperpigmentation of the skin

b. inflammatory skin disease of the sebaceous follicles marked by pimples

c. inflammatory skin rash marked by redness and itching

d. most common type of skin cancer

e. contagious bacterial skin infection caused by staphylococcus or streptococcus

f. a spreading bacterial infection of the skin and subcutaneous tissue

g. contagious infestation of the skin with an itch mite

h. noncontagious skin disorder in which red scaly plaques appear on the body surface

i. infestation with lice

j. small skin tumors cause by HPV

k. a reactivation of the varicella virus

l. athlete's foot

m. a form of skin cancer that grows very rapidly and spreads easily

n. absence or loss of hair

o. inflammation or infection of hair follicles

Anatomy Identification

1. Label each layer and structure of the skin in Figure 25-1.

A
B
C
D
E
F
G
H

S
R
Q
P
O
N
M
L
K
J
I

a. _____

b. _____

c. _____

d. _____

e. _____

_____

f. _____

_____

g. _____

_____

h. _____

_____

i. _____

_____

j. _____

_____

k. _____

_____

l. _____

_____

m. _____

_____

n. _____

_____

o. _____

_____

p. _____

_____

q. _____

_____

r. _____

_____

s. _____

_____

2. Label each lesion in Figures 25-2 through 25-11.

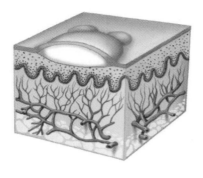

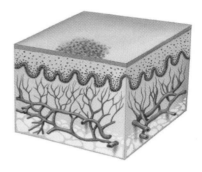

_____

_____

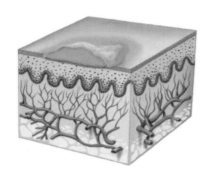

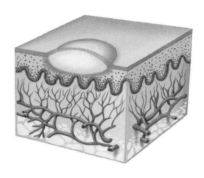

_____

_____

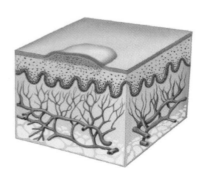

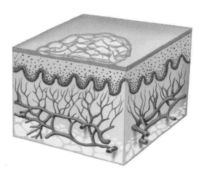

_____

_____

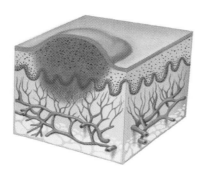

_____

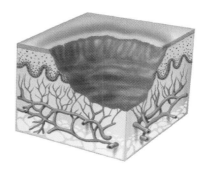

_____

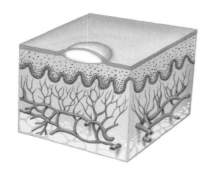

_____

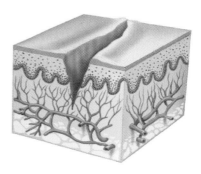

_____

Critical Thinking

1. 27-year-old Cassie Jones is seeing the dermatologist about her persistent acne. She tells you she's seen an advertisement on television about the acne drug Accutane, and she tells you she is going to ask the dermatologist to prescribe it to her. What will you ask and/or tell Cassie about the medication?

   _____

   _____

   _____

   _____

2. A 54-year-old cancer patient is visiting her primary-care physician complaining of a painful, burning rash across the trunk of her body. What condition do you think she is suffering from?

   _____

   _____

   _____

   _____

Teamwork Exercise

1. Divide into groups of three or four. Your instructor will assign a skin condition for each group to research and report on. Information in your presentation should include causative agent (if applicable), signs and symptoms, diagnosis, treatment, and prognosis. Examples of conditions can include scabies, impetigo, eczema, psoriasis, etc.

2. Divine the class into four groups. Each group will be assigned one of the following methods for allergy testing: scratch test, intradermal test, patch test, and RAST. Each group will research the actual methodology behind each test, examples of its uses, the procedure for testing, and the specificity and sensitivity of each method. After each group presents on their test method, have a class discussion about the pros and cons of each method.

PROCEDURE 25-1 – ALLERGY SKIN TESTING

Name _____

Date _____   Score _____

Instructor _____

Task
Properly perform an allergy skin prick test.

Conditions
Allergen solution
Control solution
Multiheaded skin testing device
Biohazard waste container
Marking pen
Ruler or measuring device
Tissues
Nonsterile examination gloves
Medical record or chart
Waste container

Time: _____

Standard
In the time specified and within the scoring parameters determined by the instructor, the student will successfully perform an allergy skin prick test.

Points assigned reflect importance of step to meeting the task

Important = 1 pt.
Essential = 5 pts.
Critical = 15 pts.

Automatic failure results if any of the **CRITICAL TASKS** are omitted or performed incorrectly.

(To use a pass/fail system, instructors can record "P" or "F" in the "points earned (pass/fail)" column.)

PERFORMANCE STANDARDS	PTS	PTS EARNED (Pass/Fail)	COMMENTS
1. Washed or sanitized hands and assembled supplies.	1	_____	_____
2. Greeted and identified patient and introduced yourself. Explained the procedure and asked the patient if he had taken any medications in the past 2 weeks. Also asked if the patient has applied any creams, ointments, or moisturizers to his skin today.	5	_____	_____
3. Assisted the patient onto the examination table into a position that is comfortable for the patient and convenient for testing.	1	_____	_____
4. Cleaned the skin site with water or alcohol.	5	_____	_____

PERFORMANCE STANDARDS *(cont.)*	PTS	PTS EARNED (Pass/Fail)	COMMENTS
5. Held the multiheaded skin testing device next to the patient's skin. Used the marking pen to mark the patient's skin next to each testing site.	15	_____	
6. Pressed the testing device gently against the patient's skin.	15	_____	
7. Repeated steps 6 and 7 with different prepared testing devices until all tests had been completed.	15	_____	
8. Carefully blotted any excess solution with tissue.	1	_____	
9. Set the timer for 15 minutes. Gave the patient some reading material if desired.	15	_____	
10. Noted the results and measured any positive reactions in millimeters. If wheals were not round in shape, measured the diameter in both directions and recorded the average of the two.	15	_____	
11. Removed markings from the skin with an alcohol solution or water.	5	_____	
12. Reassured the patient that any itching should resolve within 20 minutes or so.	1	_____	
13. Instructed the patient with positive reactions to remain in the office for at least 20 minutes after completion of the test.	15	_____	
14. Documented results in the medical record.	15	_____	

TOTAL POINTS	124		

DOCUMENTATION

COMMENTS

Neurology

Key Term Review *Define the following key terms:*

1. neuron

2. transaction

3. cerebral contusion

4. aural

5. myelin

6. embolic

7. bradykinesia

8. paresthesia

9. neurotransmitter

10. homeostasis

11. corpuscallostomy

12. Brudzinski sign

Key Term Review *cont.*

13. spinal fusion _____

_____

14. paresthesia _____

_____

15. affect _____

_____

16. cerebral _____

concussion _____

17. fasciculation _____

_____

18. motor nerves _____

_____

19. sensory nerves _____

_____

20. nuchal rigidity _____

_____

Review Questions

1. Discuss the functions of the neurological system.

_____

_____

_____

_____

2. Describe the role of the medical assistant in the neurologist's office.

_____

_____

_____

_____

3. Describe the structure and components of the neuron. What is the function of each component?

_____

_____

_____

_____

4. What does the central nervous system consist of?

_____

_____

_____

_____

5. Describe the function of the central nervous system.

_____

_____

_____

_____

6. What does the peripheral nervous system consist of?

_____

_____

_____

_____

7. Describe the function of the peripheral nervous system.

_____

_____

_____

_____

8. List and describe the major divisions of the brain.

_____

_____

_____

_____

9. What does the spinal cord consist of?

_____

_____

_____

_____

10. Describe the importance of the autonomic nervous system.

_____

_____

_____

_____

11. Compare and contrast paraplegia, hemiplegia, and quadriplegia.

_____

_____

_____

_____

Medical Terminology and Abbreviation Review

Give the proper medical term for the definition provided:

1. absence of speech: _____

2. nerve pain: _____

3. herniation of the brain: _____

4. slight or partial paralysis of half the body: _____

5. drooping of eyelid: _____

6. pertaining to the brain: _____

7. painful or difficult swallowing: _____

8. absence of sensation: _____

9. glue-like tumor: _____

10. increased sensation: _____

11. absence of growth: _____

12. paralysis of eye or eyes: _____

13. pertaining to the meninges: _____

14. tumor of nerve cells: _____

15. herniation of the meninges and spinal cord: _____

16. small head: _____

17. inflammation of the meninges: _____

18. inflammation of many nerves: _____

Define the following abbreviations:

1. MS: _____

2. ALS: _____

3. TIA: _____

4. PNS: _____

5. CNS: _____

6. EEG: _____

7. MRI: _____

8. CSF: _____

9. ICP: _____

10. CT: _____

Disease/Condition Review

Match the disease/condition with its definition:

Disease/condition

1. _____ stroke

2. _____ multiple sclerosis

3. _____ transient ischemic attack

4. _____ amyotrophic lateral sclerosis

5. _____ sciatica

6. _____ migraine headache

7. _____ carpal tunnel syndrome

8. _____ epilepsy

9. _____ Huntington chorea

10. _____ shingles

11. _____ meningitis

12. _____ Parkinson disease

13. _____ spinal stenosis

14. _____ poliomyelitis

15. _____ Bell palsy

Definition

a. Chronically progressive, degenerative neuromuscular disorder that destroys motor neurons of the body; also called Lou Gehrig disease.

b. Disorder of the seventh cranial nerve that causes temporary weakness or paralysis of one side of the face

c. Syndrome that is characterized by pain or numbness of the median nerve in the hand and forearm and caused by nerve compression and inflammation due to cumulative trauma from repetitive motion

d. Chronic disorder of the brain marked by recurrent seizures, which are repetitive, abnormal electrical discharges within the brain

e. Hereditary nervous disorder that leads to bizarre, involuntary movements and dementia

f. Infection of the meninges, the spinal cord, and the cerebrospinal fluid, usually caused by an infectious illness

g. Familial disorder marked by episodes of throbbing, severe headache that is commonly unilateral and, sometimes, disabling

Disease/condition	Definition *cont.*

h. Chronic, degenerative disease of the central nervous system that results in movement disorders and changes in cognition and mood

i. Inflammation of the spinal cord caused by a virus, possibly resulting in spinal and muscle deformity and paralysis

j. Severe pain of the sciatic nerve that radiates from the buttocks to the feet

k. Unilateral, painful vesicles that appear on the upper body and are caused by the herpes zoster virus

l. Disorder that involves narrowing of an area of the spine that puts pressure on the spinal cord and nerve roots

m. Sudden loss of neurological function due to vascular injury to the brain; also called cerebrovascular accident (CVA) and brain attack.

n. Temporary impairment of neurological functioning due to a brief interruption in blood supply to a part of the brain

o. Chronic autoimmune disease that affects the central nervous system, causing inflammation and degeneration of the myelin sheath that protects nerve fibers.

Anatomy Identification

1. Identify each structure of the neuron in Figure 26-1.

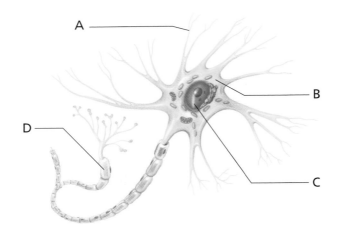

a. _____

_____

b. _____

_____

c. _____

_____

d. _____

_____

2. Identify each section of the brain in Figure 26-2.

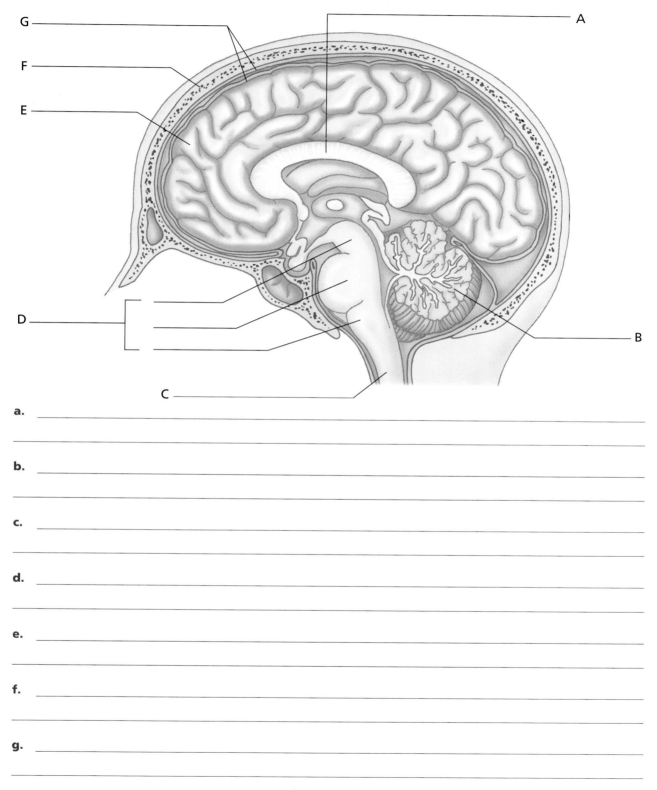

a. _____

_____

b. _____

_____

c. _____

_____

d. _____

_____

e. _____

_____

f. _____

_____

g. _____

_____

3. Identify each type of nerve in Figure 26-3.

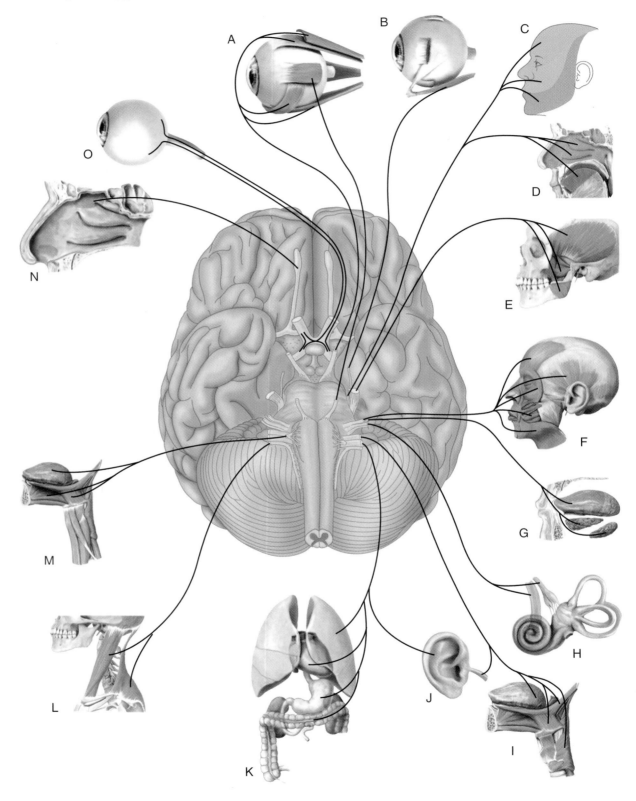

Student Activity Manual to Accompany The Professional Medical Assistant   © copyright 2009 F.A. Davis Company

a. _____

_____

b. _____

_____

c. _____

_____

d. _____

_____

e. _____

_____

f. _____

_____

g. _____

_____

h. _____

_____

i. _____

_____

j. _____

_____

k. _____

_____

l. _____

_____

m. _____

_____

n. _____

_____

o. _____

_____

Critical Thinking

1. Dr. Greer has ordered an MRI on Mr. Galgiastre. As the medical assistant, you are responsible for explaining the procedure as well as the patient preparation to Mr. Galgiastre. What are the specifics you would cover with Mr. Galgiastre?

   _____

   _____

   _____

   _____

2. Janice Resnick, a 42-year-old computer software technician, is in complaining of pain in her hands and wrists. As you continue to interview Janice, what specific questions would you ask her regarding her chief complaint? What condition could her symptoms suggest?

   _____

   _____

   _____

   _____

3. Jilley Chavez, a 15-year-old soccer player, is being seen for her third sports-related concussion in a year. The physician explained to Jilley that she cannot play contact sports for 6 months due to her history of concussions. After the physician leaves Jilley breaks down and starts crying, saying that she needs to continue to play soccer and does not care what the physician has told her. Explain to Jilley why she should follow the physician's orders.

   _____

   _____

   _____

   _____

Teamwork Exercises

1. Divide the class into groups of two or three. Allow each group to take one of the conditions/diseases within the chapter and prepare a 10-minute PowerPoint presentation on the symptoms, diagnosis, treatment, and prognosis for the condition/disease.

2. Divide the class into groups of two or three. Your instructor will each group one of the following diagnostic procedure:

   a. MRI

   b. CAT scan

   c. lumbar puncture

   d. myelogram

   e. electroencephalogram

   For each procedure, develop a patient information sheet explaining the procedure as well as the patient preparation/instructions for the procedure.

PROCEDURE 26-1 – ASSISTING WITH A NEUROLOGICAL EXAM

Name _____   Date _____   Score _____

Instructor _____

Task

Properly prepare the patient for and assist the physician with a complete neurological examination.

Conditions

Examination table
Drape
Patient examination gown
Specific supplies and equipment including but not
  limited to:
neurology reflex hammer
safety pin
otoscope
ophthalmoscope
penlight
tongue blade
tuning fork
pinwheel
cotton ball
items for testing heat and cold sensation per physician's
  instructions
small containers of sweet and salty solutions per
  physician's instructions
items for odor identification per physician's instructions.

Time: _____

Standard

In the time specified and within the scoring parameters determined by the instructor, the student will success-fully assist with a neurological examination

Points assigned reflect importance of step to meeting the task

Important = 1 pt.
Essential = 5 pts.
Critical = 15 pts.

Automatic failure results if any of the **CRITICAL TASKS** are omitted or performed incorrectly.

(To use a pass/fail system, Instructors can record "P" or "F" in the "points earned (pass/fail)" column.)

PERFORMANCE STANDARDS	PTS	PTS EARNED (Pass/Fail)	COMMENTS
1. Completed preliminary steps as for any general physical examination. Assisted the patient into positions as instructed by the physician. Arranged the drape for warmth and privacy.	5	_____	_____
2. As the physician examined the patient, was prepared to hand him items as needed, such as the oto-scope, ophthalmoscope, penlight, and tongue depressor.	5	_____	_____

PERFORMANCE STANDARDS (cont.)	PTS	PTS EARNED (Pass/Fail)	COMMENTS
3. Dimmed the lights if directed when the physician examined the patients' eyes.	1	_____	
4. Throughout the remainder of the examination, continued to assist the patient in assuming the positions directed by the physician and continued to hand needed items to the physician.	5	_____	
5. Followed standard precautions and took care when receiving any potentially contaminated items from the physician (such as the tongue depressor, speculum, or swabs) to handle them in a manner that prevented exposure to you.	15	_____	
6. Disposed of all waste in appropriate containers.	1	_____	
7. Placed any obtained specimens in appropriately labeled containers.	15	_____	
8. Upon completion of the examination, assisted the patient down from the table and instructed her to get dressed. Left the room for a few minutes so the patient could change in privacy unless she required your assistance.	15	_____	
9. Scheduled any ordered follow-up tests or appointments.	5	_____	
10. Directed the patient back to the reception area. Assisted her if needed.	1	_____	
11. Documented patient education, instructions, or scheduled tests in the medical record.	15	_____	
12. Cleaned, sanitized, and restocked the examination room as needed.	1	_____	

TOTAL POINTS	84		

DOCUMENTATION

COMMENTS

PROCEDURE 26-2 – ASSISTING WITH LUMBAR PUNCTURE

Name _____

Date _____   Score _____

Instructor _____

Task

Properly prepare an individual for and assist with lumbar puncture to collect a specimen for CSF analysis.

Conditions

Local anesthetic
Disposable lumbar puncture tray
Mayo-type supply stand
Biohazard waste container
Marker to label specimen tubes
Sterile gloves
Syringe and needle
Patient examination gown
Drape

Time: _____

Standard

In the time specified and within the scoring parameters determined by the instructor, the student will successfully assist with lumbar puncture.

Points assigned reflect importance of step to meeting the task

> Important = 1 pt.
> Essential = 5 pts.
> Critical = 15 pts.

Automatic failure results if any of the **CRITICAL TASKS** are omitted or performed incorrectly.

(To use a pass/fail system, Instructors can record "P" or "F" in the "points earned (pass/fail)" column.)

PERFORMANCE STANDARDS	PTS	PTS EARNED (Pass/Fail)	COMMENTS
1. Greeted and identified your patient and introduced yourself.	1	_____	_____
2. Reviewed the nature of the procedure and determined whether the patient had any questions.	1	_____	_____
3. Checked to make sure a consent form had been signed.	5	_____	_____
4. Instructed the patient to empty his bladder.	1	_____	_____
5. Gave the patient an examination gown. Instructed him to put it on with the opening in the back and then lie down on the examination table on his left side.	1	_____	_____
6. Provided the patient with a pillow for his head and a second pillow to place between his knees if desired.	1	_____	_____

PERFORMANCE STANDARDS (cont.)	PTS	PTS EARNED (Pass/Fail)	COMMENTS
7. Positioned the patient in a fetal position and covered him with a drape.	1	_____	_____ _____
8. Washed your hands, assembled the supplies, and set up a sterile field, including needed sterile supplies.	15	_____	_____ _____ _____
9. Performed sterile skin preparation on the patient's lumbar area.	15	_____	_____ _____
10. Assisted the physician as needed with the procedure, including:	15	_____	_____
a. Held the anesthetic vial upside down at an angle so the physician could aspirate fluid from it or pour it into a sterile cup on the sterile field.			_____ _____ _____ _____
b. Provided reassurance to the patient and assisted him in holding still in the fetal position			_____ _____
c. Held the top of the manometer if requested by the physician.			_____ _____
d. If pressure readings were taken, instructed the patient to refrain from talking or holding his breath.			_____ _____ _____
e. If directed by the physician, assisted the patient in straightening his legs			_____ _____
f. Marked the specimens sequentially according to the order in which they were collected (for example, "#1," "#2," and "#3").			_____ _____ _____
g. Completed the laboratory requisition form and packaged the specimens for transport.			_____
11. After the physician had completed the procedure and applied an adhesive bandage to the site, positioned the patient in a prone or supine position as directed by the physician.	5	_____ _____	_____ _____ _____

PERFORMANCE STANDARDS (cont.)	PTS	PTS EARNED (Pass/Fail)	COMMENTS
12. Instructed the patient to lie flat for the required number of hours.	1	_____	_____
13. Measured and recorded the patient's vital signs, provided liquids, and evaluated the patient for discomfort according to facility policy.	5	_____	_____
14. Disposed of supplies, taking care to place sharps and contaminated items in appropriate biohazard waste containers.	5	_____	_____
15. Cleaned the room per facility protocol and sanitized your hands.	1	_____	_____
16. Documented data in the patient's chart.	15	_____	_____

TOTAL POINTS	98		

DOCUMENTATION

COMMENTS

Cardiology and Lymphatics

Key Term Review   *Define the following key terms:*

1.   ablation _____

2.   blood pressure _____

3.   ligation _____

4.   phagocytosis _____

5.   lumen _____

6.   systole _____

7.   cardioversion _____

8.   angioplasty _____

9.   artifact _____

10.   depolarization _____

11.   diastole _____

12.   systemic
circulation _____

Key Term Review *cont.*

13.   perfusion   _____

_____

14.   apical pulse   _____

_____

15.   pressure point   _____

_____

16.   arteries   _____

_____

17.   pulse points   _____

_____

18.   mitral valve   _____

_____

19.   cardiac cycle   _____

_____

20.   aorta   _____

_____

21.   palpation   _____

_____

22.   lymph   _____

_____

Review Questions

1. Discuss the function and structure of the three different types of blood vessels of the body.

_____

_____

_____

_____

2. List and describe the layers of the heart.

_____

_____

_____

_____

3. What is the function of heart valves?

_____

_____

_____

_____

4. List the valves of the heart and note their locations.

_____

_____

_____

_____

5. Discuss the major vessels of the heart and their functions.

_____

_____

_____

_____

6. Compare and contrast the two chambers of the heart.

_____

_____

_____

_____

7. Describe the functions of the lymphatic system.

_____

_____

_____

_____

8. List and describe the structures associated with the lymphatic system.

_____

_____

_____

_____

9. What is the apical pulse?

_____

_____

_____

_____

10. Discuss the importance of the SA node in the heart's conduction system.

_____

_____

_____

_____

11. What does blood pressure measure?

_____

_____

_____

_____

12. What is the medical assistant's role in ECG?

_____

_____

_____

_____

13. What is the importance of standardizing an ECG machine?

_____

_____

_____

_____

14. For each chest lead, provide the proper location placement.

    a. V1

    b. V2

    c. V3

    d. V4

    e. V5

    f. V6

15. What is the purpose of a Holter monitor?

_____

_____

_____

_____

16. Describe three different cardiovascular diseases patients may present within the medical office.

_____

_____

_____

_____

17. Match the following lab test with the reason for ordering:

Lab Test

1. CPK _____

2. lipid panel _____

3. PT _____

4. digoxin _____

5. CBC _____

Reason for Ordering

a. measures the amount of a certain heart drug in a patient's system.

b. monitors levels of Coumadin in the blood

c. test used to determine a person's risk of CVD

d. measures a cardiac enzyme that is released during an MI

e. measures the blood's ability to fight off infection

Medical Terminology and Abbreviation Review

Give the proper medical term for the definition provided:

1. creating or producing blood: _____

2. condition of rapid heartbeat: _____

3. narrowing or stricture of the aorta: _____

4. vomiting of blood: _____

5. swelling of a vessel: _____

6. clotting cell: _____

7. thick, fatty tumor: _____

8. record of heart electricity: _____

9. destruction of blood: _____

10. rupture of a vein: _____

11. suture of a vessel: _____

12. swelling caused by lymph fluid: _____

13. deficiency of red blood cells: _____

14. pertaining to the atria and ventricles _____

15. a condition of white blood cells: _____

16. disease of the gland: _____

17. bursting forth of blood: _____

18. pertaining to above the ventricles: _____

19. enlargement of the spleen: _____

20. inflammation of a vein in the presence of a clot: _____

Define the following abbreviations:

1. PND: _____

2. ASHD: _____

3. HTN: _____

4. PTT: _____

5. RA: _____

6. PCP: _____

7. INR: _____

8. AIDS: _____

9. BP: _____

10. WBC: _____

11. HIV: _____

12. CABG: _____

13. RV: _____

14. PT: _____

15. PVC: _____

Disease/Condition Review

Match the disease/condition with its definition:

Disease/Condition

1. ischemia _____

2. endocarditis _____

3. anemia __b__

4. hypertension _____

5. myocardial infarction _____

6. shock _____

7. Hodgkin disease _____

8. AIDS _____

9. cardiomyopathy _____

10. lymphosarcoma _____

11. arrhythmia __d__

12. mononucleosis _____

13. orthopnea _____

14. pulmonary embolism _____

15. postphlebitic syndrome _____

Definition

a. malignant lymphoma characterized by giant Reed-Sternberg cells

b. reduction in the mass of circulating red blood cells

c. cancer of the lymphatic tissue not related to Hodgkin disease

d. irregular heartbeat

e. any of several diseases that affects the heart muscle

f. infection or inflammation of the valves and inner lining of the heart

g. blood pressure is higher than 140/90 on three separate readings that are several weeks apart

h. temporary reduction of blood supply to a localized area of tissue

i. loss of living heart muscle as a result of coronary artery occlusion

j. labored breathing that occurs when lying flat and is relieved by sitting upright

k. obstruction of a pulmonary artery from an embolus

l. syndrome marked by inadequate perfusion and oxygenation of cells, tissues, and organs due to low blood pressure

Disease/condition

m. late-stage infection with HIV

n. acute infection with the Epstein-Barr virus, which causes sore throat, fever, fatigue, and enlarged lymph nodes

o. condition sometimes followed by deep vein thrombosis in which individuals experience chronic edema and aching

p. chronic autoimmune disease that affects the central nervous system, causing inflammation and degeneration of the myelin sheath that protects nerve fibers

Anatomy Identification

1. Label each structure of the heart in Figure 27-1.

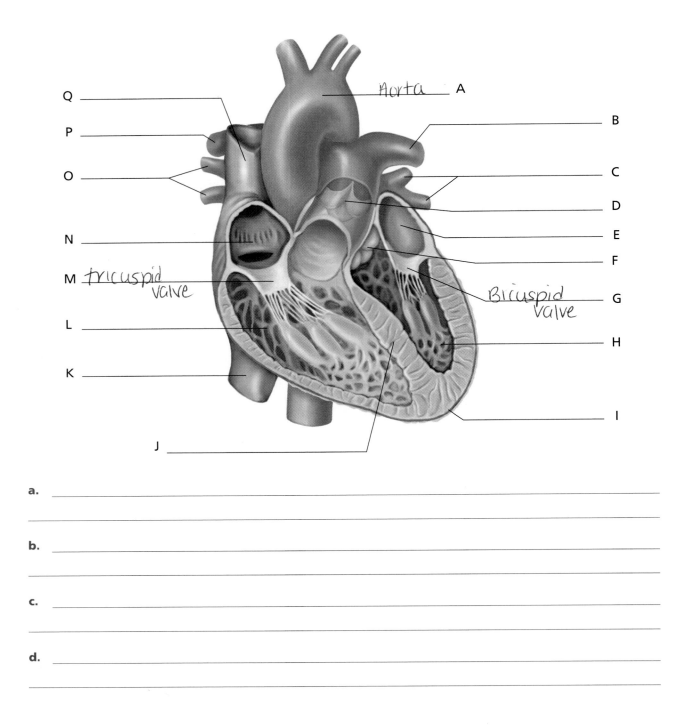

Q _____

P _____

O _____

N _____

M *tricuspid valve* _____

L _____

K _____

J _____

A ___ *Aorta* ___

B _____

C _____

D _____

E _____

F _____

G ___ *Bicuspid valve*

H _____

I _____

a. _____

_____

b. _____

_____

c. _____

_____

d. _____

_____

e. _____

_____

f. _____

_____

g. _____

_____

h. _____

_____

i. _____

_____

j. _____

_____

k. _____

_____

l. _____

_____

m. _____

_____

n. _____

_____

o. _____

_____

p. _____

_____

q. _____

_____

2. Label the structures of the lymphatic vessels in Figure 27-2.

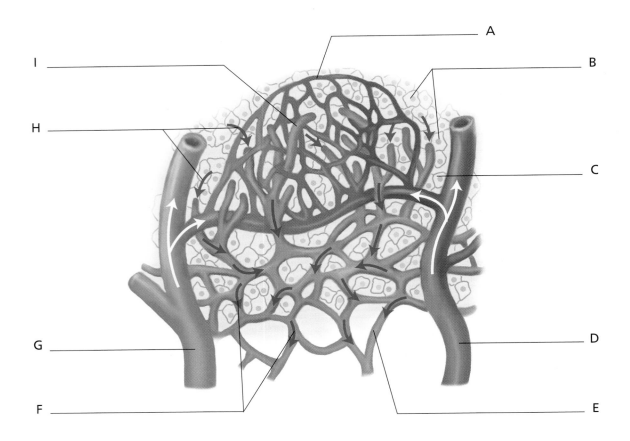

a.
_____
_____

b.
_____
_____

c.
_____
_____

d.
_____
_____

e.
_____
_____

f.
_____
_____

g.
_____
_____

h.
_____
_____

i.
_____
_____

Critical Thinking

1. Mr. Sandro has been experiencing lightheadedness and heart palpitations. Dr. Green has ordered Mr. Sandro to wear a Holtor monitor for the next 48 hours. You are the medical assistant in charge of applying the monitor and providing instructions to Mr. Sandro. Explain the procedure for properly applying the Holter monitor. What patient instructions will you give Mr. Sandro?

_____

_____

_____

_____

2. The clinic you are employed at is looking into doing a CLIA-waived test for HIV antibodies. As the clinical medical assistant, you are asked to research the testing kits that are available and prepare a report that includes a synopsis of each kit, specimen required for each, ease of procedure, as well as the kit you would recommend the clinic to use. Prepare a report detailing the criteria mentioned above.

_____

_____

_____

_____

Teamwork Exercises

1. For this exercise, it is important to prepare the women of the class ahead of time to wear sports bras or bikini tops to class, since the exercise will require students to disrobe. Have a patient gown handy for the students. Divide into groups of three or four. Each group will take turns being the patient, the person reading the ECG machine operating manual, and the person performing the ECG procedure based on the reading of the instructions. While one student is reading the ECG manual, another will actually walk through the procedure for performing the ECG, using another student as the patient.

2. Divide the class into groups of two or three. Allow each group to take one of the conditions/diseases within the chapter and prepare a 10 minute PowerPoint presentation on the symptoms, diagnosis, treatment, and prognosis for the condition/disease.

PROCEDURE 27-1 – PERFORMING A 12-LEAD ECG

Name _____

Date _____ Score _____

Instructor _____

Task
Obtain an accurate 12-lead ECG recording.

Conditions
ECG machine with cable and paper
10 disposable, self-adhesive electrodes
Examination gown
Drape

Time: _____

Standard
In the time specified and within the scoring parameters determined by the instructor, the student will successfully obtain an accurate 12-lead ECG recording.

Points assigned reflect importance of step to meeting the task

Important = 1 pt.
Essential = 5 pts.
Critical = 15 pts.

Automatic failure results if any of the **CRITICAL TASKS** are omitted or performed incorrectly.

(To use a pass/fail system, instructors can record "P" or "F" in the "points earned (pass/fail)" column.)

PERFORMANCE STANDARDS	PTS	PTS EARNED (Pass/Fail)	COMMENTS
1. Washed or sanitized hands and assembled supplies.	5	_____	_____
2. Greeted and identified patient, introduced self, and explained the procedure.	5	_____	_____
3. Instructed the patient to remove socks or pantyhose as well as clothing above the waist including undergarments Assisted the patient as necessary.	5	_____	_____
4. Positioned the patient on the examination table in the supine position. Draped her.	5	_____	_____

PERFORMANCE STANDARDS (cont.)	PTS	PTS EARNED (Pass/Fail)	COMMENTS
5. Turned on the machine. Entered the patient's name, date, time, patient's current cardiac medications into the machine or wrote the information on the tracing paper.	15	_____	_____
6. Cleaned the patient's skin with alcohol at each site where an electrode will be placed and clipped hair if necessary.	1	_____	_____
7. Applied self-adhesive electrodes to a dry, clean, intact, fleshy area on the extremities across from one another and to the cleaned areas on the chest.	1	_____	_____
8. Connected the lead wires to the electrodes using the alligator clips. Made sure the correct leads are connected to the correct electrodes. Did not cross lead wires	15	_____	_____
9. Pressed the AUTO button on the ECG machine. The machine runs automatically once the AUTO button is pressed. Watched for artifacts and made corrections as needed to get an acceptable tracing.	15	_____	_____
10. Disconnected the lead wires from the electrodes and then removed the electrodes from the patient.	5	_____	_____
11. Assisted the patient off of the examination table and with dressing as needed.	1	_____	_____
12. Cleaned and returned the ECG machine to storage.	1	_____	_____
13. Mounted the ECG tracing in the patient's chart or gave it to the physician as directed.	15	_____	_____

PERFORMANCE STANDARDS (cont.)	PTS	PTS EARNED (Pass/Fail)	COMMENTS
14. Documented the procedure in the patient's chart	5	_____	_____ _____
15. Washed or sanitized hands.	5	_____	_____

TOTAL POINTS	99		

DOCUMENTATION

_____

_____

_____

_____

COMMENTS

_____

_____

_____

_____

Pulmonology

Key Term Review

Define the following key terms:

1. pneumonectomy

2. circumoral cyanosis

3. antitussive

4. dyspnea

5. expectorant

6. purulent

7. wedge resection

8. hemoptysis

9. thoracentesis

10. aspiration

11. forced vital capacity

12. nasal cannula

Key Term Review *cont.*

13.   rhonchi _____

_____

14.   hypoxic drive _____

_____

15.   crackles _____

_____

Review Questions

1. Explain what happens during an inhalation.

_____

_____

_____

_____

2. What happens during exhalation?

_____

_____

_____

_____

3. Describe the flow of air as it enters through the upper airway.

_____

_____

_____

_____

4. Describe the difference between a hemothorax and a pneumothorax.

_____

_____

_____

_____

5. List six respiratory disorders that are considered as chronic obstructive pulmonary disease.

_____

_____

_____

_____

6. Describe some specific respiratory symptoms that COPD patients experience.

_____

_____

_____

_____

7. Describe some signs and symptoms of tuberculosis.

_____

_____

_____

_____

8. Compare and contrast the various types of lung cancer.

_____

_____

_____

_____

9. What are some pulmonary function tests that a medical assistant may perform in the medical office?

_____

_____

_____

_____

10. What are some of the pulmonary treatments that patients can perform at home?

_____

_____

_____

_____

Medical Terminology and Abbreviation Review

Give the proper medical term for the definition provided:

1. pertaining to the nose and the stomach: _____

2. pertaining to the mouth: _____

3. dilation or expansion of the bronchus: _____

4. surgical repair of cartilage: _____

5. breathing in the upright position: _____

6. surgical excision of the lungs: _____

7. surgical puncture of the thorax: _____

8. inflammation of the bronchus: _____

9. surgical incision into the trachea: _____

10. pain in the pleura: _____

Define the following abbreviations:

1. VC: _____

2. COPD: _____

3. TB: _____

4. URI: _____

5. stat: _____

6. ABGs: _____

7.   SOB: _____

8.   PND: _____

9.   SARS: _____

10. ARDS: _____

Disease/Condition Review

Match the disease/condition with its definition:

Disease/Condition

1. emphysema _____

2. asthma _____

3. croup _____

4. influenza _____

5. upper respiratory infection _____

6. cystic fibrosis _____

7. pharyngitis _____

8. pleural effusion _____

9. epistaxis _____

10. allergic rhinitis _____

Definition

a. an acute childhood viral disease marked by barking seal-like cough and respiratory distress

b. inflammation of the nasal membranes caused by allergens

c. a nosebleed

d. chronic degenerative genetic disease that causes frequent respiratory infections and an increase in airway secretions

e. a common chronic obstructive respiratory disease

f. collection of infected fluid in the pleural cavity

g. the common cold

h. inflammation of the pharynx

i. narrowing of the airways caused by inflammation

j. contagious acute viral respiratory infection

Anatomy Identification

1. Label the structures of the respiratory system in Figure 28-1.

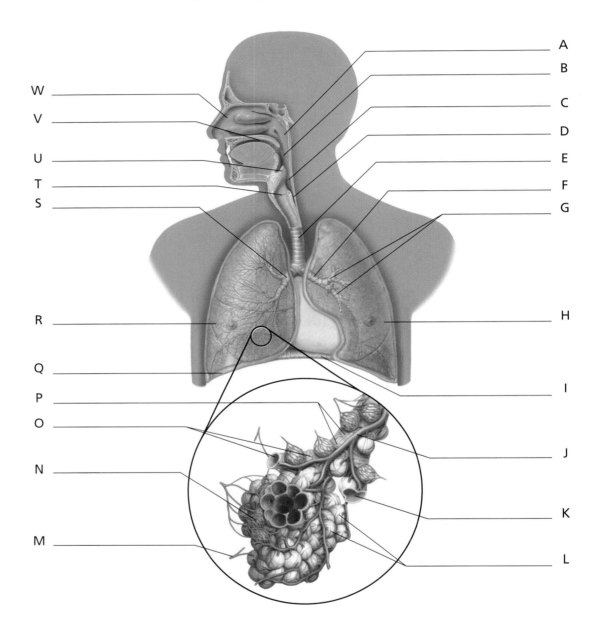

A
B
C
D
E
F
G

H

I

J

K

L

W
V
U
T
S

R

Q
P
O
N

M

a. _____

_____

b. _____

_____

c. _____

_____

d. _____

_____

e. _____

_____

f. _____

_____

g. _____

_____

h. _____

_____

i. _____

_____

J. _____

_____

k. _____

_____

l. _____

_____

m. _____

_____

n. _____

_____

o. _____

_____

p. _____

_____

q. _____

_____

r. _____

_____

s. _____

_____

t. _____

_____

u. _____

_____

v. _____

_____

w. _____

_____

Critical Thinking

1. Mrs. Phillips has brought her 12-year-old daughter, Jill, in because she is concerned that something is wrong with Jill since she has had the same cold symptoms for the past 6 weeks. Jill's symptoms include sneezing, nasal congestion, runny nose, and postnasal drip. She says the symptoms have gotten worse since their family got a new cat. What do you think could be the cause of Jill's symptoms?

_____

_____

_____

_____

2. Nellie Klarzak is an 81-year-old emphysema patient who is currently on home oxygen. As Nellie is setting down her purse, you noticed that she has a pack of cigarettes in it. The physician has told Nellie she must stop smoking, but apparently she has not. How would you handle this situation?

_____

_____

_____

_____

Teamwork Exercises

1. Working in pairs, take turns performing quality control and patient testing using a spirometer. Role-play one student as the medical assistant and one as the patient. Switch roles so that both students can act as the medical assistant.

2. As the administrative medical assistant responsible for insurance pre-certifications and authorizations, you are asked by Clara Brennan, the clinical medical assistant, to work with David Martinson in obtaining authorization from his medical insurance for a home nebulizer. David's insurance company is Blue Cross PPO. Research his insurance and provide David with the information he needs to get approval for his nebulizer.

PROCEDURE 28-1 – PERFORMING RESPIRATORY TESTING

Name _____   Date _____   Score _____

                                          Instructor _____

Task
Assist a patient in the use of a spirometer for respiratory testing.

Conditions
Spirometer with recording paper
Disposable tubing
Disposable mouthpiece
Disposable nose clips
Biohazardous waste container
Patient's medical record

Time: _____

Standard
In the time specified and within the scoring parameters determined by the instructor, the student will successfully assist a patient in the use of a spirometer to complete respiratory testing.

Points assigned reflect importance of step to meeting the task

Important = 1 pt.
Essential = 5 pts.
Critical = 15 pts.

Automatic failure results if any of the **CRITICAL TASKS** are omitted or performed incorrectly.

(To use a pass/fail system, instructors can record "P" or "F" in the "points earned (pass/fail)" column.)

PERFORMANCE STANDARDS	PTS	PTS EARNED (Pass/Fail)	COMMENTS
1. Greeted and identified patient. Introduced self and explained the procedure.	5	_____	_____
2. Washed or sanitized hands.	5	_____	_____
3. Assembled supplies and equipment. Applied new disposable tubing and mouthpiece.	5	_____	_____
4. Obtained the patient's height and weight.	5	_____	_____
5. Entered the patient's age, sex, height, and weight into the computer.	5	_____	_____

PERFORMANCE STANDARDS *(cont.)*	PTS	PTS EARNED (Pass/Fail)	COMMENTS
6. Asked the patient to loosen tight clothing and sit upright near the machine.	1	_____	
7. Described and demonstrated the breathing maneuver to the patient.	5	_____	
8. Gently applied the nose clips to patient's nose and coached in performing the maneuver using these instructions:	5	_____	
a. Take in as deep a breath as you possibly can.	15	_____	
b. Put the mouthpiece in your mouth with your lips snugly around it.	15	_____	
c. Blow out forcefully as hard as you can for as long as you can until your lungs feel completely empty.	15	_____	
9. Repeated the maneuver until three optimal readings had been obtained.	5	_____	
10. Removed the nose clips, disposable mouthpiece, and tubing. Discarded them all in the biohazardous waste container. Allowed the patient to rest for a few minutes.	5	_____	
11. Sanitized your hands, printed the report, and entered all data in the patient's medical record, including his name, the date, the time, the name of the test, and your signature	5	_____	
12. Cleaned the spirometer according to the manufacturer's instructions and put away all equipment.	5	_____	

TOTAL POINTS	101		

DOCUMENTATION

COMMENTS

Student Activity Manual to Accompany The Professional Medical Assistant

PROCEDURE 28-2 – TEACHING A PATIENT TO USE AN MDI

Name _____

Date _____ Score _____

Instructor _____

Task
Teach a patient how to use a metered-dose inhaler (MDI).

Conditions
Metered-dose inhaler
Patient's medical record

Time: _____

Standard
In the time specified and within the scoring parameters determined by the instructor, the student will successfully teach a patient to use an MDI.

Points assigned reflect importance of step to meeting the task

Important = 1 pt.
Essential = 5 pts.
Critical = 15 pts.

Automatic failure results if any of the **CRITICAL TASKS** are omitted or performed incorrectly.

(To use a pass/fail system, instructors can record "P" or "F" in the "points earned (pass/fail)" column.)

PERFORMANCE STANDARDS	PTS	PTS EARNED (Pass/Fail)	COMMENTS
1. Greeted and identified patient. Introduced self and explained the procedure.	5	_____	_____
2. If possible, asked the patient to watch an MDI demonstration video.	1	_____	_____
3. Washed or sanitized your hands.	5	_____	_____
4. Using a placebo MDI or one prescribed for the patient, pointed out the mouthpiece and cover and the medication canister. Indicated how the canister is depressed to initiate a puff of medication.	15	_____	_____
5. Instructed the patient to use purse-lipped breathing. Removed the cap from the mouthpiece and shook the MDI for 5 to 10 seconds.	15	_____	_____

PERFORMANCE STANDARDS (cont.)	PTS	PTS EARNED (Pass/Fail)	COMMENTS
6. Handed the MDI to the patient and instructed patient to hold it upside down 1 to 1½ inches in front of open mouth.	5	_____	_____
7. Instructed the patient to exhale and then, just after beginning to inhale, to depress the canister. The patient should have continued to inhale slowly for 5 to 6 seconds.	15	_____	_____
8. Instructed the patient to hold his breath for 8 to 10 seconds, if possible, and then to exhale through pursed lips.	5	_____	_____
9. If more than one puff is prescribed, instructed the patient to wait for several minutes before repeating the procedure.	5	_____	_____
10. Documented the session in the patient's medical record.	5	_____	_____

TOTAL POINTS	76		

DOCUMENTATION

COMMENTS

PROCEDURE 28-3 – ADMINISTERING OXYGEN VIA NASAL CANNULA

Name _____   Date _____   Score _____

Instructor _____

Task

Administer oxygen to a patient using a nasal cannula.

Conditions

Nasal cannula
Oxygen tubing
Oxygen source
Oxygen flow meter
Appropriate room signs
Patient's medical record

Time: _____

Standard

In the time specified and within the scoring parameters determined by the instructor, the student will successfully administer oxygen to a patient using a nasal cannula.

Points assigned reflect importance of step to meeting the task

Important = 1 pt.
Essential = 5 pts.
Critical = 15 pts.

Automatic failure results if any of the **CRITICAL TASKS** are omitted or performed incorrectly.

(To use a pass/fail system, instructors can record "P" or "F" in the "points earned (pass/fail)" column.)

PERFORMANCE STANDARDS	PTS	PTS EARNED (Pass/Fail)	COMMENTS
1. Greeted and identified patient. Introduced self and explained the procedure.	5	_____	_____ _____
2. Washed or sanitized your hands.	5	_____	_____
3. Connected the nasal cannula to the oxygen tubing (unless tubing is packaged preconnected). Attached the tubing to the oxygen source and set it at the prescribed level. Checked for oxygen flow out of the nasal cannula.	15	_____	_____ _____ _____ _____ _____ _____
4. Placed the tips of the cannula into the patient's nares with the curved prongs pointing downward.	15	_____	_____ _____

PERFORMANCE STANDARDS *(cont.)*	PTS	PTS EARNED (Pass/Fail)	COMMENTS
5. Placed the tubing on either side of patient's head and wrapped it behind the patient's ears so that the tubing laid forward on his chest. Adjusted the plastic slide so that the tubing was comfortably snug under the patient's chin.	15	_____	_____ _____ _____ _____ _____
6. Documented the procedure in the patient's medical record.	5	_____	_____ _____

TOTAL POINTS	60		

DOCUMENTATION

COMMENTS

Endocrinology

Key Term Review

Define the following key terms:

1. glucometer

2. endocrinology

3. venous

4. goiter

5. polydipsia

6. growth hormone

7. endocrinologist

8. hyperglycemia

9. fasting

10. peripheral

11. negative feedback system

Key Term Review *cont.*

12.   exophthalmos   _____

13.   hypothyroidism   _____

14.   glucosuria   _____

15.   hypertrophy   _____

16.   hyposecretion   _____

17.   hyperthyroidism   _____

18.   polyuria   _____

19.   polyphagia   _____

20.   hyperglycemia   _____

Review Questions

1. For the following endocrine system structures, provide their function and the hormone(s) they secrete:

   a. pituitary gland:

   _____

   _____

   _____

   _____

b. thyroid gland:

_____

_____

_____

c. adrenal glands:

_____

_____

_____

_____

d. pancreas:

_____

_____

_____

_____

e. pineal gland:

_____

_____

_____

_____

f. thymus gland:

_____

_____

_____

g. ovaries:

_____

_____

_____

_____

h. testes:

_____

_____

_____

_____

2. Describe the negative feedback mechanism of the endocrine system.

_____

_____

_____

_____

3. Explain what a target organ is.

_____

_____

_____

_____

Medical Terminology and Abbreviation Review

Give the proper medical term for the definition provided:

1. enlargement of the testes: _____

2. disease of a gland: _____

3. surgical fixation of the testes: _____

4. pertaining to the adrenal gland: _____

5. prolapse of the ovary: _____

6. excessive calcium in the blood: _____

7. sugar in the urine: _____

8. specialist in the study of toxins: _____

9. inflammation of the thyroid: _____

10. creating glucose: _____

Define the following abbreviations:

1. TSH: _____

2. PTH: _____

3. CA: _____

4. Ca: _____

5. ADH: _____

6. DM: _____

7. FBS: _____

8. NIDDM: _____

9. GH: _____

10. K: _____

11. Na: _____

Anatomy and Physiology Review

Match the proper hormone with its function:

Hormone

1. cortisol _____

2. growth hormone _____

3. aldosterone _____

4. thyroid stimulating hormone _____

5. epinephrine _____

6. insulin _____

7. melatonin _____

8. follicle stimulating hormone _____

9. parathyroid hormone _____

10. calcitonin _____

Function

a. secreted by the adrenal gland, responsible for increasing absorption of sodium in the kidneys

b. produced by the pineal gland, influences sleep-wake cycles

c. secreted by the pituitary gland to stimulate thyroid function

d. also known as somatotropin

e. secreted by thyroid gland, responsible for calcium-phosphorus balance in the blood

f. secreted by pancreas to aid in the utilization of glucose in the body

g. secreted by the adrenal glands, the body's natural steroid

h. responsible for the "fight or flight" response

i. secreted by the parathyroid gland, responsible for calcium-phosphorus balance in the blood

j. acts on an ovary to produce an ovum in females and on the testes to produce sperm in males

Anatomy Identification

1. Label the endocrine glands shown in Figure 29-1.

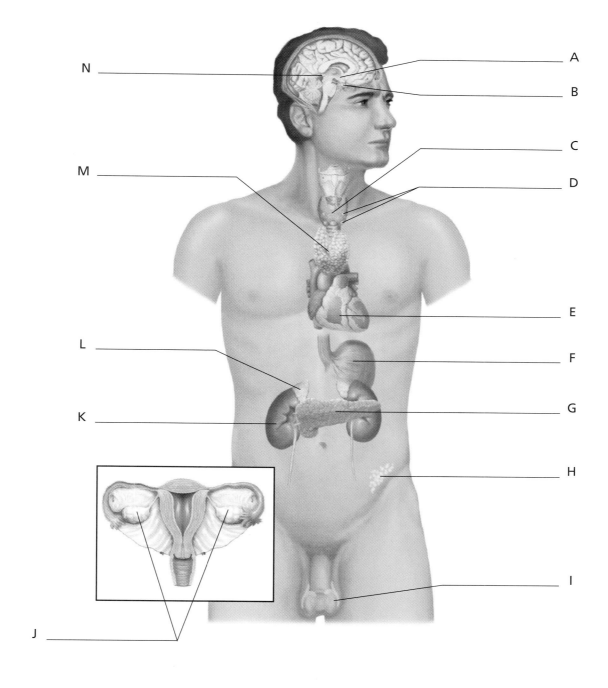

a. _____

_____

b. _____

_____

c. _____

_____

d. _____

_____

e. _____

_____

f. _____

_____

g. _____

_____

h. _____

_____

i. _____

_____

J. _____

_____

k. _____

_____

l. _____

_____

m. _____

_____

n. _____

_____

Critical Thinking

1. This is your third week externing in an endocrinologist's office, and this is the first day your site supervisor has allowed you to take patients into the examination room and perform vitals and a patient history on your own. Sally Andrews is your first patient of the day. She has been referred to the endocrinologist by her primary care physician. You notice Sally has exophthalmos. The physician has asked you to draw some blood for a TSH, T3, and T4. Which disease do you think Sally may be suffering from?

_____

_____

_____

_____

2. Jimmy Barnes, 19, is a newly diagnosed patient with diabetes mellitus. He is in today for a checkup and review of his blood glucose levels. He shares with you that he is having difficulties with remembering to test his blood sugar and managing his diet. The nurse practitioner has asked you to provide Jimmy some patient education with regards to self-care. What advice can you give Jimmy?

_____

_____

_____

_____

Teamwork Activity

1. Working in pairs, take turns performing quality control and patient testing on a glucose monitoring machine. Role-play one student as the medical assistant and one as the patient. Switch roles so that both students can act as the medical assistant.

2. Working in groups of two or three, your instructor will assign an endocrine disease for the group to research. Provide the following information on your disease:

   a. overview on disease

   b. signs and symptoms

   c. how its diagnosed

   d. treatment

   e. prognosis

PROCEDURE 29-1 – TEACHING A PATIENT TO PERFORM DAILY FOOT CARE

Name _____   Date _____   Score _____

                                          Instructor _____

Task
Teach a patient to perform daily foot care.

Conditions
Warm water
Mild soap
Three or more towels
Soft wash cloth
Moisturizing lotion
Hand mirror
Emery board
Clean, dry socks
Shoes
Foot rest
Examination gloves
Wash basins (2)
Patient's medical record

Time: _____

Standards
In the time specified and within the scoring parameters determined by the instructor, the student will successfully teach the patient to perform daily foot care.

Points assigned reflect importance of step to meeting the task

Important = 1 pt.
Essential = 5 pts.
Critical = 15 pts.

Automatic failure results if any of the **CRITICAL TASKS** are omitted or performed incorrectly.

(To use a pass/fail system, instructors can record "P" or "F" in the "points earned (pass/fail)" column.)

PERFORMANCE STANDARDS	PTS	PTS EARNED (Pass/Fail)	COMMENTS
1. Introduced self and explained the purpose of the teaching session and the importance of routine foot care, including these points:	5	_____	_____ _____ _____
a. Daily skin care helps the diabetic patient maintain healthy, intact skin.	1	_____	_____ _____
b. Daily care enables the patient to detect skin problems early so that the physician can initiate timely intervention.	1	_____	_____ _____
c. Maintaining healthy skin and detecting problems early help the diabetic patient prevent limb loss caused by nonhealing wounds and infections.	1	_____	_____ _____ _____

PERFORMANCE STANDARDS *(cont.)*	PTS	PTS EARNED (Pass/Fail)	COMMENTS
2. Instructed the patient to wash his hands with lukewarm water and soap, rinse them in lukewarm water, and dry them thoroughly. Explained that hand washing helps prevent cross-contamination of microorganisms from the hands to the feet.	5	_____	_____
3. Instructed the patient to sit in a chair and remove his shoes and socks.	1	_____	_____
4. Washed or sanitized hands and assembled supplies:	5	_____	_____
a. Placed a towel or absorbent pad on the floor beneath patient's feet (other supplies may rest on this towel).	1	_____	_____
b. Placed both basins near the patient's feet (one half full of lukewarm water with a small amount of soap added and one half full of clean rinse water).	1	_____	_____
c. Placed a footrest near the patient's feet and a towel or absorbent pad on top of it.	1	_____	_____
5. Instructed the patient to place his left foot in the basin of soapy water and let it soak for a minute or two. Explained that this allows soil particles to soften and loosen up.	15	_____	_____
6. Put on examination gloves. Used a clean, soft washcloth to wash the patient's foot, gently scrubbing all surfaces, including between the toes. Was extra gentle with any areas that were reddened, tender, or had broken skin.	5	_____	_____
7. Guided the patient's foot from the basin of soapy water to the basin of rinse water. Gently rubbed all surfaces. Explained to the patient that all of the soap must be removed.	5	_____	_____

PERFORMANCE STANDARDS *(cont.)*	PTS	PTS EARNED (Pass/Fail)	COMMENTS
8. Placed the patient's clean foot on the padded footrest and gently patted all surfaces dry. Examined the skin in all areas while patting dry. Explained that dry skin is less likely to break down or harbor microorganisms, and clean skin is easier to examine.	15	_____	_____
9. Held the hand mirror below the sole of the patient's foot and asked him to examine his foot. Explained the importance of seeing every surface of his foot. Told the patient to inspect all surfaces of the foot, including the toes, toenails, and between the toes. Explained that diabetic patients with peripheral neuropathy may have injuries they do not feel.	15	_____	_____
10. Inspected the patient's toenails for length and jagged edges. Using the emery board, filed the toenails as needed to shorten and smooth the ends. (Be sure not to shorten them too much, however.) Informed the physician if the patient has extremely thick, hypertrophied toenails. Explained that excessively long or jagged nails could result in injury from pressure or tearing. Instructed the patient to report any areas of redness, broken skin, or ulcerations to the physician as soon as possible	15	_____	_____
11. Applied a small amount of moisturizing lotion to the patient's clean foot but not between the toes. Explained that moisturized skin is less likely to crack but that the area between the toes tends to harbor moisture and could become a breeding ground for microorganisms.	5	_____	_____

PERFORMANCE STANDARDS *(cont.)*	PTS	PTS EARNED (Pass/Fail)	COMMENTS
12. Removed the examination gloves. Examined the patient's clean socks for areas of wear or hidden seams. Explained that such areas could place excessive pressure on the patient's foot.	5	_____	_____
13. Examined the patient's left shoe, including these steps:			_____
a. Examined the inside for any foreign objects or wear or wrinkles in the shoe lining. Explained that the inside of the shoe should be examined each time it is put on because pressure ulcers can develop quickly from pressure caused by foreign objects or wrinkles.	1	_____	_____
b. Examined the sole of the shoe. Explained that a flat, nonskid surface provides a good base of support and is less likely to slip when walking.	1	_____	_____
c. Explained that shoes should be worn at all times, even in the house, to prevent foot injury from stubbing the toes or stepping on objects.	1	_____	_____
d. Explained that new shoes must be broken in slowly and carefully to prevent blisters or other areas of pressure or friction.	1	_____	_____
e. Explained that slippers with nonskid soles should be kept by the bed and worn when getting up during the night, and a nightlight should be kept on to prevent foot injury from stubbing the toes or stepping on objects.	1	_____	_____
14. Assisted the patient as needed in putting his left sock and shoe on.	1	_____	_____

PERFORMANCE STANDARDS (cont.)	PTS	PTS EARNED (Pass/Fail)	COMMENTS
15. Instructed the patient to repeat steps 6 to 15 with his other foot, providing cueing as needed.	15	_____	_____ _____
16. Washed hands and document the procedure in the patient's medical record	5	_____	_____ _____

TOTAL POINTS	128		

DOCUMENTATION

COMMENTS

Gastroenterology

Key Term Review *Define the following key terms:*

1.   saliva

2.   glucagon

3.   absorption

4.   bolus

5.   villi

6.   rugae

7.   gastroenterology

8.   mastication

9.   defecation

10.   chyme

11.   saliva

12.   cardiac sphincter

Key Term Review *cont.*

13. alimentary canal _____

14. uvula _____

15. digestion _____

16. deglutition _____

17. insulin _____

18. peristalsis _____

19. enema _____

20. epiglottis _____

Review Questions

1. What is the function of the gastrointestinal tract?

    _____

    _____

    _____

    _____

2. List the structures of the gastrointestinal system.

    _____

    _____

    _____

    _____

3. What are the accessory structures of the gastrointestinal system?

_____

_____

_____

_____

4. Describe the function of the cardiac sphincter.

_____

_____

_____

_____

5. Which structures does the abdominal cavity hold?

_____

_____

_____

_____

6. Describe the functions of the liver.

_____

_____

_____

_____

7. Describe the functions of the pancreas and its involvement in blood glucose regulation.

_____

_____

_____

_____

8. What is the function of the gallbladder?

_____

_____

_____

_____

9. List some commonly used patient interview questions for a GI exam.

_____

_____

_____

_____

10. What is the purpose of performing an occult blood test?

_____

_____

_____

11. Describe some dietary restrictions given to a patient who needs to collect a specimen for occult blood testing.

_____

_____

_____

_____

12. Describe the purpose of a sigmoidoscopy examination.

_____

_____

_____

_____

13. What is the purpose of performing a cleansing enema?

_____

_____

_____

_____

14. What is the purpose of performing an upper endoscopy?

_____

_____

_____

_____

15. Describe some symptoms of gastric ulcers.

_____

_____

_____

_____

16. Describe the functions of the lower GI tract.

_____

_____

_____

_____

17. List three common sites of abdominal hernias.

_____

_____

_____

_____

18. What are some contributing factors to a patient getting diverticular diseases such as diverticulosis and diverticulitis?

_____

_____

_____

_____

19. What are some complications of Crohn disease?

_____

_____

_____

_____

20. List some risk factors for cholelithiasis.

_____

_____

_____

_____

21. Compare and contrast the five different types of viral hepatitis regarding transmission, symptoms, diagnosis, treatment, and prognosis.

_____

_____

_____

_____

22. Describe celiac disease and its symptoms.

_____

_____

_____

_____

23. Compare and contrast anorexia nervosa with bulimia.

_____

_____

_____

_____

24. Compare and contrast food poisonings caused by _E. coli_ 0157:H7, _Salmonella_, or _Campylobacter_ regarding transmission, symptoms, and treatment.

_____

_____

_____

_____

25. List the blood tests that are considered as liver function tests.

_____

_____

_____

_____

26. Compare and contrast the upper GI x-ray with the lower GI x-ray regarding organs/ structures being viewed, and patient preparation.

_____

_____

_____

_____

Medical Terminology and Abbreviation Review

Give the proper medical term for the definition provided:

1.   pertaining to the tongue: _____

2.   a salivary stone: _____

3.   inflammation of the liver: _____

4.   abnormally frequent discharge or flow
      of watery fecal matter from the bowel: _____

5.   a hernia of the esophagus: _____

6.   pertaining to the tongue and pharynx: _____

7.   loss of appetite: _____

8.   condition of gallstones: _____

9.   dilation of the pylorus: _____

10.   inflammation of the gums: _____

11.   tumor of the bile duct: _____

12.   following a meal: _____

13.   the vomiting of blood: _____

14.   intermittent painful contractions
      of the intestines: _____

15. surgery to create an opening from the ileum to outside of the body: _____

16. indigestion: _____

17. enlargement of the liver: _____

18. inflammation of the lip: _____

19. secretion of bile by the liver: _____

20. procedure to view the sigmoid colon: _____

Define the following abbreviations:

1. SBO: _____

2. ac: _____

3. po: _____

4. ALT: _____

5. PUD: _____

6. IBS: _____

7. BE: _____

8. AST: _____

9. GERD: _____

10. NPO: _____

11. pc: _____

12. BM: _____

13. GI: _____

14. LFT: _____

15. NG: _____

Disease/Condition Review

Match the disease/condition with its definition:

Disease/Condition

1. diverticulosis _____
2. food poisoning _____
3. Crohn disease _____
4. gastritis _____
5. dysphagia _____
6. GERD _____
7. abdominal hernia _____
8. viral hepatitis _____
9. celiac disease _____
10. diverticulitis _____
11. flatulence _____
12. pyrosis _____
13. hiatal hernia _____
14. pyloric stenosis _____
15. anorexia nervosa _____
16. hemorrhoids _____
17. acute appendicitis _____
18. acute pancreatitis _____
19. ulcerative colitis _____
20. cholelithiasis _____

Definition

a. heartburn

b. illness that is most commonly caused by *E. coli* 0157:H7, *Salmonella*, or *Campylobacter*

c. condition of the formation of tiny pouch-like herniations in the wall of the large intestines.

d. chronic inflammation of innermost lining of rectum and colon

e. inflammation of the liver, caused by various viruses

f. accumulation of gas in lower intestines

g. varicose veins of the anal area

h. inflammation of the lining of the stomach

i. difficult swallowing

j. the backflow of acidic gastric contents into the esophagus

k. diverticula that has become clogged with feces and becomes inflamed and infected

l. narrowing of the pyloric sphincter

m. physical and psychological eating disorder involving an intense fear of weigh gain and self-imposed food restrictions

Disease/Condition	Definition *cont.*

21. IBS _____

22. bulimia _____

n. protrusion of intestines through the abdominal wall

o. inflammation of tubelike appendage that hangs from the cecum

p. inflammation and edema deep into layers of the lining of any part of the GI tract

q. condition of gallstones

r. inflammation of the pancreas

s. intolerance to gluten

t. pattern of alternating constipation and diarrhea along with other GI symptoms

u. protrusion of stomach upward through the diaphragm

v. physical and psychological disorder involving obsessively eating huge quantities of food with purging behaviors

Anatomy Identification

1. Label the structures of the digestive system in Figure 30-1.

S _____

R _____

Q _____

P _____

O _____

N _____

M _____

L _____

K _____

A

B

C

D

E

F

G

H

I

J

a. _____

b. _____

c. _____

d. _____

Student Activity Manual to Accompany The Professional Medical Assistant *417*

e. _____

_____

f. _____

_____

g. _____

_____

h. _____

_____

i. _____

_____

J. _____

_____

k. _____

_____

l. _____

_____

m. _____

_____

n. _____

_____

o. _____

_____

p. _____

_____

q. _____

_____

r. _____

_____

s. _____

_____

Critical Thinking

1. Follow the path food takes from when it enters the mouth to when the digestive tract eliminates food.

   _____

   _____

   _____

   _____

2. Mr. Jameson has been referred to the gastroenterologist for symptoms of heartburn and gastritis. As you take a patient history from Mr. Jameson, you notice that he pulled out a package of over-the-counter acid relievers and consumed three of the tablets. What type of questions would you ask Mr. Jameson?

   _____

   _____

   _____

   _____

3. Jenn Ho, an 18-year-old college student, has just been diagnosed with gluten enteropathy. Discuss with Jenn what a gluten-free diet consists of and develop a meal plan for her.

   _____

   _____

   _____

   _____

Teamwork Exercises

1. Divide into pairs, and using the proper specimen collection containers, role-play with your partner the proper procedure for collecting a fecal specimen for occult blood testing. In the patient instructions, be sure to include reasons for collecting the specimen and any diet restrictions.

2. Dividing into pairs, role-play with your partner the instructions for administering a cleansing enema.

3. Divide into groups of two or three. Your instructor will assign each group a method (blood test, breath test, or endoscopy) for identifying *H. pylori* in an effort to diagnose peptic ulcers. Each group will research the method assigned and give a report to the class on the following features of the test:

   a. test methodology

   b. specimen used

   c. sensitivity and specificity of test

   d. procedure

   e. additional relevant facts

4. Divide into groups of two or three. Your instructor will assign each group a different cancer of the GI system. Each group will develop a fact sheet containing a description of the cancer, symptoms, diagnosis, treatment, prevention, and Internet sites for support groups and/or official disease associations.

PROCEDURE 30-1 – INSTRUCTING A PATIENT ON COLLECTING A STOOL SPECIMEN

Name _____   Date _____   Score _____

Instructor _____

Task Instruct a patient on how to collect a stool specimen.	**Standard** In the time specified and within the scoring parameters determined by the instructor, the student will successfully instruct a patient on collecting an adequate stool specimen for laboratory analysis.

Conditions
Specimen container with lid
Laboratory request form
Patient's medical record
Pen
Plastic wrap

Time: _____

Standard
In the time specified and within the scoring parameters determined by the instructor, the student will successfully instruct a patient on collecting an adequate stool specimen for laboratory analysis.

Points assigned reflect importance of step to meeting the task

> Important = 1 pt.
> Essential = 5 pts.
> Critical = 15 pts.

Automatic failure results if any of the **CRITICAL TASKS** are omitted or performed incorrectly.

(To use a pass/fail system, instructors can record "P" or "F" in the "points earned (pass/fail)" column.)

PERFORMANCE STANDARDS	PTS	PTS EARNED (Pass/Fail)	COMMENTS
1. Assembled the items next to the patient.	1	_____	_____
2. Identified the patient and explained the physician's orders for a stool sample.	5	_____	_____
3. Instructed the patient to defecate onto the plastic wrap.	5	_____	_____
4. Instructed the patient to obtain 3 to 4 tablespoons of stool from the plastic wrap and to place it in the specimen container.	15	_____	_____
5. Explained to the patient that he should be sure to avoid getting any toilet paper or urine in the container.	5	_____	_____

PERFORMANCE STANDARDS *(cont.)*	PTS	PTS EARNED (Pass/Fail)	COMMENTS
6. Told the patient to write his name along with the date and time on the container and to seal the container.	5	_____	_____ _____
7. Told the patient to bring the sample in the closed container to the office for laboratory testing.	1	_____	_____ _____
8. Instructed the patient to keep the sample refrigerated if he cannot transport it to the office within 2 hours.	5	_____	_____ _____ _____
9. Asked the patient if he understands the instructions. Answered any questions he had.	1	_____	_____ _____
10. Documented in the patient's medical record all patient education performed as well as the patient's understanding of the procedure.	5	_____	_____ _____ _____

TOTAL POINTS	48		

DOCUMENTATION

COMMENTS

PROCEDURE 30-2 – PERFORMING AN OCCULT BLOOD TEST

Name _____   Date _____   Score _____

Instructor _____

Task
Perform an occult blood test on a stool specimen.

Conditions
Nonsterile disposable gloves
Hemoccult slides with stool samples (stool cards)
  provided by the patient
Developer
Timer or clock
Biohazard bag
Patient's medical record
Pen

Time: _____

Standards
In the time specified and within the scoring parameters determined by the instructor, the student will successfully test a stool specimen for occult blood.

Points assigned reflect importance of step to meeting the task

Important = 1 pt.
Essential = 5 pts.
Critical = 15 pts.

Automatic failure results if any of the **CRITICAL TASKS** are omitted or performed incorrectly.

(To use a pass/fail system, instructors can record "P" or "F" in the "points earned (pass/fail)" column.)

PERFORMANCE STANDARDS	PTS	PTS EARNED (Pass/Fail)	COMMENTS
1. Washed hands and applied gloves.	1	_____	_____
2. Opened the test side of the Hemoccult paper slide.	1	_____	_____
3. Placed two drops of developer onto the sections of the reagent paper. Was sure to avoid touching the paper with the dropper.	15	_____	_____
4. Immediately began timing for 1 minute. At 30 seconds, watched the slide for color changes around the edges of the stool sample.	15	_____	_____
5. At 60 seconds, compared the test areas with the control area.	15	_____	_____

PERFORMANCE STANDARDS (cont.)	PTS	PTS EARNED (Pass/Fail)	COMMENTS
6. Placed an additional drop of developer between the positive and negative control areas to ensure that the controls were in good condition.	15	_____	_____ _____ _____
7. Recorded the results in the patient's medical record.	5	_____	_____ _____
8. Disposed of the cards and sample container in the biohazard bag.	5	_____	_____ _____

TOTAL POINTS	72		

DOCUMENTATION

COMMENTS

PROCEDURE 30-3 – ASSISTING WITH FLEXIBLE SIGMOIDOSCOPY

Name

Date _____ Score _____

Instructor _____

Task
Assist the physician and the patient during sigmoidoscopy.

Conditions
Nonsterile disposable gloves
Flexible sigmoidoscope
Water-soluble lubricant
Sterile specimen container with preservative
4 × 4 gauze squares
Tissue wipes
Drape
Biopsy forceps
Biohazard waste container
Patient's medical record
Pen

Time: _____

Standard
In the time specified and within the scoring parameters determined by the instructor, the student will successfully assist the physician in a flexible sigmoidoscopy examination.

Points assigned reflect importance of step to meeting the task

Important = 1 pt.
Essential = 5 pts.
Critical = 15 pts.

Automatic failure results if any of the **CRITICAL TASKS** are omitted or performed incorrectly.

(To use a pass/fail system, instructors can record "P" or "F" in the "points earned (pass/fail)" column.)

PERFORMANCE STANDARDS	PTS	PTS EARNED (Pass/Fail)	COMMENTS
1. Washed or sanitized hands.	1	_____	
2. Assembled supplies, making sure supplies were situated for easy access by the physician. Checked the light source on the sigmoidoscope.	5	_____	
3. Greeted and identified the patient and explained the examination procedure.	5	_____	
4. Asked the patient if he needed to empty his bladder prior to the examination.	5	_____	

PERFORMANCE STANDARDS (cont.)	PTS	PTS EARNED (Pass/Fail)	COMMENTS
5. Gave the patient a gown and drape and asked him to remove all clothing from the waist down. Instructed him to put the gown on with the opening in the back and to sit on the examination table with the drape over his lap.	15	_____	_____
6. Knocked before reentering the room.	1	_____	_____
7. When the physician was ready to proceed, positioned the patient in the Sims (left lateral) position.	5	_____	_____
8. Draped the patient so that the corner of the drape could be lifted to expose the anus.	5	_____	_____
9. Asked the patient if he was comfortable. Asked him to breathe slowly and deeply, and encouraged him to relax the muscles of the anus and rectum.	1	_____	_____
10. Lubricated the physician's gloved hand just before the digital rectal examination.	5	_____	_____
11. Lubricated the end of the sigmoidoscope before handing it to the physician.	5	_____	_____
12. Assisted the physician with suction as required.	1	_____	_____
13. Asked the patient if he was comfortable.	1	_____	_____
14. Assisted the physician with collection of a biopsy as needed. Handed the biopsy forceps to the physician and held the specimen container to receive specimens. Did not touch the inside of the container.	15	_____	_____

PERFORMANCE STANDARDS (cont.)	PTS	PTS EARNED (Pass/Fail)	COMMENTS
15. Placed the cover on the specimen container and placed the container on the counter for transport to the laboratory.	5	_____	_____ _____ _____
16. When the examination was complete, applied clean gloves and cleaned the patient's anal area with tissues.	1	_____	_____ _____ _____ _____
17. Removed gloves and washed hands.	5	_____	_____
18. Assisted the patient to a sitting position and allowed him to rest. Asked him if he felt faint or dizzy. If he did, allowed him to sit and observed him until he felt better.	5	_____	_____ _____ _____ _____
19. Assisted the patient off of the examination table and allowed him to dress and use the restroom.	1	_____	_____ _____
20. Prepared the laboratory requisition form and accompanying specimens.	5	_____	_____ _____
21. Cleaned the examination room.	1	_____	_____
22. Documented the procedure in the patient's medical record.	5	_____	_____ _____

TOTAL POINTS	98		

DOCUMENTATION

COMMENTS

PROCEDURE 30-4 – PERFORMING A CLEANSING ENEMA

Name _____ Date _____ Score _____

Instructor _____

Task
Perform a cleansing enema.

Conditions
Disposable nonsterile gloves
Prepackaged disposable enema
Water-soluble lubricant
Mayo tray
Biohazard waste container
Towel
Drape
Tissues
Patient's medical record
Pen

Time: _____

Standard
In the time specified and within the scoring parameters determined by the instructor, the student will successfully administer a cleansing enema.

Points assigned reflect importance of step to meeting the task

Important = 1 pt.
Essential = 5 pts.
Critical = 15 pts.

Automatic failure results if any of the **CRITICAL TASKS** are omitted or performed incorrectly.

(To use a pass/fail system, instructors can record "P" or "F" in the "points earned (pass/fail)" column.)

PERFORMANCE STANDARDS	PTS	PTS EARNED (Pass/Fail)	COMMENTS
1. Washed hands and assembled supplies.	5	_____	_____
2. Explained the procedure to the patient.	1	_____	_____
3. Asked the patient to disrobe from the waist down and to put on a gown with the opening toward the back. Provided a drape and asked him to sit on the examination table with the drape across his lap.	5	_____	_____
4. Assisted the patient into the Sims position (lying on his left side and bringing his right knee up toward the waist).	5	_____	_____
5. Removed the cover of the enema container and inspected the container.	1	_____	_____

PERFORMANCE STANDARDS (cont.)	PTS	PTS EARNED (Pass/Fail)	COMMENTS
6. Warmed the enema solution to body temperature in warm water at the sink.	1	_____	_____ _____
7. Applied a small amount of lubricant to the tip of the container.	1	_____	_____ _____
8. Adjusted the drape sheet to expose the buttocks.	1	_____	_____ _____
9. With one hand, separated the buttocks to expose the anus. Held the enema bottle with the other hand and inserted it into the anus. Pointed the tip of the bottle toward the patient's abdomen.	15	_____	_____ _____ _____ _____ _____
10. Advised the patient to breathe deeply and slowly and to relax his abdomen.	5	_____	_____ _____ _____
11. Squeezed the bottle slowly and expressed all of the solution into the patient's body.	15	_____	_____ _____
12. Told the patient that you will withdraw the enema tip and then did so slowly.	5	_____	_____ _____
13. Provided the patient with a tissue to hold against the anus and asked him to retain the liquid as long as possible.	5	_____	_____ _____ _____ _____
14. Discarded the enema container and tissues in a biohazardous waste container.	5	_____	_____ _____
15. Allowed the patient to lie quietly for 5 to 10 minutes and then directed him to the restroom. Asked him to allow you to check the results before flushing them. If the results seemed inadequate, consulted with the physician and repeated the procedure if necessary.	5	_____	_____ _____ _____ _____ _____ _____

PERFORMANCE STANDARDS (cont.)	PTS	PTS EARNED (Pass/Fail)	COMMENTS
16. While the patient was in the restroom, cleaned the examination room in preparation for the examination or sigmoidoscopy.	5	_____	_____ _____
17. Washed hands.	1	_____	_____ _____
18. Documented the procedure in the patient's medical record.	5	_____	_____ _____ _____

TOTAL POINTS	86		

DOCUMENTATION

COMMENTS

Urology and the Male Reproductive System

Key Term Review

Define the following key terms:

1. catheterization

   _____

   _____

2. anuria

   _____

   _____

3. urgency

   _____

   _____

4. lithotripsy

   _____

   _____

5. cystoscopy

   _____

   _____

6. peritoneal dialysis

   _____

   _____

7. filtrate

   _____

   _____

8. dysuria

   _____

   _____

9. renal colic

   _____

   _____

10. micturition reflex

    _____

    _____

11. vasectomy

    _____

    _____

Key Term Review *cont.*

12. urinalysis _____

_____

13. oliguria _____

_____

14. hemodialysis _____

_____

15. stent _____

_____

Review Questions

1. Discuss the various functions of the kidneys.

_____

_____

_____

_____

2. List three causes of renal failure.

_____

_____

_____

_____

3. Compare and contrast bacterial cystitis with bacterial urethritis.

_____

_____

_____

_____

4. List four microorganisms that are commonly the cause of a urinary tract infection.

_____

_____

_____

_____

5. Describe some symptoms of a urinary tract infection.

_____

_____

_____

_____

6. List some risk factors for renal cancer.

_____

_____

_____

_____

7. List some causes/contributing factors for renal calculi.

_____

_____

_____

_____

8. List some causes of nephritic syndrome.

_____

_____

_____

_____

9. Discuss some diseases of the male reproductive system.

_____

_____

_____

_____

10. What are the recommended screening tests for prostate cancer?

_____

_____

_____

_____

11. List some risk factors for testicular cancer.

_____

_____

_____

_____

12. List some causes of erectile dysfunction.

_____

_____

_____

_____

Medical Terminology and Abbreviation Review

Give the proper medical term for the definition provided:

1. inflammation of the glans penis _____

2. visual inspection of the bladder _____

3. disease of the testes _____

4. incision into a vessel _____

5. blood in the urine _____

6. surgical fixation of the urethra _____

7. abnormal condition of kidney stones _____

8. bacteria in the urine _____

9. enlargement of the testes _____

10.   pus in the urine   _____

11.   producing sperm   _____

12.   surgical removal of the testes   _____

13.   deficiency of urine   _____

14.   pertaining to the peritoneum   _____

15.   instrument used to measure urine   _____

Define the following abbreviation:

1.   UA   _____

2.   ARF   _____

3.   ED   _____

4.   KUB   _____

5.   TURP   _____

6.   BPH   _____

7.   BUN   _____

8.   DRE   _____

9.   UTI   _____

10.   TSE   _____

11.   IVP   _____

12.   HPV   _____

13.   PSA   _____

14.   CRF   _____

15.   PKD   _____

Disease/Condition Review

Match the disease/condition with its definition:

Disease/condition

1. _____ hydronephrosis

2. _____ prostatitis

3. _____ bacterial cystitis

4. _____ polycystic kidney disease

5. _____ nephritic syndrome

6. _____ pyelonephritis

7. _____ nephroblastoma

8. _____ glomerulonephritis

9. _____ balanoposthitis

Definition

a. inflammation of the bladder

b. inflammation of the kidney and renal pelvis

c. inflammation of the glomeruli

d. inflammation of the prostate gland

e. inflammation of the skin covering the glans penis

f. also known as Wilms tumor

g. disorder marked by increase glomerular permeability to proteins resulting in massive protein loss in the urine, edema, hypoalbuminemia, and hyperlipidemia

h. condition caused by obstructed urinary outflow in which tissues of the renal pelvis are stretched due to pressure from urine accumulation

i. group of hereditary progressive disorders in which cysts form in the kidneys

Anatomy Identification

1. Label the structures of the urinary system in Figure 31-1.

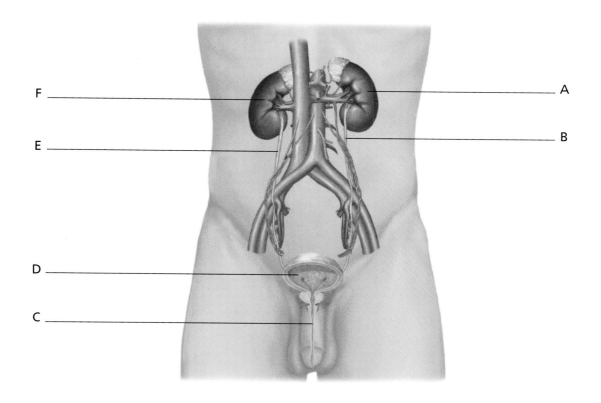

a. _____

b. _____

c. _____

d. _____

e. _____

f. _____

2. Label the structures of the male reproductive system in Figure 31-2.

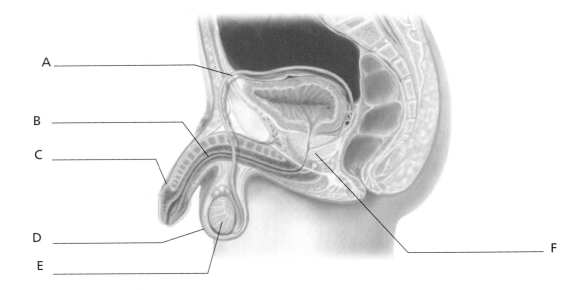

A

B

C

D

E

F

a. _____

_____

b. _____

_____

c. _____

_____

d. _____

_____

e. _____

_____

f. _____

_____

Critical Thinking

1. You are a medical assistant in a urology practice. The physician has just performed a vasectomy on James Brickman, and you are asked to provide Mr. Brickman with instructions for submitting post-vasectomy semen specimens. Describe the procedure for collection of these specimens.

_____

_____

_____

_____

2. Tomas Swenson is at the urology clinic complaining about painful urination and thick penile discharge. While taking his medical history you ask about his sexual history. He states that he tends to "sleep around." What conditions may the physician suspect? What type of diagnostic tests may the physician order?

_____

_____

_____

_____

Teamwork Activity

1. Divide into groups of two or three. Your instructor will assign each group a different cancer of the urinary system. Each group will develop a fact sheet containing a description of the cancer, symptoms, diagnosis, treatment, prevention, and Internet sites for support groups and/or official disease associations.

2. Divide into groups of two or three. Your instructor will assign each group one of the following procedures. Each group will develop a patient education brochure on the procedure, which will also include patient preparation for the procedure.

   a. cystoscopy

   b. intravenous pyelography

   c. renal computed tomography

   d. renal angiography

   e. cystourethrography

PROCEDURE 31-1 – TEACHING A PATIENT TO PERFORM TSE

Name _____   Date _____   Score _____

                                                  Instructor _____

Task
Teach a male patient to perform a testicular self-examination (TSE).

Conditions
TSE pamphlet
Examination model
TSE shower card

Time: _____

Standard
In the time specified and within the scoring parameters determined by the instructor, the student will successfully teach a male patient to perform a testicular self-examination.

Points assigned reflect importance of step to meeting the task

Important = 1 pt.
Essential = 5 pts.
Critical = 15 pts.

Automatic failure results if any of the **CRITICAL TASKS** are omitted or performed incorrectly.

(To use a pass/fail system, instructors can record "P" or "F" in the "points earned (pass/fail)" column.)

PERFORMANCE STANDARDS	PTS	PTS EARNED (Pass/Fail)	COMMENTS
1. Greeted and identified patient. Introduced self and explained the procedure.	5	_____	_____
2. Washed or sanitized hands and assembled supplies.	5	_____	_____
3. Explained the rationale for regular performance of TSE, including: **a.** Testicular cancer commonly goes undetected in early stages because many patients experience no discomfort. **b.** Regular monthly exam allows him to note any changes in a timely manner. **c.** Examinations should begin during puberty. **d.** Examination is easiest during a warm bath or shower.	15	_____	_____

PERFORMANCE STANDARDS (cont.)	PTS	PTS EARNED (Pass/Fail)	COMMENTS

4. Using the examination model, demonstrated examination of the testes:
 	
  a. Held scrotum in palms of hand and felt one testicle.
  b. Applied gentle pressure while rolling the testicle between the fingers.
  c. Noted any hard, painless lumps.
	15	_____	_____

5. Using the examination model, demonstrated examination of the epididymis:
 	
  a. Located the circular cord behind the testis.
  b. Felt for any hard lumps.
	15	_____	_____

6. Using the examination model, demonstrated examination of the vas deferens:
 	
  a. Located the firm, movable, smooth tube that runs upward from the epididymis.
  b. Felt for any hard lumps.
	15	_____	_____

7. Repeated the demonstration of examination on the other side.	15	_____	_____
8. Had the patient demonstrate TSE using the model.	1	_____	_____
9. Gave the patient a TSE pamphlet and shower card. Instructed him to hang the card in his shower.	5	_____	_____
10. Recorded TSE education in patient's medical record.	5	_____	_____
TOTAL POINTS	96		

DOCUMENTATION

COMMENTS

PROCEDURE 31-2 – PERFORMING URINARY CATHETERIZATION

Name _____   Date _____   Score _____

Instructor _____

Task
Perform urinary catheterization on a patient.

Conditions
Light source
Laboratory slip
Ink pen
Nonsterile waterproof underpad
Sterile urethral catheterization kit containing:
  Straight catheter
  Drapes
  Tray
  Gloves
  Lubricant
  Povidone-iodine swabs or cotton balls and
    povidone-iodine solution
  Specimen container and label

Time: _____

Standard
In the time specified and within the scoring parameters determined by the instructor, the student will successfully perform catheterization on a patient to empty the bladder or collect a urine specimen.

Points assigned reflect importance of step to meeting the task

Important = 1 pt.
Essential = 5 pts.
Critical = 15 pts.

Automatic failure results if any of the **CRITICAL TASKS** are omitted or performed incorrectly.

(To use a pass/fail system, instructors can record "P" or "F" in the "points earned (pass/fail)" column.)

PERFORMANCE STANDARDS	PTS	PTS EARNED (Pass/Fail)	COMMENTS
1. Washed or sanitized hands and assembled supplies.	5	_____	_____
			_____
2. Greeted and identified patient. Introduced self and explained the procedure.	5	_____	_____
			_____
			_____
3. Asked the patient about allergy to iodine. If the patient was allergic, omitted the povidone-iodine from this procedure.	1	_____	_____
			_____
			_____
			_____
4. Instructed the patient to remove clothing below the waist, including undergarments. The patient was permitted to keep socks on if desired. Assisted the patient as needed.	1	_____	_____
			_____
			_____
			_____
			_____

PERFORMANCE STANDARDS (cont.)	PTS	PTS EARNED (Pass/Fail)	COMMENTS
5. Assisted the patient into the dorsal recumbent position and draped the patient for warmth and privacy, leaving the genital area exposed.	5	_____	
6. For the female patient who is unable to lie completely flat or abduct her hips, considered an alternative side-lying position, which required a second assistant to support the patient's upper leg.	1	_____	
7. Adjusted the light source on the genital area. If an adjustable lamp was not available, had an assistant hold a flashlight.	1	_____	
8. Placed the nonsterile waterproof underpad under the patient's buttocks.	1	_____	
9. Provided perineal hygiene as needed:			
a. Applied nonsterile gloves.	1	_____	
b. Washed the perineal area with warm water and soap.	1	_____	
c. Dried the perineal area with a towel.	1	_____	
d. Removed and disposed of gloves.	1	_____	
e. Washed hands.	1	_____	
10. Opened the catheter kit on a clean, dry, uncluttered surface using sterile technique, preferably using a Mayo stand or other small wheeled table.	5	_____	
11. Kept the plastic bag that contained the kit nearby to use as a waste receptacle.	15	_____	
12. Removed the sterile gloves from the kit and put them on.	1	_____	
13. If the physician's order did not include a specimen, removed the specimen container, lid, and label and set them aside.	1	_____	

PERFORMANCE STANDARDS (cont.)	PTS	PTS EARNED (Pass/Fail)	COMMENTS
14. If the order did request a specimen, placed the label aside and put the specimen container and lid on a sterile surface within easy reach.	1	_____	_____
15. Opened the sterile lubricant package. Grasped the catheter and applied the lubricant to the distal 1 to 2 inches of the catheter. Placed the catheter back inside the urine collection tray. Disposed of the lubricant wrapper.	5	_____	_____
16. Opened the povidone-iodine swab packet and pulled the swabs most of the way from their package. If the kit contained cotton balls rather than swabs, placed them in the sterile container and poured the povidone-iodine solution over them.	1	_____	_____
17. Grasped the sterile drape so that two of the corners were wrapped around the student's hands. Placed the drape with the waterproof side down just under the patient's buttocks. Asked the patient to lift her buttocks slightly if possible.	1	_____	_____
18. Grasped the fenestrated drape and allowed it to unfold without touching a nonsterile surface. Placed it over the patient's genital area so that the genitals were visible through the window.	1	_____	_____
19. Moved the sterile tray by holding the inside with fingers extended outward against the sides and placed it on the sterile drape near the client's buttocks.	1	_____	_____
20. If the order requested a specimen, placed the specimen container upright next to the urine collection tray on the sterile drape.	1	_____	_____

PERFORMANCE STANDARDS (cont.)	PTS	PTS EARNED (Pass/Fail)	COMMENTS

Female patients

21. With the nondominant hand, separated the *inner* labia as widely as possible. This hand, considered contaminated, remained in place until the catheter was fully inserted. — 5 — _____

22. With the dominant hand, grasped the povidone-iodine swabs (or soaked cotton balls) and wiped from top to bottom on one side of the inner labia. — 5 — _____

23. Grasped another swab (or cotton ball) and wiped from top to bottom on the other side of the inner labia. — 5 — _____

24. Grasped another swab (or cotton ball) and wipe from top to bottom over the urinary meatus. — 5 — _____

25. Grasped the catheter approximately 3 inches from its tip and positioned the other end in the collection tray. — 1 — _____

26. Asked the client to cough or bear down. — 1 — _____

27. Held the catheter at a slight upward angle (pointing toward the patient's umbilicus). Inserted the lubricated tip into the urethra approximately 2 inches or until urine began to flow into the collection tray. Released the labia with the nondominant hand and grasped the catheter, without letting go of it. — 15 — _____

Male patients

28. With nondominant hand, grasped the penis gently yet firmly and used gentle traction in an upward direction. This hand, now contaminated, remained in place until the catheter was fully inserted. — 5 — _____

PERFORMANCE STANDARDS *(cont.)*	PTS	PTS EARNED (Pass/Fail)	COMMENTS
29. With the dominant hand, grasped the povidone-iodine swabs (or soaked cotton balls) and wiped in a circular pattern from the meatus outward. Repeated this step two more times.	5	_____	_____
30. Grasped the catheter approximately 3 inches from its tip and positioned the other end in the collection tray.	1	_____	_____
31. Asked the client to cough or bear down.	1	_____	_____
32. Inserted the lubricated tip of the catheter into the urethra until urine began to flow into the collection tray.	15	_____	_____
33. Released the penis with nondominant hand and grasped the catheter to hold it securely for the remainder of the procedure.	1	_____	_____

All patients

	PTS	PTS EARNED (Pass/Fail)	COMMENTS
34. If the order required a specimen, followed these steps:			_____
a. Used the dominant hand to temporarily crimp the catheter.	1	_____	
b. Moved it over the specimen container.	1	_____	
c. Uncrimped the catheter and allowed urine to flow into the specimen container.	1	_____	_____
d. Crimped the catheter once more and moved it back over the collection tray.	1	_____	_____
e. Resumed draining urine into the collection tray until the patient's bladder was empty.	1	_____	_____
35. When urine flow had stopped, gently removed the catheter from the urethra and disposed of it.	1	_____	_____

PERFORMANCE STANDARDS (cont.)	PTS	PTS EARNED (Pass/Fail)	COMMENTS
36. Disposed of supplies, removed gloves, and washed hands.	5	_____	_____
37. Secured the lid to the specimen container. Noted the total amount of urine collected in both containers and then discarded the excess urine in an approved manner.	1	_____	_____
38. Assisted the patient off of the examination table and with dressing if necessary.	1	_____	_____
39. Wrote the patient identification data on the specimen label and affixed it to the side of the specimen container, not to the lid.	5	_____	_____
40. Completed the laboratory slip, packaged it with the specimen in the approved manner, and sent it to the laboratory according to facility policy.	5	_____	_____
41. Documented the procedure in the patient's medical record	5	_____	_____

TOTAL POINTS	151		

DOCUMENTATION

COMMENTS

Obstetrics and Gynecology

Key Term Review   *Define the following key terms:*

1.   lactation _____

2.   prenatal _____

3.   abortion _____

4.   dilation _____

5.   adenomyosis _____

6.   zygote _____

7.   blastocyte _____

8.   effacement _____

9.   fetus _____

10.   colposcopy _____

11.   ovaries _____

Key Term Review *cont.*

12. perineum _____

13. gestation _____

14. menstruation _____

15. coitus _____

16. gravidity _____

17. Bartholin gland _____

18. placenta _____

19. postpartum _____

20. endometrium _____

21. menarche _____

22. fundus _____

23. episiotomy _____

24. hormone _____

Review Questions

1. Describe the two branches of medicine referred to as women's health.

   _____

   _____

   _____

   _____

2. Describe some duties a medical assistant would perform in an OB/GYN office.

   _____

   _____

   _____

   _____

3. List the major structures of the female reproductive system.

   _____

   _____

   _____

   _____

4. Describe the functions of the following structures:

   a. ovaries

   _____

   _____

   _____

   b. fallopian tubes

   _____

   _____

   _____

c. uterus

_____

_____

_____

_____

d. vagina

_____

_____

_____

_____

e. mammary glands

_____

_____

_____

_____

5. Discuss the importance of the hormones estrogen and progesterone.

_____

_____

_____

_____

6. Describe the three phases and the hormones released during each phase of the menstrual cycle.

_____

_____

_____

_____

7. Discuss the symptoms of menopause. What are some treatments for women in menopause?

_____

_____

_____

_____

8. How soon after fertilization does a zygote reach the uterus?

_____

_____

_____

_____

9. When does a zygote develop into an embryo? When does the embryo become a fetus?

_____

_____

_____

_____

10. What are some early signs and symptoms of pregnancy?

_____

_____

_____

_____

11. What developments occur to the fetus during the third trimester?

_____

_____

_____

_____

12. What are some signs a pregnant woman may experience during the beginning of her labor?

_____

_____

_____

_____

13. Describe what occurs during the first, second, and third stages of labor.

_____

_____

_____

_____

14. What is the medical assistant's function during a woman's initial prenatal visit?

_____

_____

_____

_____

15. What are the baseline laboratory tests that may be ordered during the initial prenatal visit?

_____

_____

_____

_____

16. Which type of examinations will the physician perform during the initial prenatal visit?

_____

_____

_____

_____

17. What are the purposes for scheduling routine prenatal visits?

_____

_____

_____

_____

18. List some foods a woman should avoid during her pregnancy.

_____

_____

_____

_____

19. List some common complications of pregnancy.

_____

_____

_____

_____

20. What are some teratogens woman must avoid during pregnancy? What are the affects these teratogens have on developing embryo and fetus?

_____

_____

_____

_____

21. What information can the medical assistant provide to a mother who is unsure about breast-feeding her newborn infant?

_____

_____

_____

_____

22. Describe the various diagnostic tests that can be performed during pregnancy. For each test, provide the gestation time this test would be performed at.

_____

_____

_____

_____

23. Describe the cancer staging system and how it is used.

_____

_____

_____

_____

24. Provide the proper positions a medical assistant would place a patient in for the following examinations:

a. breast exam

_____

_____

_____

_____

b. pelvic exam

_____

_____

_____

_____

c. performing of vital signs

_____

_____

_____

_____

25. When is the best time for a woman to perform a breast self-exam?

_____

_____

_____

_____

26. What role does the medical assistant play in assisting during a routine gynecological exam?

_____

_____

_____

_____

27. What is the importance of having an annual Pap smear?

_____

_____

_____

_____

28. For which conditions may cervical cryosurgery be performed?

_____

_____

_____

_____

29. Discuss the colposcopy procedure. Why would it be performed?

_____

_____

_____

_____

30. What are some patient preparation tips that should be discussed with a patient prior to having a mammogram?

_____

_____

_____

_____

31. Discuss the connection between HPV and cervical cancer. How can cervical cancer be diagnosed?

_____

_____

_____

_____

32. What is a Bartholin's gland cyst, and how might it be treated?

_____

_____

_____

_____

33. Discuss some surgical and nonsurgical treatments for infertility.

_____

_____

_____

_____

34. What are some complications of PID?

_____

_____

_____

_____

Medical Terminology and Abbreviation Review

Give the proper medical term for the definition provided:

1. first menstrual period: _____

2. prolapse of the vagina: _____

3. difficult or painful childbirth: _____

4. repair of a relaxed or prolapsed vagina: _____

5. pain associated with menstruation: _____

6. pus in the fallopian tubes: _____

7. concerning the ovary and oviducts: _____

8. surgical removal of the uterus: _____

9. reparative surgery on the perineum: _____

10. hernia of the fallopian tubes: _____

11. milk production: _____

12. radiographic imaging of the breast: _____

13. a woman who has had one pregnancy to 20 weeks duration or longer: _____

14. occurring before birth: _____

15. prior to sexual intercourse: _____

16. woman who has delivered more than one viable infant: _____

17. the mucous membrane that lines the uterus: _____

18. transabdominal puncture of the amniotic sac: _____

19.   abnormal absence of menstruation: _____

20.   woman during her first pregnancy: _____

Disease/Condition Review

Match the disease/condition with its definition:

Disease/Condition

1. ectopic pregnancy _____

2. pelvic inflammatory disease _____

3. chlamydia _____

4. abortion _____

5. placenta abruption _____

6. fibrocystic breasts _____

7. candidiasis _____

8. gestational diabetes _____

9. uterine fibroids _____

10. eclampsia _____

11. syphilis _____

12. endometriosis _____

13. toxic shock syndrome _____

14. placenta previa _____

15. ovarian cysts _____

Definition

a. condition occurring during pregnancy that is characterized by hypertension, proteinuria, edema, seizures, coma, and death

b. a condition of developing diabetes during pregnancy

c. the growth of endometrial tissue outside the uterus

d. an STD caused by the *Chlamydia trachomatis* bacterium

e. fluid-filled sacs that grow on the ovaries

f. a disorder caused by a bacterial endotoxin; can be associated with tampon use

g. zygote development in the fallopian tube instead of the uterus

h. sudden premature detachment of placenta from the uterine wall

i. vaginitis caused by a yeast

j. acute or chronic infection of the female reproductive system

k. presence of multiple cystlike or fibrous lumps in the breasts

Disease/condition

Definition *cont.*

l. condition in which the placenta implants in the lower segment of the uterus, which may result in obstruction of the fetus during delivery

m. STD characterized by painless ulcers and can develop into full body rash and systemic complications

n. Noncancerous tumors of the uterus

o. Spontaneous therapeutic loss of pregnancy

Anatomy Identification

1. Label the internal structures of the female reproductive system in Figure 32-1.

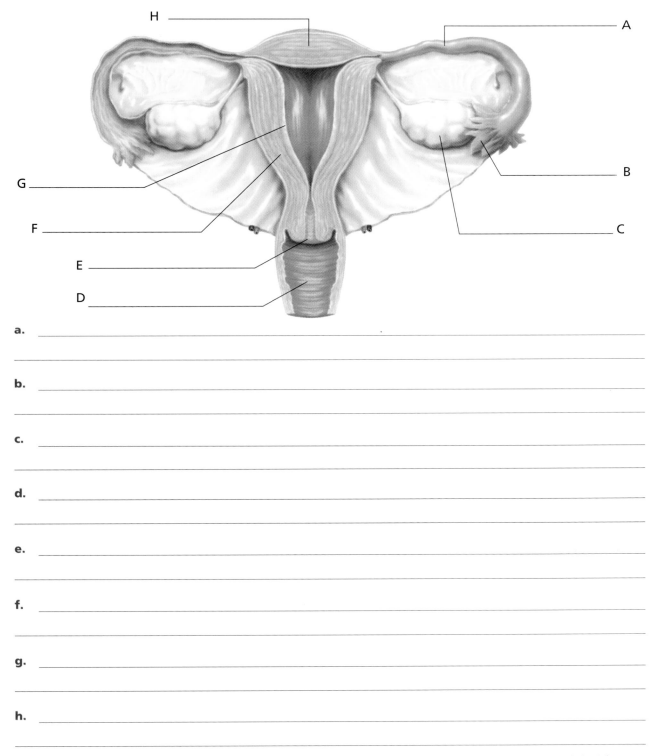

a. _____

_____

b. _____

_____

c. _____

_____

d. _____

_____

e. _____

_____

f. _____

_____

g. _____

_____

h. _____

Critical Thinking

1. Jillian St. George is in for her first prenatal visit. You are discussing Jillian's dietary needs and concerns as well as her need for prenatal vitamins. Jillian is hesitant to take the prenatal vitamins since her friends who took them during their pregnancies complained about having to take them every day. What would you say to Jillian?

_____

_____

_____

_____

2. Anna Guiloti is being scheduled for chemotherapy and radiation treatments for breast cancer. What advice can you provide to Anna regarding these treatments, and what she can do to prevent or control some of the side effects of these treatments?

_____

_____

_____

_____

3. Rissa O'Neil is in for her initial prenatal visit. The date of her last menstrual period was March 20, 2009. Calculate her estimated due date.

_____

_____

_____

_____

Teamwork Activity

1. Divide into groups of two or three. Your instructor will assign each group a different cancer of the female reproductive system. Each group will develop a fact sheet containing a description of the cancer, symptoms, diagnosis, treatment, prevention, and Internet sites for support groups and/or official disease associations.

2. Divide into pairs. Role-play taking a medical history for an initial prenatal visit and a routine gynecological visit.

3. Divide into groups of two or three. Your instructor will assign a different type of birth control method. Your group will develop a poster board or fact sheet on the method assigned. Be sure to include the methods effective rate, contraindications, and side effects. Also provide manufacturer's Web site or procedural information.

PROCEDURE 32-1 – PROVIDING INSTRUCTION ON BREAST SELF-EXAMINATION

Name _____   Date _____   Score _____

Instructor _____

Task
Instruct the patient on how to conduct a breast self-examination.

Conditions
Breast model, written patient instructions brochure, or both
Patient's medical record
Pen

Time: _____

Standard
In the time specified and within the scoring parameters determined by the instructor, the student will successfully instruct the patient on how to conduct a breast self-examination.

Points assigned reflect importance of step to meeting the task

Important = 1 pt.
Essential = 5 pts.
Critical = 15 pts.

Automatic failure results if any of the **CRITICAL TASKS** are omitted or performed incorrectly.

(To use a pass/fail system, instructors can record "P" or "F" in the "points earned (pass/fail)" column.)

PERFORMANCE STANDARDS	PTS	PTS EARNED (Pass/Fail)	COMMENTS
1. Greeted and identified the patient.	1	_____	_____
2. Discussed the importance of performing a breast self-examination as a way to detect breast lumps.	5	_____	_____
3. Explained to patient that she should perform a breast self-examination monthly and that the best time to conduct the examination is in the middle of her menstrual cycle. Suggested to the patient that she use a calendar.	5	_____	_____

PERFORMANCE STANDARDS (cont.)	PTS	PTS EARNED (Pass/Fail)	COMMENTS
4. Instructed the patient to stand in front of a mirror with her shoulders straight and arms on her hips. Told her to look at each breast for changes in size, shape, or color; dimpling or puckering; redness; rash; swelling; changes in nipple shape; or discharge from the nipple.	15	_____	_____
5. Told the patient that she should next raise her arms and repeat step 4 to get a clear view of her breasts.	15	_____	_____
6. Instructed patient to inspect her nipples for discharge by squeezing them.	15	_____	_____
7. Explained to the patient that she should also inspect her breasts by lying down on a bed and palpating each breast for lumps.	15	_____	_____
a. The patient was instructed to palpate the left breast with the first two fingers of the right hand and the right breast with the first two fingers of the left hand.	5	_____	_____
b. The patient was told to cover the entire breast, using the same starting point and going in a back-and-forth motion. Suggested to the patient she could start at the nipple and go in a circular motion from inside to outside or that she could start at the upper portion of the armpit and move back and forth, covering the entire breast.	5	_____	_____
c. Instructed the patient to check for lumps in her armpits as well as the area above the breast around the collarbone.	5	_____	_____

PERFORMANCE STANDARDS (cont.)	PTS	PTS EARNED (Pass/Fail)	COMMENTS
8. Explained to the patient that she should be looking for a small, hard, round lump. Explained to the patient that as she performs the procedure on a regular basis, she would begin to see a pattern in her breasts and feeling a lump would become easier.	15	_____	_____
9. If available, used a breast model to demonstrate the proper technique for inspecting for lumps. Allowed the patient to feel simulated lumps in breast model.	5	_____	_____
10. Gave the patient an instruction brochure to take home.	1	_____	_____
11. Asked the patient if she had any questions and reminded her to call the office immediately if she should feel a lump, and that early detection and treatment can prevent the spread of breast cancer.	5	_____	_____
12. Documented the patient education in the patient's medical record.	5	_____	_____

TOTAL POINTS	117		

DOCUMENTATION

COMMENTS

PROCEDURE 32-2 – PREPARING A PATIENT FOR AND ASSISTING WITH A GYNECOLOGICAL EXAMINATION

Name _____   Date _____   Score _____

Instructor _____

Task
Prepare a patient for and assist with a gynecological examination that includes a Papanicolaou (Pap) test.

Conditions
3 pairs of gloves
Lubricant
Tissues
Patient gown and drape
Disposable vaginal speculum
Light source
Pap test container
Cytology requisition form
Biohazard specimen transport bag
Specimen collection swab, cytobrush, or cervical scraper
Biohazardous waste container
Pen
Patient's medical record

Time: _____

Standards
In the time specified and within the scoring parameters determined by the instructor, the student will successfully prepare a patient for a gynecological examination, assist the physician with the examination, and prepare for and process a Pap test.

Points assigned reflect importance of step to meeting the task

Important = 1 pt.
Essential = 5 pts.
Critical = 15 pts.

Automatic failure results if any of the **CRITICAL TASKS** are omitted or performed incorrectly.

(To use a pass/fail system, instructors can record "P" or "F" in the "points earned (pass/fail)" column.)

PERFORMANCE STANDARDS	PTS	PTS EARNED (Pass/Fail)	COMMENTS
1. Washed or sanitized your hands and assemble the supplies, making sure supplies were situated for easy access by the physician. Labeled the specimen bottle and completed the cytology requisition form, being sure to list the source of the specimen (vaginal or cervical).	15	_____	_____ _____ _____ _____ _____
2. Greeted and identified the patient and explained the examination procedure.	5	_____	_____ _____

PERFORMANCE STANDARDS (cont.)	PTS	PTS EARNED (Pass/Fail)	COMMENTS
3. Instructed the patient on how to collect a urine specimen, if required. If a urine specimen was not required, asked the patient if she needed to void.	5	_____	_____
4. Obtained and recorded proper patient history, vital signs, and height and weight.	15	_____	_____
5. Instructed the patient to remove all clothing and advised her on the proper way to put on the gown (with the opening in the front) and to wrap the drape around her waist. Left the room unless patient required assistance.	5	_____	_____
6. Notified the physician when the patient was ready for examination.	1	_____	_____
7. Knocked before reentering the room.	1	_____	_____
8. Assisted the patient into the supine position for breast examination and then into the lithotomy position for the gynecological examination, redraping as necessary.	5	_____	_____
9. Checked the light source for the physician and made sure the supplies were readily available.	1	_____	_____
10. Put on gloves and assisted the physician in the examination as needed.	1	_____	_____
11. Lubricated or warmed the speculum according to office policy and handed it to the physician. Supported patient as necessary.	5	_____	_____
12. Handed the cytobrush or other specimen collection swab to physician.	1	_____	_____

PERFORMANCE STANDARDS (cont.)	PTS	PTS EARNED (Pass/Fail)	COMMENTS
13. Opened the bottle so the physician could insert the cytobrush into the bottle. Swirled the cytobrush in the solution 10 times. Withdrew the cytobrush from the bottle, being sure to tap it against the side of the bottle.	15	_____	_____
14. Disposed of the cytobrush in the biohazardous waste container.	5	_____	_____
15. Secured the lid to the bottle.	1	_____	_____
16. If a wet mount sample was required, followed these steps:			_____
a. Handed the cotton-tipped applicator to the physician.	1	_____	_____
b. After the physician took a sample of the vaginal discharge, took the applicator from the physician and immediately put it into a test tube containing 0.5 mL of sterile saline solution.	5	_____	_____
c. Vigorously mixed the applicator in the test tube, pressing the tip of the applicator against the sides of the test tube	1	_____	_____
d. Placed a drop of the solution onto a microscopic slide and added a cover slip.	1	_____	_____
e. Placed the slide on the microscope for the physician to view.	1	_____	_____
17. If a KOH preparation was required, follow the steps for a wet mount and added a few drops of 10% potassium hydroxide (KOH) to the microscope slide before adding a cover slip.	1	_____	_____
18. Applied lubricant to the physician's gloved index and middle fingers. Supported the patient as necessary while the physician performed the bimanual examination.	1	_____	_____

PERFORMANCE STANDARDS (cont.)	PTS	PTS EARNED (Pass/Fail)	COMMENTS
19. After the physician completed the bimanual examination, handed a new pair of gloves to the physician for the rectal examination.	1	_____	_____
20. When the physician had completed the examination, assisted the patient out of the stirrups and back onto the examination table. Provided tissues to the patient.	5	_____	_____
21. Explained to the patient that she may get dressed and told her where to dispose of the gown and drape.	5	_____	_____
22. Explained to the patient how the office would communicate the test results to her, based on office policy. Released the patient.	1	_____	_____
23. Processed the bottle and cytology requisition form for proper transport to the laboratory.	15	_____	_____
24. Washed hands.	1	_____	_____
25. Documented the examination and Pap test, as well as other tests if performed, in the patient's medical record.	5	_____	_____
26. Cleaned up the examination room according to proper disposal techniques.	1	_____	_____

TOTAL POINTS	126		

DOCUMENTATION

COMMENTS

Pediatrics

Key Terms   *Define the following key terms:*

1.   adolescence   _____

_____

2.   cerumen   _____

_____

3.   infant   _____

_____

4.   neonate   _____

_____

5.   circumcision   _____

_____

6.   pediatrics   _____

_____

7.   pediatrician   _____

_____

8.   vaccine   _____

_____

Review Questions

1. List the terms used to identify pediatric patients, and give the appropriate age range for each category.

   _____

   _____

   _____

   _____

2. Discuss ways a medical assistant can minimize the fear of the doctor's office for pediatric patients.

   _____

   _____

   _____

   _____

3. Discuss some typical developmental milestones for pediatric patients.

   _____

   _____

   _____

   _____

4. What are the five categories tested in an APGAR?

   _____

   _____

   _____

   _____

5. Discuss what activities occur during a well child visit.

   _____

   _____

   _____

   _____

6. List some questions a medical assistant may ask the parent or caregiver during a well child visit.

_____

_____

_____

_____

7. List some safety tips for the medical assistant when working with pediatric patients.

_____

_____

_____

_____

8. How do pediatric vital signs differ from adult vital signs?

_____

_____

_____

_____

9. What type of thermometer has been phased out for use? Why?

_____

_____

_____

_____

10. Outline the procedure for taking an axillary temperature.

_____

_____

_____

_____

11. Compare and contrast the method for measuring an infant's height versus a 2-year-old child.

_____

_____

_____

_____

12. List some common screening tests performed in a pediatric office.

_____

_____

_____

_____

13. Discuss the importance of providing anticipatory guidance as part of a routine well child visit.

_____

_____

_____

_____

14. Discuss the differences between the common cold and the respiratory flu.

_____

_____

_____

_____

15. What are some causes of childhood diarrhea?

_____

_____

_____

_____

16. What is the PKU test? Why is it important to perform this test on all newborns?

_____

_____

_____

_____

17. What areas does the Denver Development Screening Tool assess?

_____

_____

_____

_____

18. List some screening blood tests that may be performed on pediatric patients.

_____

_____

_____

_____

19. What is the vaccine registry?

_____

_____

_____

_____

20. Compare and contrast the signs and symptoms of the flu with the common cold.

_____

_____

_____

_____

21. What is autism? What are some symptoms of autism?

_____

_____

_____

_____

22. List five foods that may help alleviate constipation in children.

_____

_____

_____

_____

23. How is failure to thrive diagnosed?

_____

_____

_____

_____

Disease/Condition Review

Match the disease/condition with its definition:

Disease/condition

1. impetigo _____

2. scoliosis _____

3. croup _____

4. allergies _____

5. cerebral palsy _____

6. conjunctivitis _____

7. thrush _____

8. RSV _____

9. eczema _____

10. chickenpox _____

Definition

a. congenital or acquired disorder characterized by poor muscle control, muscle weakness, retardation, and developmental problems

b. viral respiratory disease common in children under 2 years old

c. highly infectious skin infection caused by *Streptococcus* or *Staphylococcus* bacteria

d. inflammatory skin disease characterized by a vesicular rash on limbs or face and neck

e. viral disease caused by varicella-zoster virus, characterized by red, itchy rash

f. abnormal curvature of the spine

g. also known as pink eye

h. contagious upper respiratory tract infection characterized by a harsh, repetitive cough

i. oral fungal infection caused by *Candida albicans*

j. reaction by the body's immune system in response to exposure to an allergen

Critical Thinking Questions

1. Mrs. Al-ridjle is bringing her newborn son in for his 2-month well child visit. You are preparing the vaccine consent form, and Mrs. Al-ridjle states, due to religious reasons, that she objects to giving her son any immunizations. How do you respond?

_____

_____

_____

_____

2. You are the medical assistant responsible for phone triage, and Mr. Peters phones with concerns about his 18-month-old daughter, who has had diarrhea for the past 2 days. He is concerned she may be dehydrated. What questions will you ask Mr. Peters before scheduling an appointment?

_____

_____

_____

_____

3. Missy Perez-Rodriguez is in for a sick child visit. You notice she has what looks like fluid-filled lesions under her nose. What do you suspect she has?

_____

_____

_____

_____

4. The other medical assistant in your office, Ursula, has a 2-year-old son, Daniel, who is the same age as your son. Ursula confides in you one day during lunch that your son seems more social than Daniel and she fears Daniel may be autistic. What do you say to her?

_____

_____

_____

_____

Teamwork Exercises

1. Divide into groups of three or four. Choose a childhood disease or disorder from the chapter (or your instructor will assign one to each group). Work together to create a fact sheet on your disease. Include information such as signs and symptoms, diagnosis, treatment, and preventative measures, if any. Present your information to the rest of the class.

2. Divide into groups of three or four. Each group will be given a specific age group, such as 4 months to 12 months, 1 year to 4 years, 5 years to 10 years, or 11 years to 18 years. Work together to create a week's worth of healthy meals and snacks for your assigned age group.

PROCEDURE 33-1 – COLLECTING A URINE SAMPLE FROM AN INFANT

Name _____

Date _____   Score _____

Instructor _____

Task
Collect an uncontaminated urine specimen from an infant.

Conditions
Nonsterile disposable gloves
Antiseptic wipes
Sterile water and sterile gauze squares
Pediatric urine collection bag
Sterile urine specimen container and label

Time: _____

Standard
In the time specified and within the scoring parameters determined by the instructor, the student will successfully collect a urine specimen from an infant.

Points assigned reflect importance of step to meeting the task

Important = 1 pt.
Essential = 5 pts.
Critical = 15 pts.

Automatic failure results if any of the **CRITICAL TASKS** are omitted or performed incorrectly.

(To use a pass/fail system, instructors can record "P" or "F" in the "points earned (pass/fail)" column.)

PERFORMANCE STANDARDS	PTS	PTS EARNED (Pass/Fail)	COMMENTS
1. Washed hands.	5	_____	_____
2. Assembled the equipment and supplies and checked the order in the patient's medical record.	5	_____	_____ _____
3. Greeted the patient and caregiver. Explained the procedure to the caregiver and answered any questions.	5	_____	_____ _____
4. Applied gloves.	5	_____	_____
5. Positioned the infant in the supine position and removed the diaper. Asked the caregiver to position the infant with legs apart.	15	_____	_____ _____ _____

PERFORMANCE STANDARDS *(cont.)*	PTS	PTS EARNED (Pass/Fail)	COMMENTS
6. Cleaned the child's genitalia thoroughly with the antiseptic wipes.			
a. For a girl, cleaned the urinary meatus from front to back using a separate wipe for each side. Used a third wipe to clean directly over the urinary meatus, again from front to back Rinsed the area thoroughly with sterile water and a sterile gauze. Dried the area with sterile gauze.	15	_____	
b. For an uncircumcised boy, retracted the foreskin of the penis slightly. Cleaned the area around the meatus and urethral opening with an antiseptic wipe. Used a fresh antiseptic wipe to clean the scrotum. Rinsed the area thoroughly with sterile water and a sterile gauze square. Dried the area with sterile gauze.	15	_____	
7. Prepared the urine collection bag by removing the peel-apart packaging and the paper backing to expose the adhesive strip around the sponge ring of the bag.	5	_____	
8. Attached the collection bag firmly to the infant.			
a. For a girl, placed the round opening of the bag covering the upper half of the external genitalia, centering the opening of the bag above the urinary meatus.	15	_____	
b. For a boy, positioned the bag so that the child's penis and scrotum were projected through the opening of the bag. The loose end of the bag should have been hanging down toward the infant's feet.	15	_____	
9. Placed a clean diaper under the child.	1	_____	

PERFORMANCE STANDARDS (cont.)	PTS	PTS EARNED (Pass/Fail)	COMMENTS
10. Offered that the caregiver give the infant water in the infant's bottle or asked the mother to breastfeed the infant.	1	_____	_____
11. Asked the caregiver to stay with the infant until he voided.	5	_____	_____
12. When the infant had voided a sufficient volume of urine, washed hands, applied gloves, and gently removed the urine collection bag. Used care in removing the bag.	15	_____	_____
13. Cleaned the genital area with antiseptic wipes and re-diapered the child.	5	_____	_____
14. Poured the urine from the collection bag directly into a sterile urine specimen container.	15	_____	_____
15. Labeled the specimen container.	15	_____	_____
16. Recorded the procedure in the patient's medical record.	5	_____	_____
17. Removed gloves and washed your hands.	5	_____	_____

TOTAL POINTS	167		

DOCUMENTATION

COMMENTS

Geriatrics

Key Term Review

Define the following key terms:

1. postmenopausal

2. in-home care

3. assisted living

4. neurofibrillary tangles

5. home health-care agency

6. palliative care

7. nursing home

8. ageism

9. neuritic plaques

10. hospice

Review Questions

1. Describe the impact of the aging population on the American health-care system.

   _____
   _____
   _____
   _____

2. What are some myths about aging that you, as a medical assistant, can dispel with your patients?

   _____
   _____
   _____
   _____

3. For the following body systems, discuss some physiological changes that happens to the aging body:

   a. integumentary:

   _____
   _____
   _____
   _____

   b. nervous:

   _____
   _____
   _____
   _____

   c. cardiovascular:

   _____
   _____
   _____
   _____

d. respiratory:

_____

_____

_____

_____

e. digestive:

_____

_____

_____

_____

f. urinary:

_____

_____

_____

_____

g. reproductive:

_____

_____

_____

_____

h. endocrine:

_____

_____

_____

i. musculoskeletal:

_____

_____

_____

_____

4. Differentiate among dementia, delirium, and depression.

_____

_____

_____

_____

5. Identify some self-care measures that you can discuss with your patients to prevent or minimize the risk of developing dementia.

_____

_____

_____

_____

6. Discuss some dos and don'ts when communicating with patients who have dementia.

_____

_____

_____

_____

7. Discuss some risk factors for osteoporosis.

_____

_____

_____

_____

8. Compare and contrast cataracts, glaucoma, and macular degeneration.

_____

_____

_____

_____

9. Describe why pain management for geriatric patients should be a priority.

_____

_____

_____

_____

10. What are some medication safety tips that a medical assistant can discuss with their elderly patients?

_____

_____

_____

_____

Critical Thinking

1. Mrs. Molly Gilligan is an active 69-year-old woman who has been diagnosed with a vertebral fracture due to osteoporosis. What patient teaching tips can you discuss with her regarding her condition?

_____

_____

_____

2. Bill Connor is an 80-year-old patient complaining of having to get up in the middle of the night two or three times to urinate. What may be the cause of Mr. Connor's symptoms?

_____

_____

_____

3. Mr. and Mrs. Vargas are regular patients at the clinic, although it has been over a year since their last visit. They visit the clinic one morning because Mrs. Vargas is concerned about her husband and states, "He seems confused much of the time and can't seem to understand or remember half of the things I tell him." Make a list of all of the potential causes of Mr. Vargas's confusion and memory problems.

_____

_____

_____

_____

Teamwork Activity

1. Divide into groups of two or three. Each group will be assigned one of the following topics that can be found on the AARP Web site.

    a. health

    b. money

    c. leisure

    d. family

    e. make a difference

Within each topic, each student in the group will read a different article from the AARP Web site. Discuss with your group the article you selected and why. Provide a brief synopsis of your article. As a class, discuss your general topic and what you learned and how you may be able to apply your knowledge to your role as a medical assistant.

2. Divide into groups of two or three. Your instructor will assign each group one of the following facilities:

    a. senior center

    b. visiting nurses association

    c. assisted living facility

    d. rehabilitative facility

    e. skilled nursing facility

Each group will locate at least three of their assigned facility that are within a 20-mile radius of their area. Write a report of the services provided by each facility, the different employment opportunities (types of health-care professions they may employ), contact information, and Web sites. Compare and contrast the types of services offered by the individual places. For example, if you researched three senior centers in three different towns, does one site offer more bus trips than the others? Out of the three assisted living facilities, does one offer more choices in dining rooms or restaurants?

Office Project

Invite members of the local senior center to have breakfast or lunch with your entire class. Depending on your college's facilities, the event can be catered or pot luck. Involve every student in the planning of the event, assigning duties as needed. During the event, each student should have a conversation with a senior and ask them about their experiences growing up, attending school and/or college, work ethic, family, aging issues, etc. Each student will write an essay about his or her conversation.

Orthopedics

Key Term Review   *Define the following key terms:*

1.   flexion   _____

   _____

2.   tendon   _____

   _____

3.   abduction   _____

   _____

4.   ultrasound   _____

   _____

5.   aponeurosis   _____

   _____

6.   hyperextension   _____

   _____

7.   gait   _____

   _____

8.   thermotherapy   _____

   _____

9.   range of motion   _____

   _____

10.   adduction   _____

   _____

11.   bone   _____

   _____

12.   cryotherapy   _____

   _____

Key Term Review *cont.*

13. modality _____

_____

14. atrophy _____

_____

15. rotation _____

_____

16. myofascia _____

_____

17. ligament _____

_____

18. inversion _____

_____

19. circumduction _____

_____

20. muscle testing _____

_____

21. ambulation _____

_____

22. contracture _____

_____

23. extension _____

_____

24. hemiplegia _____

_____

Review Questions

1. Describe the three types of muscle tissue.

   _____

   _____

   _____

   _____

2. Discuss some of the injuries that a medical assistant might see working in an orthopedic office.

   _____

   _____

   _____

   _____

3. Discuss the differences between muscles, tendons, and ligaments.

   _____

   _____

   _____

   _____

4. Identify and name body movements used in range of motion exercises.

   _____

   _____

   _____

   _____

5. Discuss uses of the following therapies:

   a. ice:

   _____

   _____

   _____

   _____

b. moist heat:

_____

_____

_____

_____

c. dry heat:

_____

_____

_____

_____

d. warm moist compressions:

_____

_____

_____

_____

6. Describe the physiological effects of the following therapies:

   a. TENS:

_____

_____

_____

_____

   b. ultrasound:

_____

_____

_____

_____

7. Discuss the various assistive devices patients may use to aid in ambulation.

_____

_____

_____

_____

Medical Terminology and Abbreviation Review

Match the word element with its definition:

Word element	Definition
1. kyph/o _____	**a.** neck
2. poster/o _____	**b.** cartilage
3. stern/o _____	**c.** clavicle
4. chondr/o _____	**d.** skull
5. ischi/o _____	**e.** cold
6. dors/o _____	**f.** back
7. therm/o _____	**g.** ischium
8. -plegia _____	**h.** humped
9. cervic/o _____	**i.** paralysis
10. crani/o _____	**j.** toward the back
11. cleid/o _____	**k.** vertebra
12. thorac/o _____	**l.** chest
13. vertebr/o _____	**m.** hot
14. cry/o _____	**n.** to break
15. spondyl/o _____	**o.** union, together

Match the abbreviation with its meaning:

Abbreviation	Meaning

Abbreviation

1. WNL _____
2. ALS _____
3. DJD _____
4. LP _____
5. TENS _____
6. MVA _____
7. ORIF _____
8. RA _____
9. PT _____
10. ROM _____
11. NSAID _____
12. MD _____
13. DTR _____
14. ADL _____
15. TMJ _____

Meaning

a. activities of daily living

b. range of motion

c. nonsteroidal anti-inflammatory drug

d. amyotrophic lateral sclerosis

e. deep tendon reflex

f. degenerative joint disease

g. lumbar puncture

h. muscular dystrophy

i. open reduction and internal fixation

j. rheumatoid arthritis

k. motor vehicle accident

l. transcutaneous electric nerve stimulation

m. temporal mandibular joint

n. within normal limits

o. physical therapy

Disease/Condition Review

For the following musculoskeletal pathologies, provide a description of the pathology and possible treatments:

Table 35-1

Pathology	Description	Treatment
carpal tunnel syndrome		
scoliosis		
fibromyalgia		
osteoarthritis		
anterior cruciate ligament tear		
dislocation		
rheumatoid arthritis		
herniated disk		
tennis elbow		
tendonitis		
kyphosis		
osteoporosis		
strain		
sprain		

Anatomy Review

1. Identify the following fracture types in Figures 35-1 through 35-7.

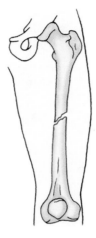

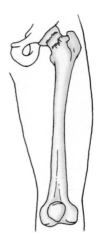

_____

_____

_____

_____

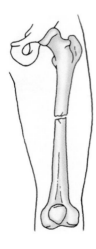

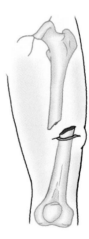

_____

_____

_____

_____

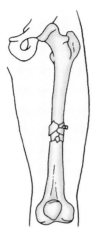

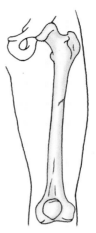

_____

_____

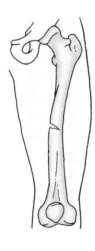

_____

_____

Student Activity Manual to Accompany The Professional Medical Assistant *505*

Critical Thinking

1. Lynn Giovanni, a 15-year-old high school soccer player, has just had surgery to repair a torn ACL. She is visiting the orthopedic surgeon for a postoperative appointment. As the medical assistant, you are responsible for setting up her physical therapy schedule. As you interview her about her availability for appointments, she appears distraught. You ask her what the matter is, and she says she is worried about going to physical therapy, that it would harm her leg even more. How would you respond to Lynn?

   _____

   _____

   _____

   _____

2. Explain how the body reacts to the application of heat and cold to soft tissue injuries.

   _____

   _____

   _____

   _____

Teamwork Exercises

1. In groups of two, refer to the movements measured by goniometry. Take turns performing the listed range of motion movements with your partner.

2. Divide the class into three groups. Assign each group one of the following patient education topics and create patient brochures. Exchange the brochures and follow the directions provided. Evaluate the instructions of your classmates. Be sure to provide constructive criticism.

   Topics: cast care, wheelchair transfer, and crutch walking.

PROCEDURE 35-1 – TRANSFERRING A PATIENT FROM A WHEELCHAIR TO AN EXAMINATION TABLE

Name _____   Date _____   Score _____

Instructor _____

Task
Move a patient from a wheelchair to an examination table safely.

Conditions
Gait belt
Stool with rubber tips and a handle for gripping

Time: _____

Standard
In the time specified and within the scoring parameters determined by the instructor, the student will successfully transfer a patient from a wheelchair to an examination table.

Points assigned reflect importance of step to meeting the task

Important = 1 pt.
Essential = 5 pts.
Critical = 15 pts.

Automatic failure results if any of the **CRITICAL TASKS** are omitted or performed incorrectly.

(To use a pass/fail system, instructors can record "P" or "F" in the "points earned (pass/fail)" column.)

PERFORMANCE STANDARDS	PTS	PTS EARNED (Pass/Fail)	COMMENTS
1. Washed hands.	5	_____	_____
2. Introduced self and addressed the patient by name. Explained to the patient that she will be helped onto the examination table.	5	_____	_____
3. Placed the wheelchair next to the examination table and locked the brakes. Placed the patient with her stronger side (if applicable) closest to the examination table	15	_____	_____
4. Placed the gait belt securely (but not too tightly) around the patient's waist.	15	_____	_____
5. Moved the footrests up and out of the way, and asked the patient to place her feet on the floor.	5	_____	_____

PERFORMANCE STANDARDS *(cont.)*	PTS	PTS EARNED (Pass/Fail)	COMMENTS
6. Positioned the stool in front of the examination table as close to the wheelchair as possible	5	_____	
7. Asked the patient to move to the front edge of the wheelchair.	5	_____	
8. Stood directly in front of the patient with feet hip-width apart. Bending at the hips and knees, grasped the gait belt on both sides. Instructed the patient to use the armrests of the wheelchair to push upward if she were able.	15	_____	
9. Gave the patient a signal to push off with her arms and good leg while the student lifted the gait belt.	5	_____	
10. Told the patient to allow the student and the gait belt to support her while she moved her stronger foot to step onto the stool. Did not let go of the gait belt.	15	_____	
11. Told the patient to pivot her back to the examination table to sit. Made sure that the patient's buttocks were high enough to get onto the table. Supported the patient's weaker, outer leg.	15	_____	
12. Instructed the patient to grasp the stool handle and placed the other hand on the examination table.	15	_____	
13. Helped the patient adjust her position on the examination table as necessary. Made sure that the patient was balanced and comfortable.	5	_____	
14. Moved the wheelchair out of the way.	5	_____	

TOTAL POINTS	130		

DOCUMENTATION

COMMENTS

PROCEDURE 35-2 – TRANSFERRING A PATIENT FROM AN EXAMINATION TABLE TO A WHEELCHAIR

Name _____   Date _____   Score _____

Instructor _____

Task
Move a patient from an examination table to a wheel-chair safely.

Conditions
Gait belt
Stool with rubber tips and a handle for gripping

Time: _____

Standard
In the time specified and within the scoring parameters determined by the instructor, the student will successfully transfer a patient from an examination table to a wheelchair.

Points assigned reflect importance of step to meeting the task

Important = 1 pt.
Essential = 5 pts.
Critical = 15 pts.

Automatic failure results if any of the **CRITICAL TASKS** are omitted or performed incorrectly.

(To use a pass/fail system, instructors can record "P" or "F" in the "points earned (pass/fail)" column.)

PERFORMANCE STANDARDS	PTS	PTS EARNED (Pass/Fail)	COMMENTS
1. Washed hands.	5	_____	_____
2. Introduced self (if not assisting the patient previously) and addressed the patient by name. Explained to the patient that she would be helped back to the wheelchair.	5	_____	_____ _____ _____ _____ _____
3. Positioned the wheelchair next to the examination table and locked the brakes. The chair should have been positioned closest to the patient's stronger side.	15	_____	_____ _____ _____ _____ _____
4. Positioned the stool next to the examination table.	5	_____	_____ _____

PERFORMANCE STANDARDS (cont.)	PTS	PTS EARNED (Pass/Fail)	COMMENTS
5. Assisted the patient into a sitting position (if not sitting already) and put the gait belt on the patient. The belt should be snug but not tight, and the excess belt should have been tucked in the back.	15	_____	_____
6. Placed one arm under the patient's arm and around her shoulders and the other arm under the patient's knees. Pivoted the patient so that her legs dangled over the edge of the examination table.	15	_____	_____
7. Positioned student's body directly in front of the patient without removing student's hand from the patient.	15	_____	_____
8. Grasped the patient by the gait belt on both sides. Student stood with feet apart and knees bent.	5	_____	_____
9. Instructed the patient that, upon a signal, she was to push off of the examination table and to grasp the stool handle for support. Gave the patient the signal as the student pulled her slightly toward self.	15	_____	_____
10. Keeping both hands on the gait belt, asked the patient to step onto the floor with her strong leg. Pivoted the patient so that her back was to the wheelchair.	15	_____	_____
11. Asked the patient to grasp the armrests of the wheelchair and assisted her to a seated position in the wheelchair.	5	_____	_____
12. Lowered the footrests and placed her feet on them.	5	_____	_____

PERFORMANCE STANDARDS (cont.)	PTS	PTS EARNED (Pass/Fail)	COMMENTS
13. Removed the gait belt.	5	_____	_____

TOTAL POINTS	125		

DOCUMENTATION

COMMENTS

_____

_____

_____

_____

PROCEDURE 35-3 – PERFORMING ROM EXERCISES, UPPER BODY

Name _____   Date _____   Score _____

Instructor _____

Task
Use passive range-of-motion (ROM) exercises to maintain and increase joint mobility in the upper extremities to prevent contracture.

Conditions
None

Time: _____

Standard
In the time specified and within the scoring parameters determined by the instructor, the student will successfully perform passive ROM exercises.

Points assigned reflect importance of step to meeting the task

> Important = 1 pt.
> Essential = 5 pts.
> Critical = 15 pts.

Automatic failure results if any of the **CRITICAL TASKS** are omitted or performed incorrectly.

(To use a pass/fail system, instructors can record "P" or "F" in the "points earned (pass/fail)" column.)

PERFORMANCE STANDARDS	PTS	PTS EARNED (Pass/Fail)	COMMENTS
1. Washed hands.	5	_____	_____
2. Introduced self and addressed the patient by name. Explained to the patient that her arms will be moved gently, within pain tolerance and flexibility of the limb.	5	_____	_____
Shoulder flexion			
1. Keeping the patient's arm straight, and holding the arm at the wrist and elbow, lifted the patient's arm straight over her head until it rested flat on the bed or to range-of-motion (ROM) tolerance.	15	_____	_____
2. Brought the arm back to the patient's side. Repeated according to the physician's instructions.	5	_____	_____

PERFORMANCE STANDARDS *(cont.)*	PTS	PTS EARNED (Pass/Fail)	COMMENTS

Shoulder abduction and adduction

1. Keeping the patient's arm straight by her side with the palm facing up, brought the arm out straight away from the patient's body. Was sure to support the arm at the wrist and elbow.   15   _____

2. Returned the patient's arm to her side and brought it across her body (adduction).   15   _____

3. Returned the patient's arm to her side. Repeated according to the physician's instructions.   5   _____

External and internal shoulder rotation

1. Brought the patient's arm out at a right angle from her body.   15   _____

2. Bent the elbow at a right angle, keeping the upper arm on the bed and the hand straight up.   15   _____

3. Keeping the patient's elbow bent at 90 degrees, gently pressed down on her shoulder with one hand while holding up her hand with the student's other hand.   15   _____

4. Moved her hand gently back until it touched the bed next to the patient's head.   15   _____

5. Brought her hand back down until the palm of the hand touched the bed. Repeated as necessary.   15   _____

Elbow flexion and extension

1. With the patient's arm by her side and her palm up, flexed and extended the elbow. Repeated as necessary.   15   _____

PERFORMANCE STANDARDS (cont.)	PTS	PTS EARNED (Pass/Fail)	COMMENTS

Wrist extension and flexion

1. While supporting the patient's arm above the wrist, held the palm of the hand and extended and flexed the wrist. — 15 — _____ — _____

Wrist inversion and eversion

1. Grasped the patient's wrist with one hand and grasped her hand with the other. — 15 — _____ — _____

2. Slowly bent the patient's hand toward her body, then away. — 15 — _____ — _____

Wrist supination and pronation

1. Grasped the patient's wrist with one hand and her hand with the other. — 15 — _____ — _____

2. Slowly turned the patient's hand toward her feet, then toward her head. — 15 — _____ — _____

Finger flexion and extension

1. Supported the patient's wrist with one hand. — 5 — _____ — _____

2. Covered her fingers with the other hand and curled them over to make a fist. — 15 — _____ — _____

3. Uncurled the patient's fingers and straightened them. — 15 — _____ — _____

| TOTAL POINTS | 265 | | |

DOCUMENTATION

COMMENTS

PROCEDURE 35-4 – PERFORMING ROM EXERCISES, LOWER BODY

Name _____   Date _____   Score _____

                                          Instructor _____

Task	Standard
Use passive range-of-motion (ROM) exercises to maintain and increase joint mobility in the lower extremities to prevent contracture.	In the time specified and within the scoring parameters determined by the instructor, the student will successfully perform passive ROM exercises.

Conditions
None

Time: _____

Points assigned reflect importance of step to meeting the task

> Important = 1 pt.
> Essential = 5 pts.
> Critical = 15 pts.

Automatic failure results if any of the **CRITICAL TASKS** are omitted or performed incorrectly.

(To use a pass/fail system, instructors can record "P" or "F" in the "points earned (pass/fail)" column.)

PERFORMANCE STANDARDS	PTS	PTS EARNED (Pass/Fail)	COMMENTS
1. Washed hands.	5	_____	_____
2. Introduced self and addressed the patient by name. Explained to the patient that his legs will be moved gently, within pain tolerance and flexibility of the limb	5	_____	_____ _____ _____ _____
Hip abduction and adduction			
1. Supported the patient's knee and ankle.	5	_____	_____ _____
2. Kept the patient's leg straight while moving the entire leg away from his body.	15	_____	_____ _____
3. Moved the patient's leg back toward the midline of the body.	5	_____	_____ _____

PERFORMANCE STANDARDS (cont.)	PTS	PTS EARNED (Pass/Fail)	COMMENTS
Hip and knee flexion and extension			
1. Supported the patient's knee and ankle.	5	_____	_____ _____
2. Bent the patient's knee and raised it as far toward the patient's chest as tolerated with comfort.	15	_____	_____ _____
3. Lowered and straightened the patient's leg.	5	_____	_____ _____
Hip rotation			
1. Supported the patient's leg at the knee and ankle.	5	_____	_____ _____
2. Rolled the patient's leg in a circular motion, away from the body.	15	_____	_____ _____
3. Rolled the patient's leg in a circular motion, toward the body.	5	_____	_____ _____
Ankle and dorsiflexion and plantar flexion			
1. Keeping the patient's leg flat on the bed, grasped the ankle with one hand and the heel of the foot with the other.	5	_____	_____ _____ _____
2. While holding the heel with the one hand, flexed the patient's foot and rested the bottom of the foot against the student's forearm.	15	_____	_____ _____ _____
3. Dorsiflexed the ankle by pushing the foot toward the patient's head.	15	_____	_____ _____
4. Kept hand on the patient's ankle and plantar-flexed the foot by pushing the foot down toward the foot of the bed.	15	_____	_____ _____ _____

PERFORMANCE STANDARDS (cont.)	PTS	PTS EARNED (Pass/Fail)	COMMENTS
Foot inversion and eversion			
1. Grasped the patient's ankle with one hand and the arch of his foot with the other.	5	_____	_____ _____
2. Gently turned the patient's foot inward.	15	_____	_____ _____
3. Returned the foot to midline, and then gently turned it outward.	15	_____	_____ _____

TOTAL POINTS	170		

DOCUMENTATION

COMMENTS

_____

_____

_____

_____

PROCEDURE 35-5 – ASSISTING WITH GAIT USING A GAIT BELT

Name _____   Date _____   Score _____

Instructor _____

Task
Help the patient ambulate safely.

Condition
Gait belt

Time: _____

Standard
In the time specified and within the scoring parameters determined by the instructor, the student will success-fully assist with gait using a gait belt.

Points assigned reflect importance of step to meeting the task

Important = 1 pt.
Essential = 5 pts.
Critical = 15 pts.

Automatic failure results if any of the **CRITICAL TASKS** are omitted or performed incorrectly.

(To use a pass/fail system, instructors can record "P" or "F" in the "points earned (pass/fail)" column.)

PERFORMANCE STANDARDS	PTS	PTS EARNED (Pass/Fail)	COMMENTS
1. Washed hands.	5	_____	_____
2. Introduced self and addressed the patient by name. Explained to the patient that student will assist him in standing and walking.	5	_____	_____ _____ _____
3. Locked the brakes on the wheel-chair, placed the patient's feet on the floor, and moved the foot plates out of the way.	5	_____	_____ _____ _____
4. Placed the gait belt around the patient's waist. The belt should have been snug but not tight. Any excess belt should have been tucked in the back and out of the way.	15	_____	_____ _____ _____ _____

PERFORMANCE STANDARDS (cont.)	PTS	PTS EARNED (Pass/Fail)	COMMENTS
5. Standing directly in front of the patient, grasped the gait belt from underneath on either side. Gave the patient a signal to push up on the arm rests to a standing position.	15	_____	_____
6. Steadied the patient in the standing position. Checked the patient for signs of dizziness, pallor, and trouble balancing. If necessary, took the patient's pulse.	5	_____	_____
7. If the patient looked steady and wanted to walk, student moved to the patient's side. Kept one hand on the gait belt at all times	5	_____	_____
8. Placed one hand on the patient's arm. Made sure that your hand is on the gait belt with fingers underneath, palm upward, and elbow bent.	5	_____	_____
9. Starting with the same foot as the patient, kept in step with the patient. Allowed the patient to control the pace and asked how he was feeling during walking.	5	_____	_____
10. Documented the procedure, including the date, time, and duration of ambulation, patient's response, and instructions given. Initialed the documentation.	5	_____	_____

Modification: Two-person assist with ambulation

1. Performed the preceding steps 1–5.	15	_____	_____
2. Had an assistant stand on either side of the patient. Grasped the gait belt from underneath with one hand and placed the other hand on the patient's back for support.	5	_____	_____

PERFORMANCE STANDARDS (cont.)	PTS	PTS EARNED (Pass/Fail)	COMMENTS
3. During ambulation, a person should have been on either side of the patient. Both assistants should have been slightly behind the patient. As in a one-person assist, allowed the patient to set the pace.	5	_____	_____ _____ _____ _____
4. Documented the procedure as above.	5	_____	_____ _____

TOTAL POINTS	100		

DOCUMENTATION

COMMENTS

PROCEDURE 35-6 – ASSISTING A PATIENT IN AMBULATING WITH A WALKER

Name _____   Date _____   Score _____

Instructor _____

Task
Teach a patient how to ambulate with a walker independently and safely.

Conditions
Walker
Gait belt

Time: _____

Standard
In the time specified and within the scoring parameters determined by the instructor, the student will successfully assist a patient in ambulating with a walker.

Points assigned reflect importance of step to meeting the task

Important = 1 pt.
Essential = 5 pts.
Critical = 15 pts.

Automatic failure results if any of the **CRITICAL TASKS** are omitted or performed incorrectly.

(To use a pass/fail system, instructors can record "P" or "F" in the "points earned (pass/fail)" column.)

PERFORMANCE STANDARDS	PTS	PTS EARNED (Pass/Fail)	COMMENTS
1. Washed hands.	5	_____	_____
2. Introduced self and addressed the patient by name. Explained to the patient that she will be assisted in standing and walking with the aid of a walker.	5	_____	_____
3. Locked the brakes on the wheelchair, placed the patient's feet on the floor, and moved the foot plates out of the way.	5	_____	_____
4. Placed the gait belt around the patient's waist. The belt should have been snug but not tight. Any excess belt should have been tucked in the back and out of the way.	15	_____	_____

PERFORMANCE STANDARDS (cont.)	PTS	PTS EARNED (Pass/Fail)	COMMENTS
5. Checked the walker to be sure that rubber tips were secure on all legs. Checked the hand rests for damage or sharp edges that could injure the patient. Checked the joints of the walker.	15	_____	_____ _____ _____
6. Checked the patient's shoes to make sure that any ties were secure. Checked to see if the shoes had rubber soles and were not slippery.	15	_____	_____ _____ _____
7. Checked the height of the walker. It should have been level with the tip of the patient's femur, and the patient's elbows should have been flexed at approximately 30 degrees for comfort and support.	15	_____	_____ _____ _____ _____
8. Positioned the patient inside the walker.	5	_____	_____ _____
9. Had the patient lift the walker and place all four legs of the walker in front of her so that the back legs of the walker were even with her toes.	15	_____	_____ _____ _____
10. Instructed the patient to lean forward and transfer some of her weight to her arms while stepping with her stronger foot first, then to follow with a step with the weaker leg.	5	_____	_____ _____ _____ _____
11. Held on to the back of the gait belt and checked the patient for signs of fatigue. Was ready to catch the patient if she were to fall.	5	_____	_____ _____ _____
12. If the walker had rollers, the patient could simply roll the walker in front of her at a comfortable distance and pace. If the walker did not have rollers, instructed the patient to lift the walker slightly and place it in front of her. Allowed the patient to find a comfortable distance to move at each step.	5	_____	_____ _____ _____ _____ _____ _____

PERFORMANCE STANDARDS *(cont.)*	PTS	PTS EARNED (Pass/Fail)	COMMENTS
13. Documented the date, time, and duration of ambulation; the response of the patient; and instructions given to her. Initialed the report.	5	_____	_____ _____ _____

TOTAL POINTS	115		

DOCUMENTATION

COMMENTS

_____

_____

_____

_____

PROCEDURE 35-7 – ASSISTING A PATIENT IN AMBULATING WITH A CANE

Name _____   Date _____   Score _____

Instructor _____

Task
Teach a patient how to ambulate with a cane independently and safely.

Condition
Cane

Time: _____

Standard
In the time specified and within the scoring parameters determined by the instructor, the student will successfully assist a patient in ambulating with a cane.

Points assigned reflect importance of step to meeting the task

Important = 1 pt.
Essential = 5 pts.
Critical = 15 pts.

Automatic failure results if any of the **CRITICAL TASKS** are omitted or performed incorrectly.

(To use a pass/fail system, instructors can record "P" or "F" in the "points earned (pass/fail)" column.)

PERFORMANCE STANDARDS	PTS	PTS EARNED (Pass/Fail)	COMMENTS
1. Washed hands.	5	_____	_____
2. Introduced self and addressed the patient by name. Explained to the patient that he will be assisted in walking with a cane.	5	_____	_____
3. Checked the cane to make sure that the bottom had a rubber tip, the handle was not broken, and no sharp edges were present that could injure the patient.	5	_____	_____
4. Applied the gait belt snugly (but not too tightly) around the patient's waist. Tucked in any excess belt in the back of the belt.	15	_____	_____
5. Assisted the patient to a standing position. Looked for signs of dizziness.	15	_____	_____

PERFORMANCE STANDARDS (cont.)	PTS	PTS EARNED (Pass/Fail)	COMMENTS
6. Placed the cane in the patient's hand on the side of the strong leg. The cane should have been adjusted so that the handle was at hip joint level.	15	_____	_____ _____ _____
7. During weight-bearing movements, the patient's elbow should have been flexed at 20 to 30 degrees.	5	_____	_____ _____
8. Had the patient move the cane forward 10–18 inches ahead of him, depending on his ability and size.	5	_____	_____ _____
9. Had the patient move his weak leg forward while transferring his weight to the cane.	5	_____	_____ _____
10. Had the patient move his strong leg forward past the cane. Kept hand on the gait belt and looked for signs of fatigue or dizziness.	5	_____	_____ _____ _____
11. Followed along behind the patient on his weak side. Allowed the patient to set the pace.	5	_____	_____ _____
12. Documented the date, time, duration of ambulation; patient's response; and instructions given. Initialed the report.	5	_____	_____ _____ _____

TOTAL POINTS	90		

DOCUMENTATION

COMMENTS

PROCEDURE 35-8 – ASSISTING A PATIENT IN AMBULATING WITH CRUTCHES

Name _____   Date _____   Score _____

Instructor _____

Task
Teach a patient how to ambulate with crutches independently and safely.

Condition
Crutches

Time: _____

Standard
In the time specified and within the scoring parameters determined by the instructor, the student will successfully assist a patient in ambulating with crutches.

Points assigned reflect importance of step to meeting the task

Important = 1 pt.
Essential = 5 pts.
Critical = 15 pts.

Automatic failure results if any of the **CRITICAL TASKS** are omitted or performed incorrectly.

(To use a pass/fail system, instructors can record "P" or "F" in the "points earned (pass/fail)" column.)

PERFORMANCE STANDARDS	PTS	PTS EARNED (Pass/Fail)	COMMENTS
1. Washed hands.	5	_____	_____
2. Introduced self and addressed the patient by name. Explained to the patient that she will be assisted in walking with crutches.	5	_____	_____
3. Assembled and fit the axillary crutches to the patient. Made sure that the joints of the crutches were secure; the rubber tips were on the ends, axillary pads, and hand rests; and the hand rests were in good shape (for example, no tears, missing pieces, or cracks in the wood).	5	_____	_____
4. Applied the gait belt and assisted the patient to stand; placed the crutches under her armpits.	15	_____	_____

PERFORMANCE STANDARDS (cont.)	PTS	PTS EARNED (Pass/Fail)	COMMENTS
5. Instructed the patient to carry her weight completely on her hands and not on her armpits.	5	_____	
6. Had the patient put all of her weight on the strong leg and bend her weak leg slightly so it would not drag on the floor.	5	_____	
7. Assisted the patient with the appropriate gait pattern.	5	_____	
8. Documented the date, time, duration of ambulation, and instructions given. Initialled the report.	5	_____	

Non-weight-bearing to injured leg (two crutches)

	PTS	PTS EARNED	COMMENTS
1. Instructed the patient to transfer all her weight to her hands and to step with the strong leg.	5	_____	
2. Told her to bring the crutches forward and then to swing her injured leg through without putting any weight on the injured leg. Had her repeat these steps.	5	_____	

Weight-bearing to injured leg with support of crutches (2 crutches)

	PTS	PTS EARNED	COMMENTS
1. Told the patient to transfer all her weight to her hands and to step with her strong leg. Instructed her to use the crutches and to step with her injured leg at the same time. Explained that the patient could put some weight on her injured leg, but only when she had transferred some of the weight to her hands. Asked her to repeat the steps.	5	_____	

PERFORMANCE STANDARDS *(cont.)*	PTS	PTS EARNED (Pass/Fail)	COMMENTS

Weight-bearing to injured leg with support of one crutch

	PTS	PTS EARNED	COMMENTS
1. Explained to the patient that one crutch could be used on her strong side to assist her weak side.	5	_____	_____ _____
2. Instructed the patient to step with her strong leg and then to move the weak leg and the crutch forward at the same time.	5	_____	_____ _____ _____
3. Told the patient to gauge the amount of weight to put on her weak leg according to her comfort level.	5	_____	_____ _____ _____

TOTAL POINTS	80		

DOCUMENTATION

COMMENTS

PROCEDURE 35-9 – ASSISTING WITH FIBERGLASS CAST APPLICATION

Name _____   Date _____   Score _____

                                          Instructor _____

Task
Assist the physician in cast application.

Conditions
Fiberglass casting material
Basin of warm water
Stockinette
Webril padding rolls
Bandage scissors
Rubber gloves
Sponge rubber (for padding)

Time: _____

Standard
In the time specified and within the scoring parameters determined by the instructor, the student will successfully assist with fiberglass cast application.

Points assigned reflect importance of step to meeting the task

Important = 1 pt.
Essential = 5 pts.
Critical = 15 pts.

Automatic failure results if any of the **CRITICAL TASKS** are omitted or performed incorrectly.

(To use a pass/fail system, instructors can record "P" or "F" in the "points earned (pass/fail)" column.)

PERFORMANCE STANDARDS	PTS	PTS EARNED (Pass/Fail)	COMMENTS
1. Washed hands.	5	_____	_____
2. Explained the procedure to the patient. Told him that the fiberglass cast will feel wet and cool as it is applied and that it dries and hardens quickly. Explained that it will be completely hardened and will protect the body part within 30 minutes. Answered any questions about the procedure or the patient's injury.	5	_____	_____
3. Prepared the stockinette by cutting to a length appropriate for the cast. Assisted the physician in placing the stockinette directly on the skin under the cast.	15	_____	_____
4. Assisted the physician in wrapping the cast padding (Webril) around the stockinette.	15	_____	_____

PERFORMANCE STANDARDS (cont.)	PTS	PTS EARNED (Pass/Fail)	COMMENTS
5. Assisted the physician as required.	5	_____	_____ _____
6. Minimized patient discomfort by supporting the affected area.	1	_____	_____ _____ _____

TOTAL POINTS	46		

DOCUMENTATION

COMMENTS

_____

_____

_____

_____

PROCEDURE 35-10 – ASSISTING WITH CAST REMOVAL

Name _____   Date _____   Score _____

Instructor _____

Task
Assist the physician in the removal of a cast.

Conditions
Cast cutter
Cast spreader
Bandage scissors
Bag or container for disposing of cast materials
Basin, soap, and water

Time: _____

Standard
In the time specified and within the scoring parameters determined by the instructor, the student will successfully assist with cast removal.

Points assigned reflect importance of step to meeting the task

Important = 1 pt.
Essential = 5 pts.
Critical = 15 pts.

Automatic failure results if any of the **CRITICAL TASKS** are omitted or performed incorrectly.

(To use a pass/fail system, instructors can record "P" or "F" in the "points earned (pass/fail)" column.)

PERFORMANCE STANDARDS	PTS	PTS EARNED (Pass/Fail)	COMMENTS
1. Washed hands.	5	_____	_____
2. Explained the procedure to the patient. Told him that the cutter vibrates but does not spin. Explained to the patient that he may feel some pressure and warmth but his skin would not be cut by the cast cutter.	5	_____	_____
3. Told the patient that when he sees the limb without the cast, it will appear small and the color may be gray. Reassured the patient that color and muscle tone will improve with therapy and exercise.	5	_____	_____
4. After the procedure, gave the patient written instructions and answered any questions.	5	_____	_____

PERFORMANCE STANDARDS (cont.)	PTS	PTS EARNED (Pass/Fail)	COMMENTS
5. Gently washed the extremity with soap and water and applied skin lotion.	1	_____	_____ _____
6. Cleaned the equipment.	1	_____	_____
7. Washed hands.	5	_____	_____
8. Documented cast removal and appearance of body part. Recorded that written instructions were given to the patient.	5	_____	_____ _____ _____

TOTAL POINTS	32		

DOCUMENTATION

COMMENTS

PROCEDURE 35-11 – APPLYING A TRIANGULAR ARM SLING

Name _____   Date _____   Score _____

                                          Instructor _____

Task
Apply a triangular arm sling.

Condition
Sling

Time: _____

Standard
In the time specified and within the scoring parameters determined by the instructor, the student will successfully assist with triangular arm sling application.

Points assigned reflect importance of step to meeting the task

Important = 1 pt.
Essential = 5 pts.
Critical = 15 pts.

Automatic failure results if any of the **CRITICAL TASKS** are omitted or performed incorrectly.

(To use a pass/fail system, instructors can record "P" or "F" in the "points earned (pass/fail)" column.)

PERFORMANCE STANDARDS	PTS	PTS EARNED (Pass/Fail)	COMMENTS
1. Washed hands.	5	_____	_____
2. Introduced self and addressed the patient by name.	1	_____	_____ _____
3. Placed the patient's elbow in a 90-degree position against her chest. Instructed patient that she could hold her injured arm with her opposite hand.	15	_____	_____ _____ _____ _____
4. Placed one point of the triangle at the patient's good shoulder and one point toward the affected elbow.	15	_____	_____ _____ _____
5. Slid the sling under the injured arm. Asked the patient to steady the injured arm with her other hand. Looked for signs of pain and discomfort.	15	_____	_____ _____ _____ _____

PERFORMANCE STANDARDS (cont.)	PTS	PTS EARNED (Pass/Fail)	COMMENTS
6. Pulled the bottom of the triangle up and around the injured arm next to the neck.	15	_____	_____ _____
7. Tied the ends of the sling at the side of the neck.	5	_____	_____ _____
8. Made sure that the patient held her injured arm at approximately 90 degrees	15	_____	_____ _____
9. Used a safety pin to secure the elbow end of the sling.	5	_____	_____ _____
10. Washed hands and documented the procedure.	5	_____	_____ _____

TOTAL POINTS	96		

DOCUMENTATION

COMMENTS

_____

_____

_____

_____

PROCEDURE 35-12 – ADMINISTERING ULTRASOUND

Name _____   Date _____   Score _____

Instructor _____

Task
Administer an ultrasound to a body area of a patient.

Conditions
Ultrasound
Aqueous-based gel

Time: _____

Standard
In the time specified and within the scoring parameters determined by the instructor, the student will successfully administer an ultrasound.

Points assigned reflect importance of step to meeting the task

Important = 1 pt.
Essential = 5 pts.
Critical = 15 pts.

Automatic failure results if any of the **CRITICAL TASKS** are omitted or performed incorrectly.

(To use a pass/fail system, instructors can record "P" or "F" in the "points earned (pass/fail)" column.)

PERFORMANCE STANDARDS	PTS	PTS EARNED (Pass/Fail)	COMMENTS
1. Washed hands.	5	_____	_____
2. Introduced self and addressed the patient by name.	1	_____	_____
3. Explained the procedure to the patient.	1	_____	_____
4. Asked the patient if she has any metal inside her body, such as surgical pins or screws. Ultrasound *cannot* be performed over metal.	15	_____	_____
5. Applied gel to the skin of the affected area. The gel should be kept at room temperature.	5	_____	_____
6. Touched the wand of the ultrasound to the gel on the skin. Moved the wand around the entire area to be examined.	15	_____	_____

PERFORMANCE STANDARDS (cont.)	PTS	PTS EARNED (Pass/Fail)	COMMENTS
7. Turned the timer on the machine to the appropriate time. Slowly turned up the intensity of the ultrasound from zero and asked the patient if she felt warmth or tingling. Turned the machine up to the prescribed wattage.	15	_____	
8. While turning up the machine, always kept the wand moving, as stopping the wand can cause burning inside the tissues.	5	_____	
9. When the time expired, removed the wand and cleaned it with a dry cloth or towel. Cleaned the patient's skin with a separate dry cloth or towel.	15	_____	
10. Washed hands and documented the procedure.	5	_____	

TOTAL POINTS	82		

DOCUMENTATION

COMMENTS

PROCEDURE 35-13 – TEACHING A PATIENT TO USE A TENS UNIT

Name _____   Date _____   Score _____

                                      Instructor _____

Task

Apply a transcutaneous electrical nerve stimulation (TENS) unit to a patient and teach him how to apply and regulate the TENS unit for home use.

Conditions

TENS unit
Disposable sticky pads

Time: _____

Standard

In the time specified and within the scoring parameters determined by the instructor, the student will successfully teach a patient to use a TENS unit.

Points assigned reflect importance of step to meeting the task

Important = 1 pt.
Essential = 5 pts.
Critical = 15 pts.

Automatic failure results if any of the **CRITICAL TASKS** are omitted or performed incorrectly.

(To use a pass/fail system, instructors can record "P" or "F" in the "points earned (pass/fail)" column.)

PERFORMANCE STANDARDS	PTS	PTS EARNED (Pass/Fail)	COMMENTS
1. Washed hands.	5	_____	_____
2. Introduced self and addressed the patient by name.	1	_____	_____ _____
3. Washed the patient's skin with alcohol to remove any lotion that may have caused the pads to fail to adhere to the skin.	1	_____	_____ _____ _____ _____
4. Made sure that the sticky pads were in good condition and that wires were safe (without exposed, frayed ends).	5	_____	_____ _____ _____
5. Applied the sticky pads to the patient's skin on designated body areas, as directed by the physician,	15	_____	_____ _____ _____
6. Made sure that the wires that connected to the TENS unit were secure. Turned on the TENS unit slowly.	15	_____	_____ _____ _____

PERFORMANCE STANDARDS (cont.)	PTS	PTS EARNED (Pass/Fail)	COMMENTS
7. Asked the patient to report first feeling of stimulation. Turned the machine up to a comfortable tolerance.	15	_____	_____ _____ _____
8. Explained to the patient that tolerance would increase and that he could turn up the unit as needed.	5	_____	_____ _____
9. Showed the patient that he could wear the unit on his belt or clip it to his pocket and he could turn it on or off at any time.	5	_____	_____ _____ _____
10. Answered any questions, washed hands, and documented the procedure.	5	_____	_____ _____

TOTAL POINTS	72		

DOCUMENTATION

COMMENTS

Student Activity Manual to Accompany The Professional Medical Assistant *541*

Ophthalmology and Otolaryngology

Key Term Review   *Define the following key terms:*

1.   visual acuity   _____

_____

2.   presbyopia   _____

_____

3.   cerumen   _____

_____

4.   tinnitus   _____

_____

5.   olfaction   _____

_____

6.   Ménière disease   _____

_____

7.   cataract   _____

_____

8.   hyperopia   _____

_____

9.   glaucoma   _____

_____

10.   astigmatism   _____

_____

11.   ophthalmoscope   _____

_____

Key Term Review *cont.*

12.   audiometer   _____

13.   gestation   _____

14.   myopia   _____

15.   conjunctivitis   _____

16.   accommodation   _____

17.   equilibrium   _____

18.   otoscope   _____

19.   otitis   _____

20.   sinusitis   _____

Review Questions

1. Explain the different types of specialists that deal with disorders of the eye, ear, nose, and throat.

_____

_____

_____

_____

2. What are some tests/procedures associated with the eye that the medical assistant may perform?

_____

_____

_____

_____

3. What are the structures that compose the external ear?

_____

_____

_____

_____

4. List the components of the middle ear.

_____

_____

_____

_____

5. What are the structures of the inner ear?

_____

_____

_____

_____

6. What are some factors that can affect equilibrium?

_____

_____

_____

_____

7. What are some tests/procedures associated with the ear that a medical assistant may perform?

_____

_____

_____

_____

8. What are some symptoms of Ménière disease?

_____

_____

_____

_____

9. List some underlying medical conditions that can lead to retinopathy.

_____

_____

_____

_____

10. What distance should the patient stand at when performing a distance visual acuity test?

_____

_____

_____

_____

11. On which line on the Snellen eye chart should the medical assistant begin the exam?

_____

_____

_____

_____

12. When testing a patient for near visual acuity, what distance should the patient hold the Jaeger card?

_____

_____

_____

_____

Medical Terminology and Abbreviation Review

Match the medical term with its definition:

Medical term

1. blepharoptosis _____

2. exotropia _____

3. acoustic _____

4. corneous _____

5. phacocele _____

6. rhinoplasty _____

7. audiometry _____

8. presbycusis _____

9. myringoplasty _____

10. keratocele _____

11. scleromalacia _____

12. oculomycosis _____

13. otorrhea _____

14. hyperopia _____

15. retinopathy _____

Definition

a. pertaining to hearing

b. measurement of hearing

c. drooping eyelids

d. pertaining to the cornea

e. progressive hearing loss due to aging

f. hernia of the cornea

g. surgical repair of the tympanic membrane

h. fungal infection of the eye

i. farsightedness

j. discharge from the ear

k. surgical fixation of the nose

l. any disorder of the retina

m. softening of the sclera

n. marked turning inward of the eyes

o. displacement of the crystalline lens into the chamber of the eye

Define the following abbreviations:

1. AD: _____

2. PERRLA: _____

3. BOM: _____

4. EOM: _____

5. OD: _____

6. HEENT: _____

7. OU: _____

8. ROP: _____

9. AU: _____

10. VA: _____

11. EAC: _____

12. TM: _____

13. OS: _____

14. IOP: _____

15. AS: _____

16. T&A: _____

17. SOM: _____

18. RK: _____

19. TMJ: _____

20. ARMD: _____

Disease/Condition Review

Match the disease/condition with its definition:

Disease/condition

1. otitis externa _____

2. macular degeneration _____

3. presbyopia _____

4. otitis media _____

5. vertigo _____

6. glaucoma _____

7. photophobia _____

8. rhinitis _____

9. hyperopia _____

10. exophthalmos _____

11. tinnitus _____

12. impetigo _____

Definition

a. protrusion of one or both eyeballs

b. sensation of moving around in space or having objects move around the person

c. unusual intolerance to light

d. increased intraocular pressure on the optic nerve

e. a defect in vision in which parallel rays come into focus behind the retina, causing a person to see distinctly only at long distance

f. subjective ringing, buzzing, or hissing in the ear

g. seasonal, year-round allergic inflammation of the nasal mucosa

h. bacterial skin infection, usually caused by staphylococcus or streptococcus

i. changes in pigmented cells of retina and macula, leading to fine-vision loss

j. infection or inflammation of the external auditory canal

k. presence of fluid in the middle ear

l. permanent loss of accommodation of crystalline lens of the eye

Anatomy Identification

1. Label the structures of the eye in Figure 36-1.

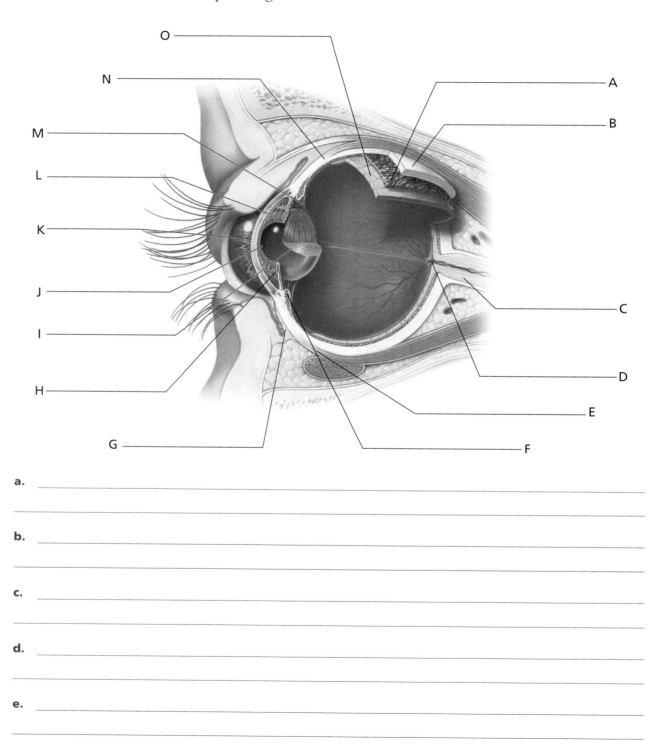

a. _____

_____

b. _____

_____

c. _____

_____

d. _____

_____

e. _____

_____

f. _____

_____

g. _____

_____

h. _____

_____

i. _____

_____

j. _____

_____

k. _____

_____

l. _____

_____

m. _____

_____

n. _____

_____

o. _____

_____

2. Label the structures of the ear in Figure 36-2.

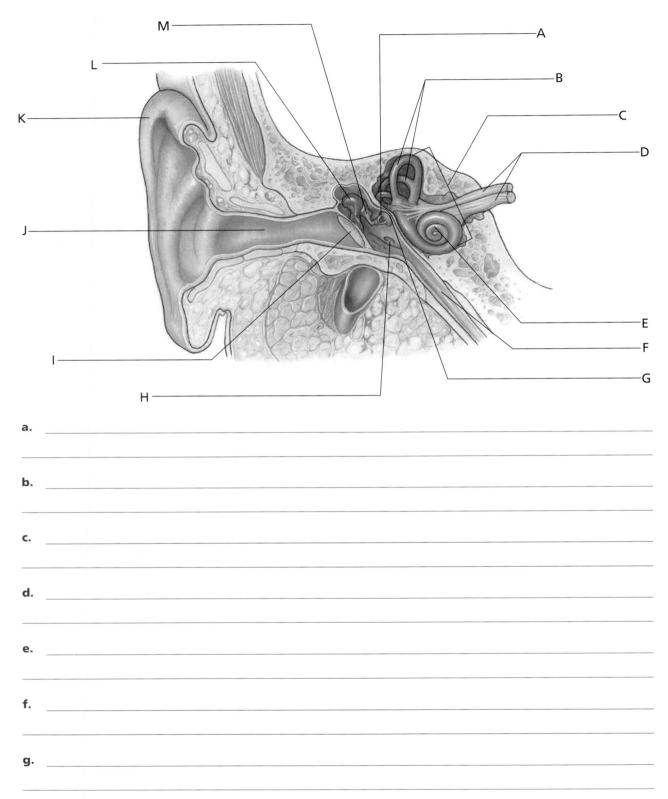

a. _____

b. _____

c. _____

d. _____

e. _____

f. _____

g. _____

Student Activity Manual to Accompany The Professional Medical Assistant   © copyright 2009 F.A. Davis Company

h. _____

_____

i. _____

_____

j. _____

_____

k. _____

_____

l. _____

_____

m. _____

_____

3. Label the structures of the nose and throat in Figure 36-3.

O

A

B

C

N

D

M

L

E

K

J

F

I

G

H

a. _____

b. _____

c. _____

d. _____

e. _____

f. _____

g. _____

_____

h. _____

_____

i. _____

_____

j. _____

_____

k. _____

_____

l. _____

_____

m. _____

_____

n. _____

_____

o. _____

_____

Critical Thinking

1. As a medical assistant who works for an ophthalmology practice, you have been asked by the local senior citizen's center to speak at their monthly luncheon information sessions on the differences between cataracts, glaucoma, and macular degeneration. Research all three diseases and develop a patient information fact sheet on your research.

   _____

   _____

   _____

   _____

2. Conjunctivitis can be caused by bacteria or a virus. Each type of infection may have different symptoms. Research both types of conjunctivitis and create a fact sheet detailing the various symptoms for bacterial versus viral conjunctivitis.

   _____

   _____

   _____

   _____

Teamwork Exercises

1. Divide into pairs. Take turns testing each other's near and distance vision. Use the procedures in the textbook to make sure you are following the proper steps. After documenting your results, compare them with your partner's.

PROCEDURE 36-1 – MEASURING DISTANCE AND VISUAL ACUITY USING THE SNELLEN CHART

Name _____   Date _____   Score _____

Instructor _____

Task
Accurately measure visual acuity using a Snellen eye chart. Document the procedure in the patient's medical record.

Conditions
Snellen eye chart
Eye occluder
Floor mark at 20 feet from the eye chart
Patient's medical record
Pen

Time: _____

Standard
In the time specified and within the scoring parameters determined by the instructor, the student will accurately measure visual acuity using a Snellen eye chart.

Points assigned reflect importance of step to meeting the task

> Important = 1 pt.
> Essential = 5 pts.
> Critical = 15 pts.

Automatic failure results if any of the **CRITICAL TASKS** are omitted or performed incorrectly.

(To use a pass/fail system, instructors can record "P" or "F" in the "points earned (pass/fail)" column.)

PERFORMANCE STANDARDS	PTS	PTS EARNED (Pass/Fail)	COMMENTS
1. Washed hands.	5	_____	_____
2. Ensured that the examination room was well lit.	1	_____	_____
3. Assembled equipment and supplies, including sanitizing the occluder and allowing it to dry completely.	5	_____	_____
4. Introduced self and addressed the patient by name.	1	_____	_____
5. Explained the procedure to the patient and answered any questions she had. Told the patient that she would be asked to read lines of letters, objects, or a rotating *E*. Explained to the patient that she should not squint during the examination. Made sure that the patient did not have an opportunity to memorize the chart.	15	_____	_____

PERFORMANCE STANDARDS (cont.)	PTS	PTS EARNED (Pass/Fail)	COMMENTS
6. Asked the patient if she was wearing contact lenses and observed for eyeglasses. Confirmed with the physician if the patient should have kept corrective eyewear on during the examination.	15	_____	_____
7. Asked the patient to stand (or sit if standing is difficult) on the floor mark, 20 feet from the Snellen chart.	15	_____	_____
8. Selected the appropriate Snellen chart for the patient. Used an object chart for preschoolers. Used a rotating *E* chart for adult patients who speak a foreign language. Was sure to explain the procedure through an interpreter or through hand motions, if necessary. Confirmed that the patient understood the procedure.	15	_____	_____
9. Positioned the center of the Snellen eye chart at the patient's eye level so that the patient didn't need to look up or down to see the chart. Stood to the side of the chart during the procedure so as not to obstruct the patient's view of the chart.	15	_____	_____
10. Asked the patient to cover her left eye with the occluder and to keep her left eye open. Assisted preschoolers with difficulty identifying left and right as needed.	5	_____	_____
11. Measured the visual acuity of the right eye.	1	_____	_____
12. Asked the patient to identify each letter, object, or direction of the *E* verbally or with a hand motion (whichever is preferred by the patient) as the student pointed to it. Started at the 20/70 line.	15	_____	_____

PERFORMANCE STANDARDS (cont.)	PTS	PTS EARNED (Pass/Fail)	COMMENTS
13. Proceeded up or down the chart as necessary.	5	_____	_____
14. If the patient was able to read the 20/70 line, proceeded down the chart, asking her to read the 20/50 line, 20/40, 20/30, 20/20, and further if possible.	5	_____	_____
15. If the patient was unable to read the 20/70 line, proceeded up the chart to the 20/100 line. If the patient was unable to read this line, asked her to read the 20/200 line.	5	_____	_____
16. Charted the results of the right eye. Recorded the smallest line that the patient could read with one or no errors.	5	_____	_____
17. Repeated the procedure for the left eye. Asked the patient to place the occluder in front of her right eye. Reminded the patient to keep her right eye open.	15	_____	_____

TOTAL POINTS	143		

DOCUMENTATION

COMMENTS

PROCEDURE 36-2 – MEASURING NEAR VISUAL ACUITY

Name _____   Date _____   Score _____

                                          Instructor _____

Task
Accurately measure near visual acuity using the Jaeger near-vision acuity card. Document the procedure in the patient's medical record.

Conditions
Jaeger card
Eye occluder
18-inch ruler or tape
Patient's medical record
Pen

Time: _____

Standard
In the time specified and within the scoring parameters determined by the instructor, the student will accurately measure near visual acuity.

Points assigned reflect importance of step to meeting the task

Important = 1 pt.
Essential = 5 pts.
Critical = 15 pts.

Automatic failure results if any of the **CRITICAL TASKS** are omitted or performed incorrectly.

(To use a pass/fail system, instructors can record "P" or "F" in the "points earned (pass/fail)" column.)

PERFORMANCE STANDARDS	PTS	PTS EARNED (Pass/Fail)	COMMENTS
1. Made sure the examination room was well lit and washed hands.	1	_____	_____
2. Assembled the equipment and supplies. Sanitized the occluder and allowed it to dry completely.	1	_____	_____
3. Introduced self and addressed the patient by name.	1	_____	_____
4. Explained the procedure to the patient and answered any questions he had.	1	_____	_____
5. Had the patient sit in a comfortable position.	1	_____	_____
6. Handed the patient the Jaeger card. Asked him to hold the card 14–16 inches away from his eyes and measured the distance.	15	_____	_____

PERFORMANCE STANDARDS (cont.)	PTS	PTS EARNED (Pass/Fail)	COMMENTS
7. Asked the patient to cover his left eye with the occluder. Instructed him not to close his left eye.	5	_____	_____ _____
8. Asked the patient to read the paragraphs on the card out loud. The patient should have started reading at the top of the card (largest print) and continued reading until he could not read the smaller print.	15	_____	_____ _____ _____ _____
9. Recorded the results of the right eye in the medical record.	5	_____	_____ _____
10. Asked the patient to cover his right eye with the occluder and repeated the test for the left eye.	15	_____	_____ _____
11. Recorded the results of the left eye in the medical record.	5	_____	_____ _____

TOTAL POINTS	65		

DOCUMENTATION

COMMENTS

PROCEDURE 36-3 – MEASURING VISUAL ACUITY USING THE ISHIHARA COLOR VISION TEST

Name _____

Date _____ Score _____

Instructor _____

Task
Accurately measure color visual acuity using the Ishihara color vision test. Document the procedure in the patient's medical record.

Conditions
Ishihara color plate book
Cotton swab
Watch with second hand
Patient's medical record
Pen

Time: _____

Standard
In the time specified and within the scoring parameters determined by the instructor, the student will accurately measure visual acuity using the Ishihara color vision test.

Points assigned reflect importance of step to meeting the task

Important = 1 pt.
Essential = 5 pts.
Critical = 15 pts.

Automatic failure results if any of the **CRITICAL TASKS** are omitted or performed incorrectly.

(To use a pass/fail system, instructors can record "P" or "F" in the "points earned (pass/fail)" column.)

PERFORMANCE STANDARDS	PTS	PTS EARNED (Pass/Fail)	COMMENTS
1. Washed hands and ensured that the examination room was well lit with natural light if possible.	5	_____	
2. Assembled the equipment and supplies.	1	_____	
3. Introduced self and addressed the patient by name.	1	_____	
4. Explained the procedure to the patient	1	_____	
5. Used the first plate in the book to explain the procedure to the patient. Told the patient that he would have 3 seconds to identify numbers verbally or to trace a winding path formed by the colored dots on the card. The patient should have kept both eyes open during the procedure.	15	_____	

	PTS	PTS EARNED (Pass/Fail)	COMMENTS

6. Held the color plate 30 inches from the patient at a right angle to the patient's line of sight.　　15　　_____

7. Asked the patient to identify the number on the plate or, using a cotton-tipped swab, to trace the winding path. Sometimes required the patient to trace the number.　　15　　_____

8. Recorded the results of each plate on a piece of paper. After all 11 plates had been tested, recorded the results in the patient's medical record. Indicated the plates that the patient read incorrectly by recording the number of the plate with an X next to it. Alternatively, simply listed the numbers of the plates read incorrectly.　　15　　_____

TOTAL POINTS	68		

DOCUMENTATION

COMMENTS

PROCEDURE 36-4 – IRRIGATING THE EYE

Name _____   Date _____   Score _____

                                                  Instructor _____

Task
Irrigate the patient's affected eye to cleanse it of a foreign object, cleanse a discharge, cleanse chemicals, apply antiseptic, or apply heat.

Conditions
Sterile irrigation solution
Sterile bulb syringe (rubber)
Kidney-shaped basin to catch irrigation solution
Sterile cotton balls
Sterile gloves
Biohazardous waste container
Patient's medical record
Pen

Time: _____

Standard
In the time specified and within the scoring parameters determined by the instructor, the student will successfully irrigate the patient's eye.

Points assigned reflect importance of step to meeting the task

Important = 1 pt.
Essential = 5 pts.
Critical = 15 pts.

Automatic failure results if any of the **CRITICAL TASKS** are omitted or performed incorrectly.

(To use a pass/fail system, instructors can record "P" or "F" in the "points earned (pass/fail)" column.)

PERFORMANCE STANDARDS	PTS	PTS EARNED (Pass/Fail)	COMMENTS
1. Washed hands.	5	_____	_____
2. Assembled equipment and supplies. Used separate equipment if both eyes were to be irrigated.	5	_____	_____ _____
3. Introduced self and addressed the patient by name.	1	_____	_____ _____
4. Explained the procedure to the patient and answered any questions she had.	1	_____	_____ _____
5. Positioned the patient in the supine position.	1	_____	_____ _____
6. Checked the expiration date on the solution bottle.	15	_____	_____ _____
7. Checked the label for the right medication three times.	15	_____	_____

PERFORMANCE STANDARDS (cont.)	PTS	PTS EARNED (Pass/Fail)	COMMENTS
8. Warmed the solution to body temperature.	1	_____	_____
9. Tilted the patient's head toward the affected eye and placed a towel on the patient's shoulder.	15	_____	_____
10. Placed the basin next to the affected eye.	5	_____	_____
11. Put on sterile gloves.	5	_____	_____
12. Moistened two or three cotton balls with the irrigation solution and cleaned the eyelids and eyelashes of the affected eye from the inner to the outer canthus. Discarded the cotton ball after each wipe.	15	_____	_____
13. Exposed the lower conjunctiva by separating the eyelid with your index finger and thumb.	5	_____	_____
14. Asked the patient to stare at a fixed spot. Was sure to keep the eye open with fingers during irrigation, as the patient's reflex is to shut the eye.	1	_____	_____
15. Irrigated the affected eye with sterile solution by resting the bulb on the bridge of the patient's nose. Was careful not to touch the tip of the bulb syringe to any part of the patient's face.	15	_____	_____
16. Allowed the stream to flow from the inner canthus to the outer canthus.	15	_____	_____
17. After irrigation, dried the eyelid and eyelashes with sterile cotton balls.	1	_____	_____
18. Discarded supplies in a biohazardous waste container if discharge or exudate is present.	5	_____	_____
19. Removed your gloves.	1	_____	_____

PERFORMANCE STANDARDS (cont.)	PTS	PTS EARNED (Pass/Fail)	COMMENTS
20. Washed hands and documented the procedure.	5	_____	_____
21. Repeated the procedure on other eye if a bilateral procedure was indicated.	15	_____	_____

TOTAL POINTS	147		

DOCUMENTATION

COMMENTS

PROCEDURE 36-5 – INSTILLING EYEDROPS

Name _____ Date _____ Score _____

Instructor _____

Task
Instill eyedrops to treat eye infections, soothe irritation, anesthetize the eye, or dilate pupils.

Conditions
Sterile eyedropper
Sterile ophthalmic medication as ordered by the
  physician
Sterile cotton balls
Sterile gloves
Biohazardous waste container
Patient's medical record
Pen

Time: _____

Standard
In the time specified and within the scoring parameters determined by the instructor, the student will successfully instill eyedrops.

Points assigned reflect importance of step to meeting the task

Important = 1 pt.
Essential = 5 pts.
Critical = 15 pts.

Automatic failure results if any of the **CRITICAL TASKS** are omitted or performed incorrectly.

(To use a pass/fail system, instructors can record "P" or "F" in the "points earned (pass/fail)" column.)

PERFORMANCE STANDARDS	PTS	PTS EARNED (Pass/Fail)	COMMENTS
1. Washed hands.	5	_____	_____
2. Assembled the necessary equipment and supplies.	1	_____	_____
3. Introduced self and addressed the patient by name.	1	_____	_____
4. Explained the procedure to the patient and answered any questions that she had. Told the patient that the instillation may temporarily blur her vision. If the medication was to dilate the pupil for examination, explained to the patient that the eye would be very sensitive to light.	5	_____	_____
5. Checked the medication label carefully against the physician's orders. Noted the name of the medication and the expiration date. Checked the label three times.	15	_____	_____

PERFORMANCE STANDARDS (cont.)	PTS	PTS EARNED (Pass/Fail)	COMMENTS
6. Positioned the patient in a sitting or supine position.	1	_____	_____ _____
7. Asked the patient to stare at a fixed spot on the ceiling. Was careful to keep the eye open with your fingers during instillation, as the patient's reflex is to shut the eye.	5	_____	_____ _____ _____ _____ _____
8. Held the eye open by placing a tissue under the eye and gently pulling down on the skin below the eye.	15	_____	_____ _____ _____
9. Placed the number of drops ordered in the lower conjunctival sac or a thin line of ointment in the lower surface of the eyelid. Was careful not to touch the tip of the eyedropper to any portion of the patient's eye.	15	_____	_____ _____ _____ _____ _____ _____
10. Asked the patient to close her eye and roll her eyeball.	5	_____	_____ _____
11. Documented the procedure in the patient's chart.	5	_____	_____ _____

TOTAL POINTS	72		

DOCUMENTATION

_____

COMMENTS

_____
_____
_____
_____
_____

PROCEDURE 36-6 – TESTING HEARING USING AN AUDIOMETER

Name _____   Date _____   Score _____

Instructor _____

Task
Use an audiometer to test a patient's hearing.

Conditions
Audiometer
Headphones
Enclosed area (such as a small room or cubicle)

Time: _____

Standard
In the time specified and within the scoring parameters determined by the instructor, the student will successfully test hearing using an audiometer.

Points assigned reflect importance of step to meeting the task

Important = 1 pt.
Essential = 5 pts.
Critical = 15 pts.

Automatic failure results if any of the **CRITICAL TASKS** are omitted or performed incorrectly.

(To use a pass/fail system, instructors can record "P" or "F" in the "points earned (pass/fail)" column.)

PERFORMANCE STANDARDS	PTS	PTS EARNED (Pass/Fail)	COMMENTS
1. Washed hands.	5	_____	_____
2. Assembled the equipment and supplies.	1	_____	_____ _____
3. Introduced self and addressed the patient by name.	1	_____	_____ _____
4. Explained the procedure to the patient and established a signal for the patient to give when she hears the tone (such as holding up a hand or finger on the same side as she hears the tone).	15	_____	_____ _____ _____ _____ _____
5. Made sure that the patient was comfortably seated and placed headphones over one of her ears.	5	_____	_____ _____ _____

PERFORMANCE STANDARDS (cont.)	PTS	PTS EARNED (Pass/Fail)	COMMENTS
6. Began with a low frequency and watched patient for an indication that she heard the sound. Pushed the button to record the results.	15	_____	_____ _____ _____
7. Gradually increased frequency until the test for the first ear was complete.	5	_____	_____ _____
8. Repeated the procedure for the other ear.	15	_____	_____ _____
9. Documented results in the patient's medical record.	5	_____	_____
10. Cleaned the equipment as directed by manufacturer's instructions.	1	_____	_____ _____

TOTAL POINTS	68		

DOCUMENTATION

COMMENTS

_____

_____

_____

_____

PROCEDURE 36-7 – IRRIGATING THE EAR

Name _____

Date _____   Score _____

Instructor _____

Task

Irrigate the patient's affected ear to relieve inflammation or cleanse it of cerumen, a foreign object, or discharge.

Conditions

Irrigation solution warmed to body temperature (98.6° F)
Ear syringe
Kidney-shaped basin to catch irrigation solution
Basin for warmed solution
Towel
Cotton balls
Gloves
Patient's medical record
Pen

Time: _____

Standard

In the time specified and within the scoring parameters determined by the instructor, the student will successfully irrigate the ear.

Points assigned reflect importance of step to meeting the task

Important = 1 pt.
Essential = 5 pts.
Critical = 15 pts.

Automatic failure results if any of the **CRITICAL TASKS** are omitted or performed incorrectly.

(To use a pass/fail system, instructors can record "P" or "F" in the "points earned (pass/fail)" column.)

PERFORMANCE STANDARDS	PTS	PTS EARNED (Pass/Fail)	COMMENTS
1. Washed hands.	5	_____	_____
2. Assembled the equipment and supplies.	1	_____	_____
3. Introduced self and addressed the patient by name.	1	_____	_____
4. Explained the procedure to the patient and informed him that he may experience minimal dizziness or discomfort during the procedure when the solution comes into contact with the tympanic membrane. Answered any questions that the patient had.	5	_____	_____
5. Checked the label of the solution three times and checked the expiration date.	15	_____	_____

PERFORMANCE STANDARDS (cont.)	PTS	PTS EARNED (Pass/Fail)	COMMENTS
6. Warmed the bottle of solution under running water. The solution should have been close to body temperature (98.6° F).	5	_____	_____
7. Poured the solution into a basin and filled the syringe with the warmed irrigation solution as prescribed by the physician. Used approximately 30–50 ml of solution at a time.	15	_____	_____
8. Positioned the patient in the sitting position, with his head tilted toward the affected ear.	1	_____	_____
9. Placed a towel on the patient's shoulder and the ear basin under the affected ear. Asked the patient to hold the basin in place.	1	_____	_____
10. Cleaned the outer ear with a wet cotton ball moistened with irrigation solution.	1	_____	_____
11. Gently pulled the auricle upward and backward to straighten the ear canal (downward and backward if the patient is 3 years old or younger).	15	_____	_____
12. Expelled air from the syringe and gently inserted the syringe tip into the affected ear. Was careful not to insert too deeply. Directed the solution upward toward the roof of the canal. Was careful to avoid occluding the external auditory canal.	15	_____	_____
13. Noted in the medical record any material that is irrigated, such as impacted cerumen, objects, dirt, and small particles of metal.	5	_____	_____
14. Refilled the syringe with more clean, warmed solution from the other basin.	5	_____	_____

PERFORMANCE STANDARDS (cont.)	PTS	PTS EARNED (Pass/Fail)	COMMENTS
15. Repeated the irrigation, allowing the solution to drain from the ear. Asked the patient how he felt. Stopped the procedure if the patient was too uncomfortable.	5	_____	_____
16. Dried the outer ear and visualized the canal with the otoscope to verify the procedure had removed the foreign body. If the foreign material was still in the canal, repeated the procedure.	5	_____	_____
17. After the procedure was complete, dried the patient's ear and face and removed the towel and basin. Had the patient lie on his affected side on the examination table. If performing a bilateral procedure, allowed the patient to rest before performing the second irrigation.	5	_____	_____
18. Gave cotton balls to the patient to wipe any further drainage. Asked the patient how he feels.	1	_____	_____
19. Disposed of supplies.	1	_____	_____
20. Washed hands.	5	_____	_____
21. Documented the procedure, noting the return and amount.	5	_____	_____
22. Provided post-care instructions to the patient. Was sure to tell the patient to call the office and speak to the physician if he feels pain or continued dizziness. Also emphasized to the patient that he should not insert a cotton applicator or any other object into the ear canal.	5	_____	_____

TOTAL POINTS	122		

DOCUMENTATION

COMMENTS

PROCEDURE 36-8 – INSTILLING EARDROPS

Name _____ Date _____ Score _____

Instructor _____

Task
Instill eardrops to soften impacted cerumen, fight infection locally with antibiotic drops, or administer analgesics to relieve pain.

Conditions
Otic medication as prescribed by the physician
Sterile ear dropper
Cotton balls
Gloves
Drape or paper towel
Patient's medical record
Pen

Time: _____

Standard
In the time specified and within the scoring parameters determined by the instructor, the student will successfully instill eardrops.

Points assigned reflect importance of step to meeting the task

Important = 1 pt.
Essential = 5 pts.
Critical = 15 pts.

Automatic failure results if any of the **CRITICAL TASKS** are omitted or performed incorrectly.

(To use a pass/fail system, instructors can record "P" or "F" in the "points earned (pass/fail)" column.)

PERFORMANCE STANDARDS	PTS	PTS EARNED (Pass/Fail)	COMMENTS
1. Washed hands.	5	_____	_____
2. Assembled equipment and supplies.	1	_____	_____
3. Introduced self and addressed the patient by name.	1	_____	_____
4. Explained the procedure to the patient.	1	_____	_____
5. Checked the label of the medication three times for correct medication and expiration date.	15	_____	_____
6. Warmed the eardrops under running warm water.	5	_____	_____
7. Positioned the patient to lie on her unaffected side or in a sitting position with her head tilted toward her unaffected ear.	15	_____	_____

PERFORMANCE STANDARDS (cont.)	PTS	PTS EARNED (Pass/Fail)	COMMENTS
8. Provided the patient with a paper towel or nonsterile drape for her shoulder.	1	_____	_____
9. Drew up the prescribed amount of medication into the sterile ear dropper.	5	_____	_____
10. Gently pulled the top of the auricle up and back (for adults) or pulled the earlobe down and back (for children ages 3 and under).	15	_____	_____
11. Squeezed the rubber bulb to instill the prescribed dose of medication into the affected ear.	15	_____	_____
12. Asked the patient to maintain the position for about 5 minutes after instillation.	5	_____	_____
13. If instructed by the physician, inserted a moistened cotton ball into the external ear canal for 15 minutes.	5	_____	_____
14. Washed hands.	5	_____	_____
15. Documented the procedure in the patient's medical record.	5	_____	_____
16. Repeated the procedure with the other ear if a bilateral procedure was ordered.	15	_____	_____
17. Taught the patient or caregiver how to instill the drops, stressing the importance of hand washing before and after instillation. As with eye-drops, made sure the patient understood that she should avoid touching the tip of the dropper to her ear or any object.	15	_____	_____

TOTAL POINTS	129		

DOCUMENTATION

COMMENTS

PROCEDURE 36-9 – OBTAINING A THROAT CULTURE

Name _____   Date _____   Score _____

Instructor _____

Task
Collect a throat or nasopharyngeal culture without contamination.

Conditions
Culturette kit
Laboratory requisition slip
Tongue depressor
Biohazardous waste container

Time: _____

Standard
In the time specified and within the scoring parameters determined by the instructor, the student will successfully obtain a throat culture.

Points assigned reflect importance of step to meeting the task

Important = 1 pt.
Essential = 5 pts.
Critical = 15 pts.

Automatic failure results if any of the **CRITICAL TASKS** are omitted or performed incorrectly.

(To use a pass/fail system, instructors can record "P" or "F" in the "points earned (pass/fail)" column.)

PERFORMANCE STANDARDS	PTS	PTS EARNED (Pass/Fail)	COMMENTS
1. Washed hands.	5	_____	_____
2. Assembled the equipment and supplies.	1	_____	_____
3. Introduced self and addressed the patient by name.	1	_____	_____
4. Explained the procedure to the patient.	1	_____	_____
5. Put on your gloves.	5	_____	_____
6. Positioned the patient facing a light source and asked the patient to open his mouth as wide as possible.	1	_____	_____
7. Asked the patient to say, "aaah."	5	_____	_____

PERFORMANCE STANDARDS (cont.)	PTS	PTS EARNED (Pass/Fail)	COMMENTS
8. Depressed the tongue and inserted a swab, rolling it firmly across the back of the throat. Took care not to contaminate the swab by touching the patient's teeth, lips, tongue, or inside of the cheek.	15	_____	
9. Inserted the swab into the plastic vial. Crushed the internal vial of the transport medium and made sure that the swab was saturated.	15	_____	
10. Placed the sample in a labeled mailing or transporting envelope and stapled it shut if necessary.	15	_____	
11. Washed hands.	5	_____	
12. Documented the procedure in the patient's medical record.	5	_____	

TOTAL POINTS	74		

DOCUMENTATION

COMMENTS

Nutrition

Key Term Review   *Define the following key terms:*

1.   metabolism   _____
                        _____

2.   glycemic index   _____

3.   fatty acid   _____

4.   lipid   _____

5.   glucose   _____

6.   calorie   _____

7.   vitamin   _____

8.   carbohydrate   _____

9.   undernutrition   _____

10.   nutrient   _____

11.   catabolism   _____
                        _____

Key Term Review *cont.*

12.   cholesterol   _____

                               _____

13.   dehydration   _____

                               _____

14.   mineral   _____

                               _____

15.   malnutrition   _____

                               _____

16.   overnutrition   _____

                               _____

17.   protein   _____

                               _____

18.   soluble fiber   _____

                               _____

19.   adenosine triphosphate   _____

                               _____

20.   emulsification   _____

                               _____

21.   insoluble fiber   _____

                               _____

Review Questions

1. What is a nutrient? What is the difference between an energy nutrient and a non-energy nutrient?

   _____

   _____

   _____

   _____

2. How is food energy measured?

   _____

   _____

   _____

   _____

3. What is a simple carbohydrate? List four simple carbohydrates.

   _____

   _____

   _____

   _____

4. What are some of the food sources of simple carbohydrates?

   _____

   _____

   _____

   _____

5. Define a complex carbohydrate. List three types of complex carbohydrates.

   _____

   _____

   _____

   _____

6. How is glycogen utilized by the body?

_____

_____

_____

_____

7. What are some of the food sources of complex carbohydrates?

_____

_____

_____

_____

8. Discuss the difference between soluble and insoluble fiber.

_____

_____

_____

_____

9. List four types of soluble fiber and give their food sources.

_____

_____

_____

_____

10. List four types of insoluble fiber and give their food sources.

_____

_____

_____

_____

11. Discuss the relationship between carbohydrates and a person's blood sugar.

_____

_____

_____

_____

12. What is the glycemic index? How is it used when determining a patient's diet?

_____

_____

_____

_____

13. What are proteins, and why are they important in the diet?

_____

_____

_____

_____

14. Discuss good sources of protein.

_____

_____

_____

_____

15. What is the effect of protein deficiency on the body?

_____

_____

_____

_____

16. What is a fatty acid? How are fatty acids classified?

_____

_____

_____

_____

17. What is the function of fatty acids in the body?

_____

_____

_____

_____

18. What is the most common form of fat in the diet and the major storage form?

_____

_____

_____

_____

19. What are some food sources of cholesterol?

_____

_____

_____

_____

20. Obesity is on the rise in the United States. Discuss some of the factors affecting obesity along with some solutions.

_____

_____

_____

_____

21. Discuss the importance of minerals in the body.

_____

_____

_____

_____

22. Give some food sources for the following minerals:

    a. phosphorus:

_____

_____

_____

_____

    b. iron:

_____

_____

_____

_____

c. magnesium:

_____

_____

_____

_____

d. calcium:

_____

_____

_____

_____

e. potassium:

_____

_____

_____

_____

f. zinc:

_____

_____

_____

_____

g. iodine:

_____

_____

_____

_____

23. Discuss the functions of water in the body.

_____

_____

_____

_____

24. For the following medical conditions, give some dietary patient teaching tips:

   a. diabetes:

      _____

      _____

      _____

      _____

   b. high blood pressure:

      _____

      _____

      _____

      _____

25. What are some of the concerns when advising adolescents on their diet?

   _____

   _____

   _____

   _____

26. What are some of the hazards of fad dieting?

   _____

   _____

   _____

   _____

27. Vitamins – sources and function. Fill in the blank areas of the vitamin table below.

Table 37-1

Vitamin	Function	Food Source
Biotin		
	Aids in the mineralization of bone	
		Spinach, broccoli, mushrooms, milk, yogurt
B_{12}		
		Mushrooms, avocado, broccoli, beef liver, whole grains
E		
B_6		
	Aids in the synthesis of blood	
	Coenzyme complex that helps to synthesize DNA	
K		
		Peas, corn, potatoes, peanut butter, shrimp, chicken, ham
A	Assists in energy metabolism	
	.	
C		

Critical Thinking

1. Stacey Jennings, a 16-year-old high school athlete, has just been diagnosed with a whey and gluten allergy. Her typical diet before the diagnosis included cheeseburgers, french fries, and pizza. This will be a major behavior modification for Stacey, and you are responsible for educating Stacey in choosing the proper food items as well as reading food labels. Discuss ways to alleviate some of Stacey's concerns as well as ways to maintain compliance with this new diet modification. Supply a list of food items, including snacks that Stacey can eat as well as those she has to stay away from.

   _____

   _____

   _____

   _____

2. Stanley Wronzek has just been diagnosed with hyperlipidemia. He is adamant about not wanting to go on statin drugs to lower his cholesterol. First, discuss with Stan the components of the lipid profile as well as the normal ranges for each test result. Next, discuss some diet and lifestyle modifications Stan will have to make to lower his cholesterol.

   _____

   _____

   _____

3. Janice Taylor, an overweight, diabetic patient, has just been diagnosed with hypertension and hyperlipidemia. What metabolic disorder does she most likely have? Discuss each condition with Janice and the importance of addressing and understanding each disorder and its effect on her body. Design a weight loss program for Janice.

   _____

   _____

   _____

4. The food pyramid has been recently modified. Discuss the changes made to the food pyramid and the reasons behind the changes.

_____

_____

_____

_____

5. You have a 6-year-old daughter in the local elementary school. When you attended your daughter's career day, when talking about the duties of a medical assistant, you mentioned that you do a lot of nutritional education with patients. The teacher and PTO have asked you to work with them in addressing some of the nutritional needs of the student body. Come up with some good ideas of promoting good eating habits and a way to implement fun activities for the students.

_____

_____

_____

_____

Teamwork Exercises

1. Divide into groups of two or three. Your group will select or your instructor will assign a fad diet for your group to research. Prepare a PowerPoint presentation or poster report on the diet. Provide the claims made by the diet and the specifics of the diet, including the type(s) of foods required. Your group should also provide their opinion of the diet as it relates to a person's health and ability to lose weight and keep it off.

2. Divide the class into three groups. Each group will be assigned a meal (breakfast, lunch, or dinner). Each group should develop at least four different healthy meals that would include proper amounts of carbohydrates, protein, calcium, and fiber. Calculate the amount of calories in your meals. Come together as a class and compare each meal. Combine the meals to see the total amount of calories for the day. (Alternately, the class can be divided into four groups, and the fourth group can work on two snacks for the day.)

Office Project

As a class, make a food pyramid poster that shows specific examples of foods within each group. If the medical assisting program has its own bulletin board, ask the program coordinator if your class can post the food pyramid on it, or find a bulletin board on your campus that would allow for the most students to see it.

Introduction to Pharmacology

Key Term Review   *Define the following key terms:*

1. contraindications

_____

_____

2. pharmacodynamics

_____

_____

3. anaphylaxis

_____

_____

4. toxicology

_____

_____

5. indication

_____

_____

6. administer

_____

_____

7. action

_____

_____

8. dispense

_____

_____

9. pharmacokinetics

_____

_____

10. therapeutic effect

_____

_____

11. prescribe

_____

_____

12. interaction

_____

_____

Key Term Review *cont.*

13. pharmacotherapeutics _____

_____

14. efficacy _____

_____

15. systemic effect _____

_____

16. dose _____

_____

17. tolerance _____

_____

18. allergy _____

_____

19. cumulative _____
medication action _____

20. over-the-counter _____

_____

Review Questions

1. Compare and contrast the DEA and the FDA.

_____

_____

_____

_____

2. List the five schedules of the Controlled Substance Act and give three drugs within each schedule.

_____

_____

_____

_____

3. List the four sources from which drugs are derived. List two drugs within each source.

_____

_____

_____

_____

4. Discuss the various drug references a medical assistant may use when looking for information on a certain drug.

_____

_____

_____

_____

5. Describe what happens to a drug from the time it enters the body until the time that it is excreted.

_____

_____

_____

_____

6. Differentiate between OTC and prescription drugs. Give three examples of each.

_____

_____

_____

_____

7. Explain the seven rights of medication administration.

_____

_____

_____

_____

8. Describe the various routes of drug administration.

_____

_____

_____

9. Discuss the medical reasons to use medications.

_____

_____

_____

_____

10. List three examples of solid medications.

_____

_____

_____

_____

11. List three examples of a liquid medication.

_____

_____

_____

_____

Matching

Match the drug with its classification:

Drug

1. heparin _____
2. Zithromax _____
3. estrogen _____
4. acyclovir _____
5. Zoloft _____
6. Xanax _____
7. norepinephrine _____
8. Flexeril _____

Classification

a. antianxiety

b. hormone

c. vasoconstrictor

d. skeletal muscle relaxant

e. antibiotic

f. nonsteroid anti-inflammatory

g. anesthetic

h. anticoagulant

9. naproxen _____

10. Xylocaine _____

i. antidepressant

j. antiviral

Match the drug with its corresponding type of name:

Drug

1. ibuprofen _____

2. Amoxil _____

3. lorazepam _____

4. acyclovir _____

5. acetylsalicylic acid _____

6. Prilosec _____

7. butanoic acid _____

8. Xylocaine _____

9. Ritalin _____

10. (chemical) _____

Name

a. Trade

b. Generic

c. Chemical

Critical Thinking

1. You are preparing an immunization injection for a 2-month-old baby. The baby's mother seems nervous and asks you about the effects these immunizations may have on the baby. How do you respond?

   _____

   _____

   _____

   _____

2. You are working at the front desk this week and are responsible for taking prescription refills orders. This morning a patient calls for a refill on her Synthroid. What questions do you ask her? After you get off the phone, what is your next step?

   _____

   _____

   _____

   _____

3. You're a medical assistant in a group practice and primarily work with Dr. Graves. One of Dr. Graves' patients, Jeff Dewhurst, has been in the office quite a few times during the past 3 months complaining of lower back pain. The doctor has been requesting that Jeff go for an MRI, to further help in the diagnosis of his back pain, but Jeff has refused and instead keeps calling for a refill of his Darvocet. Dr. Graves has made it clear that the medication will not be refilled until the MRI has been done. Today, you notice your fellow medical assistant, Tony, assisting Jeff to an exam room for Dr. Caletta. Tony sees a perplexed look on your face and asks what's the matter? You explain that you think Mr. Dewhurst may be addicted to pain killers. Tony has not taken a patient history yet on Mr. Dewhurst; how can you help Tony maximize his patient history taking of Mr. Dewhurst?

   _____

   _____

   _____

   _____

Teamwork Exercises

1. Divide into groups of two or three. Your instructor will give each group a different drug reference guide for the group to analyze for ease of use, comprehensiveness, and type of drug information. Write a review on your group's book and share with the class.

2. Divide into groups of two or three. Each group will make up note cards of drugs. On one side of the card, put a drug's trade name and on the other side, put the drug's generic name. Each team will quiz each other on the names of these drugs. If the class wants, they can give all of the cards to their instructor and the instructor can create a game for the class to play, and the team with the most drugs correct wins.

Office Project

Using the most current *Physician's Desk Reference*, research the list of medications and provide the following information: 1) description of medication, 2) condition(s) prescribed for, 3) adverse effects, and 4) contraindications.

List of Medications

1. Remicade

2. albuterol

3. Norvasc

4. Zyban

5. BuSpar

6. Suprax

7. Plavix

8. Clomid

9. Nexium

10. Flonase

Dosage Calculation and Medication Administration

Key Term Review

Define the following key terms:

1. capsule _____

   _____

2. syrup _____

   _____

3. apothecary _____

   _____

4. enteric coated _____

   _____

5. meniscus _____

   _____

6. metric _____

   _____

7. buccal _____

   _____

8. tablet _____

   _____

9. suspension _____

   _____

10. sublingual _____

    _____

Review Questions

1. Describe the seven rights of medication administration.

   _____

   _____

   _____

   _____

2. Explain the importance of strictly adhering to the seven rights of administration.

   _____

   _____

   _____

   _____

3. What factors go into choosing the appropriate route of medication administration?

   _____

   _____

   _____

   _____

4. List four types of medications that can be taken orally.

   _____

   _____

   _____

   _____

5. What are some of the factors that affect the absorption rate of oral medications?

   _____

   _____

   _____

   _____

6. Discuss the difference between oral, sublingual, and buccal routes of administration.

   _____

   _____

   _____

   _____

7. List a medication that can be administered via subcutaneous injection.

_____

_____

_____

_____

8. List three medications that can be administered via intramuscular injection.

_____

_____

_____

_____

9. List two medications that can be administered via intradermal injection.

_____

_____

_____

_____

10. What are the proper angle of needle insertion for the following injections:

   a. IM:

_____

_____

_____

_____

   b. ID:

_____

_____

_____

_____

   c. Subq:

_____

_____

_____

_____

11. Why is it important to withdraw the needle slightly prior to injecting an IM medication?

_____

_____

_____

12. Explain the difference between a Z-track injection and an IM injection.

_____

_____

_____

13. List three medications that can be delivered via the oral route.

_____

_____

_____

14. List three medications that can be delivered via a transdermal patch.

_____

_____

_____

15. Discuss the different types of suppositories. What types of medications can be delivered in this manner?

_____

_____

_____

16. Discuss four reasons for administering medications intravenously.

_____

_____

_____

17. Describe the four basic types of IV solutions.

_____

_____

_____

_____

18. What are the two most common units of measurement of medications?

_____

_____

_____

_____

19. List the units that are used in the apothecary system of measurement.

_____

_____

_____

_____

20. List the units that are used in the household system of measurement.

_____

_____

_____

_____

21. What are some factors to consider when calculating dosages for infants and children?

_____

_____

_____

_____

Abbreviation Review

Define the following abbreviations:

1. NPO: _____

2. cc: _____

3. ac: _____

4. L: _____

5. Kg: _____

6. fl: _____

7. EC: _____

8. DC: _____

9. cap: _____

10. IU: _____

11. mg: _____

12. NaCl: _____

13. mcg: _____

14. mL: _____

15. aq: _____

16. bid: _____

17. subq: _____

18. hs: _____

19. OD: _____

20. Rx: _____

21. tab: _____

22.   OS: _____

23.   OTC: _____

24.   qid: _____

25.   OU: _____

26.   sol: _____

27.   pc: _____

28.   gtt: _____

29.   MEq: _____

30.   qd: _____

Critical Thinking

1. Perform the following system conversions:

   a. 60 mg = _____ gr

   _____

   _____

   _____

   _____

   b. 15 gtt = _____ mL

   _____

   _____

   _____

   _____

   c. 4 fldr = _____ ml

   _____

   _____

   _____

   _____

d. 15 mL = _____ tbsp

e. 4 cups = _____ mL

f. 1 g = _____ gr

g. 2.2 lb = _____ kg = _____ mg

2. Perform the following dosage calculations

   a. The nurse practitioner orders 250 mcg of Lanoxin tabs. You have 0.25 mg tabs on hand. How many tabs will you administer?

   b. The physician orders Coumadin tabs 2.5 mg. You have available Coumadin 5 mg tabs. How many tabs will you administer?

c. The physician assistant orders 250 mg of Tagamet liquid. You have 300 mg/5 mL on hand. How many milliliters will you administer?

_____

_____

_____

_____

d. The physician orders 500 mg of amoxicillin liquid. You have 250 mg/5 mL on hand. How many milliliters will you administer?

_____

_____

_____

_____

e. The physician orders 750 units of heparin sodium subcutaneously. You have 1,000 units/mL on hand. How many milliliters will you administer?

_____

_____

_____

_____

f. The nurse practitioner orders atropine sulfate 0.4 mg IM. You have vials of atropine sulfate 1 mg/mL available. How many milliliters will you administer?

_____

_____

_____

_____

Teamwork Exercises

1. Divide into groups of two or three. Following the procedures in the chapter, take turns preparing and administering intradermal, subcutaneous, and intramuscular injections. As each student gets a chance to prepare and administer each type of injection, the others in the group can provide suggestions and comments as to the proper technique.

2. Dosage calculations can be a difficult concept to learn. Form into groups of two or three and practice dosage calculations together. Ask your instructor for additional dosage exercises and work the problems out as a group. Discuss how each student got to his or her answer.

PROCEDURE 39-1 – ADMINISTERING AN ORAL MEDICATION

Name _____   Date _____   Score _____

Instructor _____

Task
Properly interpret a physician's order and apply pharmacological principles to prepare and administer an oral medication.

Conditions
Medication ordered by the physician
Medication cup (for liquid administration)
Water, when appropriate
Patient's medical record

Time: _____

Standards
In the time specified and within the scoring parameters determined by the instructor, the student will success-fully read the medication order and prepare and administer an oral medication to a patient.

Points assigned reflect importance of step to meeting the task

Important = 1 pt.
Essential = 5 pts.
Critical = 15 pts.

Automatic failure results if any of the **CRITICAL TASKS** are omitted or performed incorrectly.

(To use a pass/fail system, instructors can record "P" or "F" in the "points earned (pass/fail)" column.)

PERFORMANCE STANDARDS	PTS	PTS EARNED (Pass/Fail)	COMMENTS
1. Washed hands.	5	_____	_____
2. Reviewed the "seven rights" of medication administration.	5	_____	_____ _____
3. Assembled equipment and supplies and read the medication order. If in doubt, checked with the physician.	5	_____	_____ _____
4. Selected the right drug and checked the medication label. If the medication was unfamiliar, read the package insert or used a drug reference.	15	_____	_____ _____ _____
5. Checked the expiration date of the medication.	15	_____	_____ _____
6. Read the dosage information on the label and calculated the correct dose.	15	_____	_____ _____

PERFORMANCE STANDARDS (cont.)	PTS	PTS EARNED (Pass/Fail)	COMMENTS
7. Checked the medication label again.	15	_____	_____
8. Prepared the dose needed.	15	_____	_____
a. For solids, such as capsules and tablets, poured the medication from the bottle into the bottle cap and then transferred it to a medication cup. Did not touch the medication or the inside of the cup with hands.	5	_____	_____ _____ _____ _____
b. For liquids, poured syrups and mix suspensions as directed on the bottle. Poured the medication into the medication cup, measuring the meniscus.	5	_____	_____ _____ _____ _____
9. Checked the medication label a third and final time before returning it to the cabinet.	15	_____	_____ _____
10. Carried the medication to the treatment room. Took care not to spill it (used a tray if needed).	5	_____	_____ _____
11. Administered the medication to the patient, being sure to confirm the "right" patient once more.	15	_____	_____ _____
12. Offered the patient some water, as appropriate.	1	_____	_____ _____
13. Remained with the patient until he swallowed the medication.	1	_____	_____ _____
14. Washed hands.	5	_____	_____
15. Documented the procedure in the patient's medical record.	5	_____	_____

TOTAL POINTS	147		

DOCUMENTATION

COMMENTS

PROCEDURE 39-2 – PREPARING A PARENTERAL MEDICATION FROM A VIAL

Name _____   Date _____   Score _____

Instructor _____

Task

Measure the correct amount of medication from a vial into a 3-mL hypodermic syringe for injection.

Conditions

Vial of medication ordered by physician
70% isopropyl alcohol wipes
Appropriate syringe for ordered dose
Needle with safety device appropriate for site injection
2 × 2 sterile gauze pads
Sharps container
Patient's medical record

Time: _____

Standard

In the time specified and within the scoring parameters determined by the instructor, the student will successfully measure the correct medication dose from a vial into a syringe for injection.

Points assigned reflect importance of step to meeting the task

Important = 1 pt.
Essential = 5 pts.
Critical = 15 pts.

Automatic failure results if any of the **CRITICAL TASKS** are omitted or performed incorrectly.

(To use a pass/fail system, instructors can record "P" or "F" in the "points earned (pass/fail)" column.)

PERFORMANCE STANDARDS	PTS	PTS EARNED (Pass/Fail)	COMMENTS
1. Washed hands.	5	_____	_____
2. Assembled the equipment and supplies and verified the order.	5	_____	_____ _____
3. Checked the expiration date of the medication.	15	_____	_____ _____
4. Followed the seven rights of medication administration.	15	_____	_____ _____
5. Checked the medication against the physician's order	15	_____	_____ _____
6. Checked the patient's medical record for allergies or conditions that might contraindicate the medication.	15	_____	_____ _____ _____

PERFORMANCE STANDARDS (cont.)	PTS	PTS EARNED (Pass/Fail)	COMMENTS
7. Calculated the correct dose to be given (if not already provided).	15	_____	_____ _____
8. Checked the medication against the physician's written order.	15	_____	_____ _____
9. If the vial was new, removed the hard plastic or metal cover. If it was a multidose vial that had already been used, wiped the top of the vial with an alcohol wipe.	5	_____	_____ _____ _____ _____
10. Allowed the top of the vial to dry before withdrawing the medication.	1	_____	_____ _____
11. If the medication needed mixing, rotated the vial between the palms of hands.	1	_____	_____ _____
12. Opened the peel-apart sterile packaging around the syringe and needle and assembled the needle and syringe.	1	_____	_____ _____ _____
13. If the needle and syringe were packaged separately, opened both packages using sterile technique, removed the small plastic cap covering the Luer-Lok on the syringe, and attached the needle by twisting it securely to the Luer-Lok.	1	_____	_____ _____ _____ _____ _____ _____
14. Did not allow the hub of the needle to touch anything other than the Luer-Lok.	5	_____	_____ _____
15. Removed the cover from the needle. Held the barrel of the syringe with one hand and carefully removed the cover with the other hand. Placed the needle cover on the counter.	1	_____	_____ _____ _____ _____
16. Closely inspected the needle at eye level and discarded if any burrs were present on the tip or the shaft of the needle.	1	_____	_____ _____ _____ _____

PERFORMANCE STANDARDS (cont.)	PTS	PTS EARNED (Pass/Fail)	COMMENTS
17. Drew air into the syringe. With the needle cover over the needle, drew an amount of air equal to the volume of medication to administer.	15	_____	_____ _____ _____
18. Inserted the needle into the vial. Placed the vial on the counter without holding it. Held the barrel of the syringe with one hand guiding the needle into the rubber stopper. Once the needle had penetrated the stopper, used the other hand to hold the vial. Injected the air into the vial.	5	_____	_____ _____ _____ _____ _____ _____
19. To fill the syringe, inverted the vial and syringe so that the tip of the needle was immersed in the medication. Withdrew a little more than the required volume of medication from the vial.	15	_____	_____ _____ _____ _____ _____
20. If air bubbles had formed in the syringe, inverted the syringe and tapped the barrel with finger or fingernail until the air bubble rose to the top of the liquid. Advanced the plunger to express the air out of the syringe. When the air had been expelled, measured the exact dose needed by advancing the plunger to the required mark on the barrel.	5	_____	_____ _____ _____ _____ _____ _____ _____
21. Removed the needle from the vial stopper by pulling hands away from each other. Was careful not to touch the needle.	5	_____	_____ _____ _____ _____
22. If necessary, recapped the needle by placing the needle cap on a clean, dry surface (such as the countertop), holding the syringe in one hand, and carefully guided the exposed needle into the cap without touching the needle to the cap. When the cap was on the needle, secured it by hand, touching only the cap, not the needle.	1	_____	_____ _____ _____ _____ _____ _____

PERFORMANCE STANDARDS (cont.)	PTS	PTS EARNED (Pass/Fail)	COMMENTS
23. If preparing the needle in a different room than the patient, capped and carried the needle on a tray.	5	_____	_____ _____ _____

TOTAL POINTS	167		

DOCUMENTATION

_____	_____
_____	_____
_____	_____

COMMENTS

_____

_____

_____

_____

PROCEDURE 39-3 – PREPARING A PARENTERAL MEDICATION FROM AN AMPULE

Name _____   Date _____   Score _____

Instructor _____

Task

Measure the correct amount of medication from an ampule into a 3-mL hypodermic syringe for injection.

Conditions

Ampule of medication ordered by physician
70% isopropyl alcohol wipes
Appropriate syringe for ordered dose
Needle with safety device appropriate for injection site
Filter needle (for ampule)
2 × 2 sterile gauze pads
Sharps container
Patient's medical record

Time: _____

Standard

In the time specified and within the scoring parameters determined by the instructor, the student will successfully measure the correct medication dose from an ampule into a syringe for injection.

Points assigned reflect importance of step to meeting the task

Important = 1 pt.
Essential = 5 pts.
Critical = 15 pts.

Automatic failure results if any of the **CRITICAL TASKS** are omitted or performed incorrectly.

(To use a pass/fail system, instructors can record "P" or "F" in the "points earned (pass/fail)" column.)

PERFORMANCE STANDARDS	PTS	PTS EARNED (Pass/Fail)	COMMENTS
1. Washed hands.	5	_____	_____
2. Assembled the equipment and supplies and verified the order.	5	_____	_____
3. Checked the expiration date of the medication.	15	_____	_____
4. Followed the seven rights of medication administration.	15	_____	_____
5. Checked the medication against the physician's order.	15	_____	_____
6. Checked the patient's medical record for allergies or conditions that might contraindicate the medication.	15	_____	_____

PERFORMANCE STANDARDS (cont.)	PTS	PTS EARNED (Pass/Fail)	COMMENTS
7. Calculated the correct dose to be given (if not already provided).	15	_____	_____
8. Checked the medication against the physician's written order.	15	_____	_____
9. Cleaned the ampule with an alcohol wipe and allowed it to air-dry before withdrawing the medication.	5	_____	_____
10. Using an ampule breaker or a piece of gauze wrapped around the top of the ampule, broke off the top of the ampule. Was sure to do so in the direction away from the student's body. Discarded the ampule top in the sharps container.	5	_____	_____
11. Held the barrel of the filter needle syringe with one hand and carefully removed the needle cover with the other hand. Placed the needle cover on its side on the counter.	5	_____	_____
12. Inspected the needle and discarded if any burrs were present on the tip or the shaft of the needle.	1	_____	_____
13. Inserted the filter needle into the ampule. Placing the ampule on the countertop, held the barrel of the syringe with one hand and carefully lowered the needle into the ampule so that the bevel of the needle was below the surface of the liquid.	5	_____	_____
14. Did not inject air into the ampule and did not touch the broken edge of the ampule with the needle or fingers.	5	_____	_____
15. Withdrew the entire amount of medication, if ordered. Kept the bevel of the needle under the surface of the liquid as the medication was withdrawn.	15	_____	_____

PERFORMANCE STANDARDS (cont.)	PTS	PTS EARNED (Pass/Fail)	COMMENTS
16. Using sterile technique, exchanged the filter needle for an injection needle with a safety device. Inspected the injection needle for defects and discarded if any were found. Did not touch the end of the hub of the needle or the tip of the barrel of the syringe.	5	_____	_____ _____ _____ _____ _____ _____
17. Removed the cover of the new needle. If air bubbles had formed in the syringe, inverted the syringe and tapped the barrel with finger or fingernail until the air bubble rose to the top of the liquid. Advanced the plunger. When any air had been expelled, measured the exact dose needed by advancing the plunger to the required mark on the barrel.	15	_____	_____ _____ _____ _____ _____ _____ _____ _____
18. Recapped the needle if necessary. Placed the needle cap on a clean, dry surface (such as the countertop) and, holding the syringe in one hand, carefully guided the exposed needle into the cap without touching it. When the cap was on the needle, secured it by hand, touching only the cap, not the needle.	1	_____	_____ _____ _____ _____ _____ _____ _____
19. If the needle was prepared in a different room than the patient, capped and carried the needle on a tray.	1	_____	_____ _____
20. Checked the medication label and discarded the ampule in the sharps container.	15	_____	_____ _____
21. Washed hands.	5	_____	_____ _____
TOTAL POINTS	183		

DOCUMENTATION

COMMENTS

PROCEDURE 39-4 – ADMINISTERING A SUBCUTANEOUS INJECTION

Name _____   Date _____   Score _____

Instructor _____

Task

Select the proper site and properly administer a subcu-taneous injection.

Conditions

Nonsterile disposable gloves
Medication ordered by the physician
Appropriate syringe for the ordered dose
Needle with a safety device
2 × 2 sterile gauze pads
70% isopropyl alcohol wipes
Sharps container
Biohazardous waste container
Patient's medical record

Time: _____

Standard

In the time specified and within the scoring parameters determined by the instructor, the student will success-fully select the proper site and properly administer a subcutaneous injection.

Points assigned reflect importance of step to meeting the task

Important = 1 pt.
Essential = 5 pts.
Critical = 15 pts.

Automatic failure results if any of the **CRITICAL TASKS** are omitted or performed incorrectly.

(To use a pass/fail system, instructors can record "P" or "F" in the "points earned (pass/fail)" column.)

PERFORMANCE STANDARDS	PTS	PTS EARNED (Pass/Fail)	COMMENTS
1. Washed hands.	5	_____	_____
2. Assembled the equipment and supplies and verified the order.	5	_____	_____
3. Checked the expiration date of the medication.	15	_____	_____
4. Followed the seven rights of medication administration.	15	_____	_____
5. Checked the medication against the physician's written order.	15	_____	_____
6. Checked the patient's medical record for allergies or conditions that might contraindicate the medication.	15	_____	_____
7. Calculated the correct dose to be given, if necessary.	15	_____	_____

PERFORMANCE STANDARDS (cont.)	PTS	PTS EARNED (Pass/Fail)	COMMENTS
8. Prepared the syringe with the ordered dose.	15	_____	_____
9. Followed the procedure for drawing medication into the syringe.	5	_____	_____
10. Greeted and identified the patient.	5	_____	_____
11. Explained the procedure to the patient.	5	_____	_____
12. Selected the appropriate injection site and positioned the patient.	5	_____	_____
13. Exposed the injection site and inspected the site for scars and inflammation. If scaring or inflammation were present, chose a different site. Was sure to explain to the patient why the site was changed.	5	_____	_____
14. Put on gloves.	5	_____	_____
15. Rechecked the medication against the physician's written order.	15	_____	_____
16. Prepared the injection site by cleaning it with an alcohol wipe, beginning at the center and working in an outward circular motion. Allowed the site to air dry. Did not touch the site or allow the patient to touch the site.	5	_____	_____
17. Removed the cover from the needle.	1	_____	_____
18. Rechecked the medication against the physician's written orders.	15	_____	_____
19. Secured the skin at the injection site. Grasped a generous portion of skin around the injection site between the thumb and forefinger of the non-dominant hand. Held the syringe at a 45-degree, upward angle.	15	_____	_____
20. Punctured the skin with the needle in a quick, smooth motion.	5	_____	_____

PERFORMANCE STANDARDS (cont.)	PTS	PTS EARNED (Pass/Fail)	COMMENTS
21. Checked to see if blood aspirated into the syringe. If it did, withdrew the syringe from the site, then began the procedure again with a new needle.	5	_____	_____
22. If blood did not aspirate into the syringe, released grasp of the skin and pulled back on the plunger.	5	_____	_____
23. If no blood aspirated into the syringe when pulling the plunger, injected the medication slowly.	5	_____	_____
24. Placed a gauze pad over the injection site and quickly withdrew the needle from the site at the same 45-degree angle.	1	_____	_____
25. Used a 2 × 2 sterile gauze pad to massage the injection site gently but firmly.	1	_____	_____
26. Discarded the syringe and needle in the sharps container. Removed gloves and discarded them in the biohazardous waste container, and washed hands.	5	_____	_____
27. Checked on the patient. Asked the patient how she felt and observed her for any signs of immediate emergency reaction, such as dizziness, light-headedness, or fainting.	1	_____	_____
28. Documented the procedure, including the date, time, lot number of the medication, dose given, and injection site used. Charted any reactions observed.	15	_____	_____

TOTAL POINTS	224		

DOCUMENTATION

COMMENTS

PROCEDURE 39-5 – ADMINISTERING AN INTRADERMAL INJECTION

Name _____   Date _____   Score _____

Instructor _____

Task
Select the proper site and properly administer an intradermal injection.

Conditions
Nonsterile disposable gloves
Medication ordered by the physician
Appropriate syringe for ordered dose (tuberculin syringe)
Needle with safety device (26G or 27G, 3/8–1/2 inch)
2 × 2 sterile gauze pads
70% isopropyl alcohol wipes
Written patient instructions for post-testing
Sharps container
Biohazardous waste container
Patient's medical record

Time: _____

Standard
In the time specified and within the scoring parameters determined by the instructor, the student will successfully select the proper site and properly administer an intradermal injection.

Points assigned reflect importance of step to meeting the task

Important = 1 pt.
Essential = 5 pts.
Critical = 15 pts.

Automatic failure results if any of the **CRITICAL TASKS** are omitted or performed incorrectly.

(To use a pass/fail system, instructors can record "P" or "F" in the "points earned (pass/fail)" column.)

PERFORMANCE STANDARDS	PTS	PTS EARNED (Pass/Fail)	COMMENTS
1. Washed hands.	5	_____	_____
2. Assembled the equipment and supplies and verified the order.	5	_____	_____
3. Checked the expiration date of the medication.	15	_____	_____
4. Followed the seven rights of medication administration.	15	_____	_____
5. Checked the medication against the physician's written order.	15	_____	_____
6. Checked the patient's medical record for allergies or conditions that might contraindicate the medication.	15	_____	_____

PERFORMANCE STANDARDS (cont.)	PTS	PTS EARNED (Pass/Fail)	COMMENTS
7. Calculated the correct dose to be given, if necessary.	15	_____	_____
8. Prepared the syringe with the correct dose.	15	_____	_____
9. Followed the procedure for drawing medication into the syringe.	5	_____	_____
10. Greeted and identified the patient.	5	_____	_____
11. Explained the procedure to the patient.	1	_____	_____
12. Selected the appropriate injection site and positioned the patient.	5	_____	_____
13. Rechecked the medication against the physician's written orders.	15	_____	_____
14. Exposed the injection site and inspected the site for scars and inflammation. If scaring or inflammation were present, chose a different site. Was sure to explain to the patient why the site had to be changed.	5	_____	_____
15. Put on gloves.	5	_____	_____
16. Prepared the injection site by cleaning it with an alcohol wipe, beginning at the center and working in an outward circular motion. Allowed the site to air-dry. Did not touch the site or allow the patient to touch the site.	1	_____	_____
17. Rechecked the medication against the physician's written orders.	15	_____	_____
18. Removed the cover without touching the needle. Visually inspected the injection site to be sure that the alcohol had dried before injection was administered.	1	_____	_____

PERFORMANCE STANDARDS (cont.)	PTS	PTS EARNED (Pass/Fail)	COMMENTS
19. Secured the skin at the injection site. Pulled the skin at the injection site taut with the thumb and forefinger of your nondominant hand. Positioned the needle almost parallel to the skin at an angle of 10 to 15 degrees.	15	_____	_____
20. Inserted the needle until the bevel barely penetrated the skin. Was sure that the entire bevel was below the surface of the skin.	15	_____	_____
21. Released grasp on the forearm skin and used nondominant hand to inject the medication slowly. Kept a slow, steady pressure on the plunger until all of the liquid was injected and a wheal formed. The wheal should have been 6–10 mm in diameter.	5	_____	_____
22. If no wheal formed, notified the physician immediately.	15	_____	_____
23. Withdrew the needle from the injection site at the same angle (10–15 degrees) and activated the safety device.	5	_____	_____
24. Dabbed the area with a gauze pad. Did not apply pressure to the wheal.	1	_____	_____
25. Discarded the needle in the sharps container and washed hands.	5	_____	_____
26. Asked the patient how he felt and observed him for any signs of an immediate emergency reaction, such as dizziness, light-headedness, or fainting.	5	_____	_____

PERFORMANCE STANDARDS *(cont.)*	PTS	PTS EARNED (Pass/Fail)	COMMENTS
27. Discussed the monitoring of test results with the patient. Based on the type of test and the office policy, student may have:	5	_____	_____ _____ _____ _____
a. Read the test result in the office. Using inspection (looking) and palpation (feeling) at the site of the injection, determined the presence of a reaction and the amount of induration.	15	_____	_____ _____ _____ _____ _____
b. Informed the patient of a date and time to return to the office to have the physician read the results of the injection.	5	_____	_____ _____ _____
c. Instructed the patient on reading and interpreting the injection site at home. Gave him a card with various levels of induration for comparison. Instructed the patient to call the office with the test results. Explained the importance of reading the site at the correct date and time.	5	_____	_____ _____ _____ _____ _____ _____
28. Documented the procedure in the patient's chart.	15	_____	_____ _____

TOTAL POINTS	269		

DOCUMENTATION

COMMENTS

PROCEDURE 39-6 – ADMINISTERING AN INTRAMUSCULAR INJECTION

Name _____   Date _____   Score _____

Instructor _____

Task

Select the proper site and properly administer an intra-muscular injection.

Conditions

Nonsterile disposable gloves
Medication ordered by the physician
Appropriate syringe for ordered dose
Needle with safety device
2 × 2 sterile gauze pads
70% isopropyl alcohol wipes
Sharps container
Biohazardous waste container
Patient's medical record

Time: _____

Standards

In the time specified and within the scoring parameters determined by the instructor, the student will success-fully select the proper site and properly administer an intramuscular injection.

Points assigned reflect importance of step to meeting the task

> Important = 1 pt.
> Essential = 5 pts.
> Critical = 15 pts.

Automatic failure results if any of the **CRITICAL TASKS** are omitted or performed incorrectly.

(To use a pass/fail system, instructors can record "P" or "F" in the "points earned (pass/fail)" column.)

PERFORMANCE STANDARDS	PTS	PTS EARNED (Pass/Fail)	COMMENTS
1. Washed hands.	5	_____	_____
2. Assembled the equipment and supplies and verified the order.	5	_____	_____
3. Checked the expiration date of the medication.	15	_____	_____
4. Followed the seven rights of medication administration.	15	_____	_____
5. Checked the medication against the physician's written order.	15	_____	_____
6. Checked the patient's medical record for allergies or conditions that might contraindicate the medication.	15	_____	_____
7. Calculated the correct dose to be given, if necessary.	15	_____	_____

PERFORMANCE STANDARDS (cont.)	PTS	PTS EARNED (Pass/Fail)	COMMENTS
8. Prepared the syringe with the ordered dose of the medication.	5	_____	_____
9. Followed the procedure for drawing medication into the syringe.	5	_____	_____
10. Greeted and identified the patient.	5	_____	_____
11. Explained the procedure to the patient.	1	_____	_____
12. Selected the appropriate injection site and positioned the patient.	5	_____	_____
13. Rechecked the medication against the physician's written orders.	15	_____	_____
14. Exposed the injection site and inspected the site for scars and inflammation. If scaring or inflammation is present, chose a different site. Was sure to explain to the patient why the site had to be changed.	5	_____	_____
15. Put on gloves.	5	_____	_____
16. If the patient was a child, asked the parent or caregiver to help restrain the child if necessary. If the parent or guardian was unable to assist, obtained assistance from a second health-care professional. Restrained the patient only if necessary and only for as long as necessary.	5	_____	_____
17. Prepared the injection site by cleaning it with an alcohol wipe, beginning at the center and working in an outward circular motion. Allowed the site to air-dry. Did not touch the site or allow the patient to touch the site.	1	_____	_____
18. Rechecked the medication against the physician's written orders.	15	_____	_____

PERFORMANCE STANDARDS *(cont.)*	PTS	PTS EARNED (Pass/Fail)	COMMENTS
19. Removed the cover without touching the needle. Visually inspected the injection site.	1	_____	_____ _____
20. Secured the skin at the injection site by spreading the skin around the injection site taut with the thumb and forefinger of the student's non-dominant hand.	5	_____	_____ _____ _____ _____
21. Punctured the skin quickly at a 90-degree angle and inserted the entire needle up to the hub.	15	_____	_____ _____ _____
22. Checked to see if blood aspirated into the syringe by releasing grasp of the tissues and pulling back on the plunger a little with nondominant hand. If blood had aspirated, withdrew the needle from the site, then began the procedure again with a new needle.	5	_____	_____ _____ _____ _____ _____ _____ _____
23. If blood did not aspirate into the syringe, pushed the plunger of the syringe slowly and steadily into the intramuscular tissue. Was careful to hold the needle still while administering the medication.	5	_____	_____ _____ _____ _____ _____
24. Placed a gauze pad over the injection site and withdrew the needle from the site at the same 90-degree angle.	1	_____	_____ _____ _____
25. Used a 2 × 2 sterile gauze pad to massage the injection site gently but firmly. Did not massage the injection site of heparin or insulin.	1	_____	_____ _____ _____
26. Discarded the syringe and needle in the sharps container, removed gloves and discarded them in the biohazardous waste container, and washed hands.	5	_____	_____ _____ _____ _____ _____

PERFORMANCE STANDARDS (cont.)	PTS	PTS EARNED (Pass/Fail)	COMMENTS
27. Checked on the patient. Asked the patient how she felt and observed her for any signs of immediate emergency reaction, such as dizziness, light-headedness, or fainting.	5	_____	_____
28. Documented the procedure, including the date, time, lot number of the medication, dose given, and injection site used. Charted any reactions observed.	15	_____	_____

TOTAL POINTS	210		

DOCUMENTATION

COMMENTS

Introduction to the Clinical Laboratory

Key Term Review   *Define the following key terms:*

1. physician's office laboratory (POL)   _____

2. specimen   _____

3. analyzer   _____

4. automated method   _____

5. normal ranges   _____

6. qualitative result   _____

7. requisition slip   _____

8. anatomical lab   _____

9. clinical diagnosis   _____

10. panel   _____

11. biopsy   _____

Key Term Review *cont.*

12. routine test _____

_____

13. proficiency testing _____

_____

14. manual method _____

_____

15. reagent _____

_____

16. quantitative result _____

_____

17. reference laboratory _____

_____

18. quality control _____

_____

Review Questions

1. What is the medical assistant's role in a POL?

_____

_____

_____

_____

2. What are some of the functions of a clinical laboratory?

_____

_____

_____

_____

3. Describe the life cycle of a lab test.

_____

_____

_____

_____

4. List the various departments within the clinical laboratory, and give two tests performed in each department.

_____

_____

_____

_____

5. Discuss the various personnel within the laboratory.

_____

_____

_____

_____

6. Explain the purpose of CLIA '88.

_____

_____

_____

_____

7. Define the four categories of testing as defined by CLIA '88. Provide two tests with each category.

_____

_____

_____

_____

8. What is quality control? How is it similar to quality assurance? How is it different?

_____

_____

_____

_____

9. Discuss the purpose and importance of the requisition slip.

_____

_____

_____

_____

10. Discuss the various reasons a health-care provider might order laboratory tests.

_____

_____

_____

_____

11. Discuss the medical assistant's role in proper patient preparation prior to collection of specimens.

_____

_____

_____

_____

12. What is some equipment that may be used in a laboratory? Discuss proper preventative maintenance for these pieces of equipment.

_____

_____

_____

_____

Critical Thinking

1. For each of the following laboratory tests, research if there is any special collection procedure that should be followed:

   a. bleeding time:

   _____

   _____

   _____

   _____

b. urinalysis:

_____

_____

_____

_____

c. CBC:

_____

_____

_____

_____

d. blood culture:

_____

_____

_____

_____

e. ABO blood type:

_____

_____

_____

_____

f. urine pregnancy:

_____

_____

_____

_____

g. RPR:

_____

_____

_____

_____

2. Search the Web for a college with an MLT program. Compare the curriculum with your medical assisting curriculum. Are there any similarities? Differences?

_____

_____

_____

_____

3. Log onto the CLIA Web site and go to the section on CLIA waived tests. Have any new tests been added that you have not read about in the chapter? If so, make a list of them and search the Web for companies that may sell such tests to physicians' offices.

_____

_____

_____

_____

Teamwork Exercises

1. Divide into groups of two or three students. Have each group contact a different hospital or reference laboratory to obtain an example of their laboratory requisition form. (Students can also contact local physicians' offices or clinics for copies of laboratory requisition forms.) Compare and contrast each facility's requisition forms. Look at specifics such as color coding for departments, codes for proper tube selection, and CPT billing codes. Which form seems the easiest to use?

2. Divide into groups of two or three. As a group, go around your classroom and review the different CLIA waived instruments and test kits. Read the instructor's manual and/or package insert for the instrument and/or test kit. Pay close attention to the type of specimen the instrument or test uses as well as the quality control involved, actual procedure for testing, and preventive maintenance. Develop note cards for each test for future reference.

Office Project

Create quality-control log sheets for each instrument in your classroom. Post the logs in the laboratory area nearest to the instrument. These log sheet will be used during the semester as the class practices performing testing on each instrument.

Phlebotomy

Key Term Review   *Define the following key terms:*

1.   lancet   _____
_____

2.   whole blood   _____
_____

3.   plasma   _____
_____

4.   buffy coat   _____
_____

5.   thrombocytes   _____
_____

6.   evacuated tube   _____
_____

7.   serum   _____
_____

8.   additive   _____
_____

9.   coagulate   _____
_____

10.   anticoagulant   _____
_____

11.   hemoconcentration   _____
_____

Key Term Review *cont.*

12. leukocytes _____

_____

13. hematoma _____

_____

14. antecubital space _____

_____

15. hemolysis _____

_____

16. erythrocyte _____

_____

Review Questions

1. Describe the difference between a venipuncture and a capillary puncture.

_____
_____
_____
_____

2. List and describe the supplies and equipment required for a venipuncture.

_____
_____
_____
_____

3. Explain the evacuated tube system.

_____
_____
_____
_____

4. Discuss the medical assistant's role in proper blood collection.

_____

_____

_____

_____

5. Explain the differences between plasma, serum, and whole blood.

_____

_____

_____

_____

6. For the following blood tubes, provide the additive it contains:

a. lavender:

_____

_____

_____

_____

b. light blue:

_____

_____

_____

_____

c. green:

_____

_____

_____

_____

d. yellow:

_____

_____

_____

_____

e. gray:

_____

_____

_____

_____

f. red:

_____

_____

_____

_____

7. Explain some of the special considerations a medical assistant must take when drawing blood on:

a. pediatric patients:

_____

_____

_____

_____

b. elderly patients:

_____

_____

_____

_____

c. anxious patients:

_____

_____

_____

_____

8. List the approved sites for capillary punctures.

_____

_____

_____

_____

9. Describe some of the safety precautions a medical assistant must take when drawing blood.

_____

_____

_____

_____

10. For the following blood test, give the proper tube for collection:

a. BUN

_____

_____

_____

b. FBG

_____

_____

_____

c. H&H

_____

_____

_____

_____

d. INR

_____

_____

_____

_____

e. blood culture

_____

_____

_____

_____

f. lipid panel

_____

_____

_____

_____

g. TSH

_____

_____

_____

_____

h. PTT

_____

_____

_____

_____

i. CBC

_____

_____

_____

_____

j. ammonia

_____

_____

_____

_____

Critical Thinking

1. Describe what you would do and/or say in the following situations:

   a. After inserting the tube into the holder, you think the tube has no vacuum:

   _____

   _____

   _____

   _____

   b. A hematoma is forming at site of the needle insertion:

   _____

   _____

   _____

   _____

   c. The patient states, "You have one try and one try only!":

   _____

   _____

   _____

   _____

   d. The patient states, "Use the vein in my left arm; it's the good one":

   _____

   _____

   _____

   _____

   e. The patient states, "They never get me on the first try":

   _____

   _____

   _____

   _____

f. After asking the patient if he has been fasting, he responds, "No, I didn't eat anything this morning; I only had orange juice with my pills."

_____

_____

_____

_____

2. You work in a pediatric clinic and a new mother comes in with her 1-year-old baby, who has had a fever of 102°F the past 3 days. Upon examination, the physician asks you to perform a capillary puncture to collect blood for a CBC and differential. Answer the following questions:

a. What is the setup, and which collection supplies would you use for the collection?

_____

_____

_____

b. The mother is extremely nervous about the procedure you are about to perform; how would you answer her to make her at ease?

_____

_____

_____

_____

3. Lisbeth Davenport is in the office this morning for blood work. The physician has ordered a PT, FBS, lipid panel, and a CBC. Which tubes would you chose for this draw? In which order would you draw each tube? Upon inserting the second blood tube, you notice that the blood has stopped flowing and the puncture site is beginning to form a hematoma. What would you do?

_____

_____

_____

_____

Teamwork Exercises

1. Form into groups of two or three. Your instructor will provide you with copies of a typical laboratory requisition form. Using the blank laboratory requisition form, have each student complete requisitions for the following orders. Upon completion, share forms with each other and check for completeness. Point out any inconsistencies with each student's forms.

   a. Dannie Frinsz
      D.O.B. 12-30-92
      MR# 319857
      Orders: STAT mono, CBC, liver function tests

   b. Bob Kozlowski
      D.O.B. 12-25-62
      MR # 002837
      Orders: CK, CKMB, BUN, creatinine, troponin, urinalysis

   c. Therese Boyd
      D.O.B. 10-26-72
      MR# 610938
      Orders: Type and screen

2. Divide into groups of two or three. Obtain the proper supplies for a typical venipuncture and using a fake arm have each student follow the procedure in the textbook for performing the venipuncture. The students in the group should provide assistance in the steps as needed.

PROCEDURE 41-1 – PERFORMING A VENIPUNCTURE

Name _____   Date _____   Score _____

Instructor _____

Task
Perform a venipuncture.

Conditions
Requisition slip
Blood tubes
Needles
Gauze
Alcohol cleansing pad
Tourniquet
Adapter
Adhesive bandage or surgical tape
Sharps container
Biohazardous waste container

Time: _____

Standard
In the time specified and within the scoring parameters determined by the instructor, the student will successfully perform a venipuncture.

Points assigned reflect importance of step to meeting the task

Important = 1 pt.
Essential = 5 pts.
Critical = 15 pts.

Automatic failure results if any of the **CRITICAL TASKS** are omitted or performed incorrectly.

(To use a pass/fail system, instructors can record "P" or "F" in the "points earned (pass/fail)" column.)

PERFORMANCE STANDARDS	PTS	PTS EARNED (Pass/Fail)	COMMENTS
1. Examined the requisition slip.	1	_____	_____
2. Greeted the patient and asked him to state his full name and date of birth. Checked pretesting requirements, such as fasting, nonfasting, and medication restrictions.	15	_____	_____ _____ _____ _____
3. Reassured the patient and explained the procedure.	1	_____	_____ _____
4. Selected the correct equipment and tubes for the procedure. Had extra tubes handy in case the first tube did not work.	15	_____	_____ _____ _____
5. Washed hands and put on gloves.	5	_____	_____ _____

	PTS	PTS EARNED (Pass/Fail)	COMMENTS

6. Positioned the patient's arm. The arm with the vein selected for venipuncture should have been extended and in a straight line from the shoulder to the wrist with the antecubital veins facing anteriorly. A towel may have been used to support the arm if the armrest was too low. — 5

7. Applied a tourniquet 3–4 inches above the antecubital area of the patient's arm and asked the patient to clench his fist. — 5

8. Identified the vein of choice by palpation. — 5

9. Released the tourniquet. — 1

10. Cleaned the site and allowed it to air-dry. Cleaning should have been done in a circular motion starting from the inside and moving away from the puncture site. — 5

11. Assembled the equipment. Screwed the needle into the adaptor and selected the first tube to be drawn. Positioned all items to be used during the procedure within reach. Rested the tube in the back of the adaptor without pushing it into the back of the needle. — 15

12. Reapplied the tourniquet, positioning it 3–4 inches above the antecubital space. Made sure it was snug but not tight. — 5

13. Did not touch the puncture site. — 5

14. Anchored the vein below the puncture site. Then grasped the patient's arm with student's nondominant hand, placing student's thumb 1–2 inches below the puncture site. Using thumb, drew the skin over the vein in the direction of the patient's hand. — 15

PERFORMANCE STANDARDS (cont.)	PTS	PTS EARNED (Pass/Fail)	COMMENTS
15. When the vein was securely anchored, aligned the needle with the vein and inserted the needle, bevel up, at an angle of 15 to 30 degrees, depending on the depth of the vein.	15	_____	_____
16. Once the needle was in the vein, pushed the tube into the back of the needle; blood should have started flowing into the tube.	15	_____	_____
17. Did not move the needle when changing tubes. The hand used to hold the needle assembly should have remained braced on the patient's arm while tubes were inserted or removed from the adapter.	15	_____	_____
18. Used tubes in the correct order.	5	_____	_____
19. Made certain to mix tubes gently and promptly. Rotated the tube 8 to 10 times to mix it with the anticoagulant.	5	_____	_____
20. Made certain that each evacuated tube was filled to level appropriate for that tube.	5	_____	_____
21. Released the tourniquet after inserting the last tube.	5	_____	_____
22. Was sure to remove the last tube from the adapter.	5	_____	_____
23. Placed a sterile gauze pad over the needle and quickly withdrew the needle. Did not apply pressure to the puncture site until the needle was completely removed.	5	_____	_____
24. Activated the safety needle.	1	_____	_____
25. Applied pressure with the gauze pad for 1 to 2 minutes (or longer for a patient on anticoagulation therapy).	1	_____	_____

PERFORMANCE STANDARDS (cont.)	PTS	PTS EARNED (Pass/Fail)	COMMENTS
26. Disposed of the needle and holder in a sharps container.	5	_____	_____
27. Labeled the tubes containing samples.	15	_____	_____
28. Examined the puncture site for bleeding.	1	_____	_____
29. Applied a bandage over the puncture site.	1	_____	_____
30. Disposed of all used supplies in appropriate containers.	5	_____	_____
31. Removed your gloves and washed your hands.	5	_____	_____
32. Documented the procedure in the patient's chart.	5	_____	_____

TOTAL POINTS	212		

DOCUMENTATION

COMMENTS

PROCEDURE 41-2 – PERFORMING A VENIPUNCTURE USING A WINGED INFUSION SET

Name _____   Date _____   Score _____

                                          Instructor _____

Task
Properly perform a venipuncture using a winged infusion set or butterfly system.

Conditions
Winged infusion set with push-button needle
  activation
Requisition form
Blood tubes
Alcohol wipe
Gauze
Tourniquet
Adaptor
Adhesive bandage or surgical tape
Biohazardous waste container
Sharps container

Time: _____

Standard
In the time specified and within the scoring parameters determined by the instructor, the student will successfully perform a venipuncture using a winged infusion set.

Points assigned reflect importance of step to meeting the task

> Important = 1 pt.
> Essential = 5 pts.
> Critical = 15 pts.

Automatic failure results if any of the **CRITICAL TASKS** are omitted or performed incorrectly.

(To use a pass/fail system, instructors can record "P" or "F" in the "points earned (pass/fail)" column.)

PERFORMANCE STANDARDS	PTS	PTS EARNED (Pass/Fail)	COMMENTS
1. Examined the requisition slip.	1	_____	_____
2. Greeted the patient and asked him to state his full name and date of birth. Checked pre-testing requirements, such as fasting, nonfasting, and medication restrictions.	15	_____	_____
3. Reassured the patient and explained the procedure.	5	_____	_____
4. Selected the correct equipment and tubes for the procedure.	15	_____	_____
5. Washed hands and put on gloves.	5	_____	_____

PERFORMANCE STANDARDS (cont.)	PTS	PTS EARNED (Pass/Fail)	COMMENTS
6. Positioned the patient's arm. The arm with the vein selected for venipuncture should have been extended and in a straight line from the shoulder to the wrist with the antecubital veins facing anteriorly. The arm should also have been supported in the armrest by a towel.	5	_____	_____
7. Applied a tourniquet and identified the vein of choice by palpation.	5	_____	_____
8. Released the tourniquet.	1	_____	_____
9. Cleaned the site and allow it to air-dry. Cleaning should have been done in a circular motion starting from the inside and moving away from the puncture site.	5	_____	_____
10. Assembled the winged infusion set. Peeled back the packaging at the arrows so that the back of the winged infusion set was exposed. Grasped the rear barrel of the set and removed it from the package. If the winged infusion set had a button, was careful not to activate the button when removing the set from the package.	5	_____	_____
11. Attached the adaptor to the multiple-sample Luer adaptor at the end of the tubing.	5	_____	_____
12. Assembled additional supplies and positioned self within reach all of the items to be used during the procedure.	5	_____	_____
13. Reapplied the tourniquet 3–4 inches (7.5–10 cm) above the antecubital space, making it snug but not tight.	5	_____	_____

PERFORMANCE STANDARDS *(cont.)*	PTS	PTS EARNED (Pass/Fail)	COMMENTS
14. Did not touch the puncture site.	5	_____	_____
15. Anchored the vein below the puncture site, then grasped the patient's arm with student's nondominant hand, placing thumb 1–2 inches (2.5–5 cm) below the puncture site. Using thumb, drew the skin over the vein in the direction of the patient's hand.	15	_____	_____
16. When the vein was securely anchored, grasped the wings together with thumb and index finger and inserted the needle into the vein at a 15-to-20-degree angle. (Student may have held the body of the device instead of the wings during insertion as preferred.)	15	_____	_____
17. Saw a flash of blood enter the tubing.	5	_____	_____
18. Attached the proper blood collection tube to the adaptor and watched as blood entered the tube.	5	_____	_____
19. Made certain to mix tubes with anticoagulant promptly.	5	_____	_____
20. Made certain that each evacuated tube was completely full.	5	_____	_____
21. After inserting the last tube, released the tourniquet. Removed the last tube from the adaptor before removing the needle.	5	_____	_____
22. After blood collection was complete, placed a gauze pad over the venipuncture site and, while the needle was still in the vein, grasped the body of the infusion set with thumb and middle finger and activated the button, if available, with the tip of index finger.	5	_____	_____

PERFORMANCE STANDARDS (cont.)	PTS	PTS EARNED (Pass/Fail)	COMMENTS
23. Removed the needle from the patient's arm and applied pressure to the venipuncture site with gauze.	5	_____	_____ _____
24. Disposed of the winged infusion set in a sharps container.	5	_____	_____ _____
25. Labeled the tubes containing samples.	15	_____	_____ _____
26. Examined the puncture site for bleeding.	1	_____	_____ _____
27. Applied a bandage over the puncture site and dismissed the patient.	1	_____	_____ _____
28. Disposed of all used supplies in the appropriate containers.	1	_____	_____ _____
29. Removed gloves and washed hands.	5	_____	_____
30. Documented the procedure in the patient's chart.	5	_____	_____ _____

TOTAL POINTS	180		

DOCUMENTATION

COMMENTS

PROCEDURE 41-3 – PERFORMING A CAPILLARY PUNCTURE

Name _____ Date _____ Score _____

Instructor _____

Task
Perform a capillary puncture.

Conditions
Gauze
Alcohol cleansing pad
Adhesive bandage or surgical tape
Lancets
Micro-collection tubes or capillary tubes
Sharps container
Biohazardous waste container

Time: _____

Standard
In the time specified and within the scoring parameters determined by the instructor, the student will successfully perform a capillary puncture.

Points assigned reflect importance of step to meeting the task

Important = 1 pt.
Essential = 5 pts.
Critical = 15 pts.

Automatic failure results if any of the **CRITICAL TASKS** are omitted or performed incorrectly.

(To use a pass/fail system, instructors can record "P" or "F" in the "points earned (pass/fail)" column.)

PERFORMANCE STANDARDS	PTS	PTS EARNED (Pass/Fail)	COMMENTS
1. Examined the requisition slip.	1	_____	_____
2. Greeted the patient and asked him to state his full name and date of birth. Checked pre-test requirements, such as fasting, non-fasting, and medication restrictions.	15	_____	_____ _____ _____ _____
3. Reassured the patient and explained the procedure.	5	_____	_____ _____
4. Selected the correct equipment and tubes for the procedure.	15	_____	_____ _____
5. Washed your hands and put on gloves.	5	_____	_____ _____
6. Selected the puncture site.	1	_____	_____
7. Warmed the puncture site if necessary.	1	_____	_____ _____

PERFORMANCE STANDARDS *(cont.)*	PTS	PTS EARNED (Pass/Fail)	COMMENTS
8. Cleaned the site and allowed it to air-dry. Cleaning should have been done in a circular motion starting from the inside and moving away from the puncture site.	5	_____	_____
9. Assembled the equipment. Positioned within reach all items to be used during the procedure.	5	_____	_____
10. Performed the puncture using the proper lancet.	15	_____	_____
11. Wiped away the first drop of blood.	5	_____	_____
12. Collected the sample using the proper collection tubes.	15	_____	_____
13. Mixed the sample if necessary.	1	_____	_____
14. If point-of-care testing must be done, performed the test according to the manufacturer's specifications.	15	_____	_____
15. Applied pressure to the site. Examined the site for bleeding and bandaged it according to the facility's policy.	5	_____	_____
16. Disposed of the puncture device in a sharps container.	5	_____	_____
17. Labeled the sample.	15	_____	_____
18. Removed gloves and disposed of them properly.	5	_____	_____
19. Washed hands.	5	_____	_____
20. Documented the procedure in the patient's chart.	5	_____	_____
TOTAL POINTS	**144**		

DOCUMENTATION

COMMENTS

Hematology and Coagulation Procedures

Key Term Review   *Define the following key terms:*

1.   polycythemia   _____

2.   serum   _____

3.   leukopenia   _____

4.   hemoglobin   _____

5.   anemia   _____

6.   thrombocytopenia   _____

7.   leukocytosis   _____

8.   hemostasis   _____

9.   plasma   _____

10.   hematocrit   _____

11. prothrombin time _____

_____

12. hemolysis _____

_____

Review Questions

1. What do the hematology and coagulation laboratory departments study?

_____

_____

_____

_____

2. List five types of substances that blood transports.

_____

_____

_____

_____

3. Compare and contrast whole blood, plasma, and serum.

_____

_____

_____

_____

4. Discuss the functions of red blood cells.

_____

_____

_____

_____

5. Discuss the functions of white blood cells.

_____

_____

_____

_____

6. Discuss the functions of platelets.

_____

_____

_____

_____

7. Explain how hemoglobin and hematocrit determinations are related.

_____

_____

_____

_____

8. What is the purpose of the differential portion of the CBC?

_____

_____

_____

_____

9. Explain the INR format for reporting PT results.

_____

_____

_____

_____

10. Discuss hemostasis and the role of the coagulation process involved.

_____

_____

_____

_____

Critical Thinking Questions

1. Using table 42-1 from the textbook, determine if the following blood test results are within normal range or are abnormal.

   a. HCT (male): 47%

   _____

   _____

   _____

   _____

   b. Hgb (female): 11.6 g/dL

   _____

   _____

   _____

   _____

   c. total WBC count: 34,000

   _____

   _____

   _____

   _____

   d. ESR (male): 9 mm

   _____

   _____

   _____

   _____

   e. Hgb (male): 12.6 g/dL

   _____

   _____

   _____

   _____

f. PT: 17.2 seconds

_____

_____

_____

g. neutrophil count: 54%

_____

_____

_____

h. platelet count: 100,000/uL

_____

_____

_____

i. RBC (female) – 6.7 cells/uL

_____

_____

_____

_____

j. bleeding time: 16 minutes

_____

_____

_____

_____

2. You have just obtained a new medical assisting position at a hematology practice. You want to familiarize yourself with the different types of leukemia as well as the procedures that may be performed to diagnose these conditions. Research the various types of leukemia as well as any procedures that may be used for them.

_____

_____

_____

_____

3. Mrs. Sheila Anselm has just begun Coumadin therapy and is in for the second time in two weeks to have her INR done. She asks you why she has to get this blood test done so frequently. How would you respond to her?

_____

_____

_____

_____

Teamwork Exercises

1. In groups of two or three, take turns teaching each other how to operate the various hematology/coagulation analyzers in your classroom. Include all quality-control, calibration, and preventative maintenance procedures in the demonstrations.

2. In groups of two or three, practice the microhematocrit procedure on each other.

3. Form into groups of two or three. Your instructor will assign each group one of the following coagulation disorders to research and present to the rest of the class:

   a. hemophilia A

   b. hemophilia B

   c. disseminated intravascular coagulation

   d. thrombophilic disorder

   e. idiopathic thrombocytopenia

PROCEDURE 42-1 – MEASURING HEMOGLOBIN USING THE HEMOCUE ANALYZER

Name _____   Date _____   Score _____

Instructor _____

Task
Measure hemoglobin using the HemoCue analyzer.

Conditions
HemoCue analyzer
Calibrator cuvette
Quality-control sample
Testing cuvettes
Lancet
Alcohol preparation
Gauze
Gloves
Manufacturer's manual
Biohazardous waste container

Time: _____

Standard
In the time specified and within the scoring parameters determined by the instructor, the student will successfully measure hemoglobin using a HemoCue analyzer.

Points assigned reflect importance of step to meeting the task

Important = 1 pt.
Essential = 5 pts.
Critical = 15 pts.

Automatic failure results if any of the **CRITICAL TASKS** are omitted or performed incorrectly.

(To use a pass/fail system, instructors can record "P" or "F" in the "points earned (pass/fail)" column.)

PERFORMANCE STANDARDS	PTS	PTS EARNED (Pass/Fail)	COMMENTS
1. Washed or sanitized hands and put on gloves and other personal protective equipment (PPE) as designated by the facility.	5	_____	_____
2. Assembled the supplies.	1	_____	_____
3. Greeted and identified your patient and introduced self. Explained the procedure.	5	_____	_____
4. Calibrated the analyzer by putting the calibrator cuvette into the machine.	15	_____	_____
5. Performed the necessary quality-control procedures and recorded the results.	15	_____	_____

PERFORMANCE STANDARDS (cont.)	PTS	PTS EARNED (Pass/Fail)	COMMENTS
6. Performed a capillary puncture on the patient using the proper procedure.	5	_____	_____ _____
7. Using a testing cuvette, collected the appropriate specimen from the capillary puncture.	15	_____	_____ _____
8. Wiped off the end of the cuvette in the proper manner	5	_____	_____ _____
9. Placed the cuvette in the machine.	15	_____	_____
10. Read the results.	15	_____	_____
11. Recorded the results in the patient's chart.	5	_____	_____ _____
12. Disposed of the cuvette in the biohazardous waste container.	5	_____	_____ _____
13. Disinfected the equipment, if indicated.	5	_____	_____ _____
14. Disposed of the gloves and washed or sanitized hands.	5	_____	_____ _____

TOTAL POINTS	116		

DOCUMENTATION

COMMENTS

PROCEDURE 42-2 – MEASURING HEMATOCRIT USING A MICROHEMATOCRIT CENTRIFUGE

Name _____   Date _____   Score _____

                                     Instructor _____

Task
Measure hematocrit using a microhematocrit centrifuge.

Conditions
Microhematocrit centrifuge
Heparinized capillary tubes
Lancet
Gloves
Hematocrit reader grid
Sealing clay
Alcohol preparation
Gauze
Sharps container
Biohazardous waste container

Time: _____

Standard
In the time specified and within the scoring parameters determined by the instructor, the student will successfully measure hematocrit using a microhematocrit centrifuge.

Points assigned reflect importance of step to meeting the task

Important = 1 pt.
Essential = 5 pts.
Critical = 15 pts.

Automatic failure results if any of the **CRITICAL TASKS** are omitted or performed incorrectly.

(To use a pass/fail system, instructors can record "P" or "F" in the "points earned (pass/fail)" column.)

PERFORMANCE STANDARDS	PTS	PTS EARNED (Pass/Fail)	COMMENTS
1. Washed or sanitized hands and put on gloves and other personal protective equipment (PPE) as designated by facility.	5	_____	_____
2. Assembled the supplies.	1	_____	_____
3. Greeted and identified your patient and introduced yourself. Explained the procedure.	5	_____	_____
4. Performed a capillary puncture on the patient using the proper procedure.	5	_____	_____
5. Collected the appropriate specimen from the capillary puncture using the heparinized capillary tubes.	15	_____	_____

PERFORMANCE STANDARDS (cont.)	PTS	PTS EARNED (Pass/Fail)	COMMENTS
6. Filled both tubes as required.	15	_____	_____
7. Sealed both tubes by gently pushing the end of one tube into the clay two to three times.	15	_____	_____
8. Placed both tubes in the microhematocrit centrifuge, making sure the tubes were placed directly across from each other (also called *balanced*).	15	_____	_____
9. Secured the cover to the centrifuge and started the centrifuge timer for the desired time as indicated by the manufacturer's or your instructor's specifications.	15	_____	_____
10. Listened for the timer to go off. Allowed the centrifuge to come to a complete stop before opening it.	5	_____	_____
11. Inspected the tubes, making sure they were intact and not broken.	5	_____	_____
12. Read the results. Depending on the type of microhematocrit centrifuge, the cover may have had the reading grid on it or the student may have had to use a handheld hematocrit reader grid.	15	_____	_____
13. Disposed of both capillary tubes in a biohazardous waste container.	5	_____	_____
14. Recorded the results in the patient's chart.	5	_____	_____
15. Disinfected the centrifuge, if indicated.	5	_____	_____
16. Disposed of the gloves and washed or sanitized hands.	5	_____	_____

TOTAL POINTS	136		

DOCUMENTATION

COMMENTS

PROCEDURE 42-3 – MEASURING PROTHROMBIN TIME USING A CLIA-WAIVED ANALYZER

Name _____ Date _____ Score _____

Instructor _____

Task
Measure prothrombin time using a CLIA-waived analyzer.

Conditions
Prothrombin time analyzer
Test strips
Lancet
Alcohol preparation
Gauze
Biohazardous waste container
Gloves

Time: _____

Standard
In the time specified and within the scoring parameters determined by the instructor, the student will successfully measure prothrombin time using a CLIA-waived analyzer.

Points assigned reflect importance of step to meeting the task

Important = 1 pt.
Essential = 5 pts.
Critical = 15 pts.

Automatic failure results if any of the **CRITICAL TASKS** are omitted or performed incorrectly.

(To use a pass/fail system, instructors can record "P" or "F" in the "points earned (pass/fail)" column.)

PERFORMANCE STANDARDS	PTS	PTS EARNED (Pass/Fail)	COMMENTS
1. Washed or sanitized hands and put on gloves and any other personal protective equipment (PPE) as designated by the facility.	5	_____	
2. Assembled the supplies.	1	_____	
3. Greeted and identified your patient and introduced self. Explained the procedure.	5	_____	
4. Turned the meter on.	1	_____	
5. Inserted the test strip into the meter and checked the code. The test strip code must have matched the meter code.	15	_____	

PERFORMANCE STANDARDS (cont.)	PTS	PTS EARNED (Pass/Fail)	COMMENTS
6. Performed a capillary puncture on the patient.	5	_____	_____ _____
7. Applied a large hanging drop of blood to the test strip when prompted by the meter.	15	_____	_____ _____ _____
8. Waited for results to appear on the display.	15	_____	_____ _____
9. Read the results.	15	_____	_____ _____
10. Recorded the results correctly in the patient's chart.	15	_____	_____ _____
11. Disposed of the cuvette in the biohazardous waste container.	5	_____	_____ _____
12. Disinfected the equipment, if indicated.	5	_____	_____ _____
13. Disposed of the gloves and washed or sanitized hands.	5	_____	_____ _____

TOTAL POINTS	107		

DOCUMENTATION

_____

_____

_____

COMMENTS

_____

_____

_____

_____

Student Activity Manual to Accompany The Professional Medical Assistant

Clinical Chemistry and Serological Procedures

Key Term Review

Define the following key terms:

1. methodology

2. microsample

3. antibody

4. agglutination

5. panel

6. antigen

7. atherosclerosis

8. analyte

9. photometric reflectance

Review Questions

1. What kinds of substances can be measured in a person's blood?

   _____

   _____

   _____

   _____

2. What steps should a medical assistant take prior to operating a new chemistry analyzer?

   _____

   _____

   _____

   _____

3. What types of specimen can a chemistry analyzer test?

   _____

   _____

   _____

   _____

4. What is the function of insulin?

   _____

   _____

   _____

   _____

5. What is the purpose of performing a fasting blood glucose level?

   _____

   _____

   _____

   _____

6. Why is patient prep so important for a successful glucose tolerance test?

_____

_____

_____

_____

7. What is the importance of the Hgb A1c blood test to a diabetic patient?

_____

_____

_____

_____

8. List the tests that make up a lipid panel.

_____

_____

_____

_____

9. Discuss the role of cholesterol in the body.

_____

_____

_____

_____

10. Compare and contrast HDL with LDL.

_____

_____

_____

_____

11. List the blood tests that make up the following panels:

    a. cardiac:

    _____

    _____

    _____

    _____

b. hepatic:

_____

_____

_____

_____

c. renal:

_____

_____

_____

_____

d. comprehensive metabolic:

_____

_____

_____

_____

e. thyroid:

_____

_____

_____

_____

f. basic metabolic:

_____

_____

_____

_____

12. Compare and contrast the agglutination serological method with the ELISA method of testing.

_____

_____

_____

_____

13. Discuss the differences between an antigen and an antibody.

_____

_____

_____

_____

14. How is a person's blood type determined?

_____

_____

_____

_____

15. A person with a blood type of O positive can donate to which blood type(s)?

_____

_____

_____

_____

16. List some serological tests that can be performed in a POL.

_____

_____

_____

_____

Critical Thinking

1. Using the Common Blood Chemistry Tests table from the textbook, determine if the following blood test results are within normal range or are abnormal.

    a. K+: 4.6 mmol/L:

_____

_____

_____

_____

b. cholesterol: 185 mg/dL:

_____

_____

_____

_____

c. iron: 67 ug/dL:

_____

_____

_____

_____

d. glucose: 142 mg/dL:

_____

_____

_____

_____

e. ALT: 33 units/L:

_____

_____

_____

_____

f. CO_2: 18 mmol/L:

_____

_____

_____

g. CK-MB: 12.6 ng/mL:

_____

_____

_____

_____

h. Na+: 148 mmol/L:

_____

_____

_____

_____

i. TSH: 3.7 million IU/mL:

_____

_____

_____

_____

j. Cl–: 99 mmol/L:

_____

_____

_____

_____

2. Jamie Santos is being scheduled for a 3-hour GTT, because her FBG was 136 mg/dL. Your job is to explain the procedure for the test, which includes the patient instructions prior to and during the test.

_____

_____

_____

3. You have just obtained a new medical assisting position at a diabetic clinic. You want to familiarize yourself with the different types of insulin so that you can better educate your patients. Research the various types of insulin and develop a drug card for each type.

_____

_____

_____

4. Mr. Miarecki has been diagnosed with hyperlipidemia. Your role as a medical assistant is to discuss the lifestyle changes he needs to make.

_____

_____

_____

_____

Teamwork Exercises

1. In groups of two or three, take turns teaching each other how to operate the various chemistry analyzers in your classroom. Include all quality-control, calibration, and preventative maintenance procedures in the demonstrations.

2. In groups of two, role-play being the medical assistant providing patient education for blood glucose monitoring to a newly diagnosed diabetic patient. Be sure to review all operating and maintenance procedures as well as patient documentation.

3. Form into groups of two or three. Your instructor will assign each group one of the following immunological disorders to research and present to the rest of the class:

   a. HIV/AIDS

   _____

   _____

   _____

   _____

   b. mononucleosis

   _____

   _____

   _____

   c. rheumatoid arthritis

   _____

   _____

   _____

d. lupus

_____

_____

_____

_____

e. syphilis

_____

_____

_____

_____

f. hemolytic disease of the newborn

_____

_____

_____

_____

PROCEDURE 43-1 – PERFORMING A BLOOD GLUCOSE TEST AND PATIENT EDUCATION FOR A GLUCOSE MONITORING SYSTEM

Name _____ Date _____ Score _____

Instructor _____

Task
Properly perform a capillary puncture and glucose test and instruct the patient in the care and use of a glucose monitoring system.

Conditions
Glucose monitoring system
Gloves
Alcohol wipe
Gauze
Lancet
Adhesive bandage
Test strips
Glucose control
Biohazardous waste container

Time: _____

Standards
In the time specified and within the scoring parameters determined by the instructor, the student will successfully perform a capillary puncture and glucose testing and instruct the patient in the care and use of a glucose monitoring system.

Points assigned reflect importance of step to meeting the task

Important = 1 pt.
Essential = 5 pts.
Critical = 15 pts.

Automatic failure results if any of the **CRITICAL TASKS** are omitted or performed incorrectly.

(To use a pass/fail system, instructors can record "P" or "F" in the "points earned (pass/fail)" column.)

PERFORMANCE STANDARDS	PTS	PTS EARNED (Pass/Fail)	COMMENTS
1. Washed or sanitized hands and assembled the supplies.	5	_____	
2. Put on gloves.	5	_____	
3. Identified the patient and explained the procedure.	5	_____	
4. Performed quality-control measures:			
a. Turned the meter on.	1	_____	
b. Checked the code number on the display with the code number on the test strip package, making sure they matched.	15	_____	
c. Inserted the test strip when prompted.	15	_____	

PERFORMANCE STANDARDS (cont.)	PTS	PTS EARNED (Pass/Fail)	COMMENTS
d. When APPLY SAMPLE appeared, applied one drop of quality-control reagent.	15	_____	_____
e. Read the meter for results.	5	_____	_____
f. Checked the results against the proper control range, as set by the manufacturer.	5	_____	_____
g. Repeated the process if necessary using additional control reagents, such as high or low values.	5	_____	_____
h. Recorded the results. Notified the instructor if controls were out of range.	5	_____	_____
5. Instructed the patient on how to operate the glucose monitoring system. Topics should have included:			_____
a. turning on the monitor	1	_____	_____
b. display area	1	_____	_____
c. proper code reading	1	_____	_____
d. proper testing strips	1	_____	_____
e. proper cleaning and care	1	_____	_____
6. Performed patient testing:			_____
a. Pressed the ON-OFF button.	1	_____	_____
b. Inserted the test strip.	5	_____	_____
c. Prepared the patient for capillary puncture.	5	_____	_____
d. Performed the puncture and wiped away the first drop of blood, then applied one drop of blood to the test strip without touching the test strip or smearing the blood.	15	_____	_____
e. Bandaged the patient's finger.	1	_____	_____
f. Read the results after hearing the beep.	15	_____	_____
g. Correctly recorded the results in the patient's chart.	15	_____	_____
h. Discussed with the patient the physician's orders and any necessary follow-up visits.	5	_____	_____

PERFORMANCE STANDARDS (cont.)	PTS	PTS EARNED (Pass/Fail)	COMMENTS
i. Removed the test strip and discarded all biohazardous material in the appropriate container.	5	_____	_____ _____

TOTAL POINTS	153		

DOCUMENTATION

COMMENTS

PROCEDURE 43-2 – PERFORMING CHOLESTEROL OR LIPID PANEL TESTING

Name _____   Date _____   Score _____

                                              Instructor _____

Task

Perform cholesterol or lipid panel testing using a CLIA-waived instrument.

Conditions

Cholesterol instrument
Gloves
Alcohol wipe
Gauze
Lancet
Capillary tubes and other supplies as required by manufacturer
Adhesive bandage
Test strips
Control reagents
Calibration cassette
Biohazardous waste container

Time: _____

Standard

In the time specified and within the scoring parameters determined by the instructor, the student will successfully perform cholesterol or lipid panel testing.

Points assigned reflect importance of step to meeting the task

Important = 1 pt.
Essential = 5 pts.
Critical = 15 pts.

Automatic failure results if any of the **CRITICAL TASKS** are omitted or performed incorrectly.

(To use a pass/fail system, instructors can record "P" or "F" in the "points earned (pass/fail)" column.)

PERFORMANCE STANDARDS	PTS	PTS EARNED (Pass/Fail)	COMMENTS
1. Washed or sanitized hands and assembled supplies.	5	_____	_____
2. Put on gloves.	5	_____	_____
3. Identified the patient and explained the procedure.	5	_____	_____
4. Performed quality-control measures:			_____
a. Turned the instrument on, and watched as it performed a self-test.	1	_____	_____
b. Removed the cassette from the pouch without touching the black bar or magnetic strip. Placed the cassette on a flat surface.	1	_____	_____

PERFORMANCE STANDARDS (cont.)	PTS	PTS EARNED (Pass/Fail)	COMMENTS
c. Applied a quality-control reagent to the well of the cassette. Placed the cassette in the drawer and pressed the RUN button.	15	_____	_____
d. Read the results after the beep sounded.	5	_____	_____
e. Checked the results against the control range, as set by the manufacturer.	15	_____	_____
f. Repeated the process if necessary using additional control reagents, such as high or low values.	5	_____	_____
g. Recorded the results. Notified the instructor if a control was out of range. If quality-control results were out of range, corrective action must have taken place prior to any patient testing.	5	_____	_____
5. Performed patient testing steps:			
a. Prepared the patient for capillary puncture.	1	_____	_____
b. Removed the cassette from the pouch without touching the black bar or magnetic strip. Placed the cassette on a flat surface.	1	_____	_____
c. Performed the puncture, wiped away the first drop of blood, and then collected the blood in the capillary tube.	15	_____	_____
d. Applied the sample to the well of the cassette within 5 minutes of collection.	15	_____	_____
e. Placed the cassette in the drawer and pressed the RUN button.	15	_____	_____
f. Bandaged the patient's finger.	1	_____	_____
g. Read the results after hearing the beep.	5	_____	_____
h. Recorded the results in the patient's chart.	15	_____	_____
i. Talked to the patient about the physician's orders and follow-up.	5	_____	_____

PERFORMANCE STANDARDS (cont.)	PTS	PTS EARNED (Pass/Fail)	COMMENTS
j. Removed the test strip and discarded all biohazardous material appropriately.	5	_____	_____
k. Removed the results and washed your hands.	5	_____	_____

TOTAL POINTS	145		

DOCUMENTATION

COMMENTS

Urinalysis

Key Term Review   *Define the following key terms:*

1.   turbid   _____

   _____

2.   anuria   _____

   _____

3.   renal threshold   _____

   _____

4.   dysuria   _____

   _____

5.   specific gravity   _____

   _____

6.   glycosuria   _____

   _____

7.   polyuria   _____

   _____

8.   hematuria   _____

   _____

9.   proteinuria   _____

   _____

10.   ketonuria   _____

   _____

11.　　　　nocturia　　_____

　　　　　　　　　　　_____

12.　　　　oliguria　　_____

　　　　　　　　　　　_____

Review Questions

1. For the following urinary system structures, provide their function:

   a. urethra:

   _____

   _____

   _____

   _____

   b. kidneys:

   _____

   _____

   _____

   _____

   c. urinary bladder:

   _____

   _____

   _____

   _____

   d. ureters:

   _____

   _____

   _____

   _____

2. What are some substances that are found in urine?

_____

_____

_____

_____

3. How much urine does a person normally produce in one day?

_____

_____

_____

_____

4. Provide some causes for the following urine output conditions:

   a. dysuria:

_____

_____

_____

_____

   b. nocturia:

_____

_____

_____

_____

   c. oliguria:

_____

_____

_____

_____

   d. anuria:

_____

_____

_____

_____

e. polyuria:

_____

_____

_____

_____

5. List and explain the six types of urine specimen that can be collected.

_____

_____

_____

_____

6. What are some guidelines the medical assistant must take into consideration when collecting, handling, and processing a urine specimen?

_____

_____

_____

_____

7. What are the three components of a urinalysis?

_____

_____

_____

_____

8. Describe reasons for the color of urine to be abnormal.

_____

_____

_____

_____

9. What does specific gravity measure in a urine sample?

_____

_____

_____

_____

10. What could a urine with a fruity odor indicate?

_____

_____

_____

_____

11. Explain renal threshold and how it relates to urine glucose testing.

_____

_____

_____

_____

12. What are some reasons why a urine may contain protein?

_____

_____

_____

_____

13. Explain how bilirubin is formed and its connection to urobilinogen.

_____

_____

_____

_____

14. Explain the connection between the nitrite and the leukocyte chemical components of the reagent strip. If both results are positive, what could that indicate?

_____

_____

_____

_____

15. Discuss the various components that can be seen in the microscopic evaluation of urine.

_____

_____

_____

_____

16. How are urinary casts formed?

_____

_____

_____

_____

17. What are some causes of urinary crystals?

_____

_____

_____

_____

18. Which hormone does the urine pregnancy test detect?

_____

_____

_____

_____

Critical Thinking

1. During an office staff meeting, the clinical supervisor reports that many urine specimens collected by patients have been unacceptable for testing. What are some suggestions you could provide to the clinical supervisor?

_____

_____

_____

_____

2. You are performing quality control on the urinalysis reagent strips and observe that both the normal and abnormal controls are out of range. Discuss some reasons for the out-of-range results.

_____

_____

_____

_____

3. Seventeen-year-old Stacy Hermanski was in your office this morning for a urine pregnancy test. During the afternoon, you receive a phone call from Mrs. Hermanski asking if the results of Stacy's pregnancy test are in yet. How would you respond?

_____

_____

_____

_____

Teamwork Exercises

1. Divide into pairs. Role-play with your partner the proper ways to collect a clean voided mid-stream urine for both males and females. Provide feedback after each scenario.

2. Divide into groups of two or three. Take turns performing the physical and chemical analysis of urine, making sure to perform any quality-control procedures. If your classroom has a urine analyzer, test specimens using both manual and automated methods. Compare your results.

3. Divide into groups of two or three. Take turns performing a urine pregnancy test, making sure to include any quality-control procedures.

PROCEDURE 44-1 – INSTRUCTING PATIENT ON COLLECTING A CLEAN-CATCH MIDSTREAM URINE SPECIMEN

Name _____   Date _____   Score _____

                                          Instructor _____

Task
Instruct a patient on how to collect a clean-catch, midstream urine specimen.

Conditions
Sterile screw-cap container
Computer-generated patient label
Antiseptic towelettes (2)

Time: _____

Standard
In the time specified and within the scoring parameters determined by the instructor, the student will success-fully instruct a patient on how to collect a clean-catch, midstream urine specimen.

Points assigned reflect importance of step to meeting the task

Important = 1 pt.
Essential = 5 pts.
Critical = 15 pts.

Automatic failure results if any of the **CRITICAL TASKS** are omitted or performed incorrectly.

(To use a pass/fail system, instructors can record "P" or "F" in the "points earned (pass/fail)" column.)

PERFORMANCE STANDARDS	PTS	PTS EARNED (Pass/Fail)	COMMENTS
1. Washed or sanitized hands and assembled the equipment.	5	_____	_____
2. Greeted the patient, introduced self, and explained the proper collection procedure.	1	_____	_____
For female patients			
3. For female patients, instructed the patient to:			_____
a. Wash her hands and remove her undergarments.	1	_____	_____
b. Expose the urinary meatus by spreading the labia apart with the nondominant hand.	5	_____	_____

PERFORMANCE STANDARDS (cont.)	PTS	PTS EARNED (Pass/Fail)	COMMENTS
c. Take one of the towelettes and clean one side of the urinary meatus from the front to the back on one side. Repeat the same procedure with the other towelette on the opposite side of the meatus.	5	_____	
d. Continue to keep the labia spread apart and void a small amount of urine into the toilet	5	_____	
e. Collect the next amount of urine by voiding into the sterile container.	5	_____	
f. After filling the container adequately, void the remaining urine into the toilet.	5	_____	
g. Wipe the area and wash her hands.	1	_____	
h. Securely cap the specimen container and place it in the specified area. (The area in the physician's office laboratory or hospital laboratory designated for specimens.)	5	_____	

For male patients

	PTS	PTS EARNED	COMMENTS
4. For male patients, instructed the patient to:			
a. Wash his hands and remove his underwear.	1	_____	
b. If uncircumcised, retract the foreskin and hold it back during the entire procedure.	5	_____	
c. Clean the area around the penile opening (glans penis) by starting at the tip of the penis and cleaning downward, using a separate towelette for each side.	5	_____	
d. Void a small amount of urine into the toilet. Excreting a small amount of urine before collection clears the urethra of contaminants and thus ensures accurate results.	5	_____	

PERFORMANCE STANDARDS (cont.)	PTS	PTS EARNED (Pass/Fail)	COMMENTS
e. Collect the next amount of urine by voiding into the sterile container, being careful not to touch the inside of the container with the hand or penis.	5	_____	_____
f. After filling the container adequately, void the last amount of urine into the toilet.	5	_____	_____
g. Dry the area and wash his hands.	1	_____	_____
h. Securely cap the specimen container and place it in the specified area.	5	_____	_____

TOTAL POINTS	70		

DOCUMENTATION

COMMENTS

PROCEDURE 44-2 – PERFORMING A URINALYSIS

Name _____

Date _____ Score _____

Instructor _____

Task

Perform and document a urinalysis.

Conditions

Sterile specimen cup
Computer-generated label
Urine reagent strips or Clinitek automatic urine analyzer
Clean glass microscope slide
Clean glass microscope coverslip
Microscope
Blank urine report form or the patient's chart
Paper towel
Disposable examination gloves
Plastic centrifuge tube
Gown or laboratory coat with a zipper or button closure
Biohazardous waste container

Time: _____

Standard

In the time specified and within the scoring parameters determined by the instructor, the student will successfully perform and document a urinalysis.

Points assigned reflect importance of step to meeting the task

Important = 1 pt.
Essential = 5 pts.
Critical = 15 pts.

Automatic failure results if any of the **CRITICAL TASKS** are omitted or performed incorrectly.

(To use a pass/fail system, instructors can record "P" or "F" in the "points earned (pass/fail)" column.)

PERFORMANCE STANDARDS	PTS	PTS EARNED (Pass/Fail)	COMMENTS
1. Assembled the supplies. Accurately completed the label and affixed it to the specimen cup (not to the lid).	5	_____	
2. Greeted and identified your patient. Introduced self and explained the procedure for collecting a clean-catch midstream urine specimen.	5	_____	
3. Washed or sanitized hands and applied gloves.	1	_____	
4. Obtained the urine specimen from the patient.	1	_____	
5. Observed the specimen for physical characteristics, such as color, clarity, and odor.	15	_____	

PERFORMANCE STANDARDS (cont.)	PTS	PTS EARNED (Pass/Fail)	COMMENTS
6. Recorded observations on the blank urine report form or in the patient's chart.	15	_____	_____ _____ _____
7. Poured the specimen into a conical centrifuge tube.	5	_____	_____ _____
8. Tested the urine using a chemical reagent strip, making sure all test pads had been exposed to the urine.	15	_____	_____ _____ _____
9. Tapped the side of the strip gently on a paper towel to remove excess urine.	1	_____	_____ _____
10. After waiting for the required time, according to the manufacturer's guidelines, read each reagent pad and recorded the results on the urine report form or in the patient's chart.	15	_____	_____ _____ _____ _____ _____ _____
11. Centrifuged the tube for 5 minutes at 1,500 rpm.	5	_____	_____ _____
12. Poured off the fluid and tapped the bottom of the tube to mix the remaining contents.	5	_____	_____ _____ _____
13. Placed a drop of sediment on a glass slide and covered with a coverslip.	5	_____	_____ _____
14. Placed the slide on the microscope stage.	5	_____	_____ _____
15. Notified the physician that the slide was ready for evaluation and provided the urine report form or the patient's chart so the physician could document the results.	5	_____	_____ _____ _____ _____ _____
16. Disposed of the biological materials in appropriate containers.	5	_____	_____ _____

PERFORMANCE STANDARDS (cont.)	PTS	PTS EARNED (Pass/Fail)	COMMENTS
17. Removed gloves and washed hands.	1	_____	_____
18. Recorded the procedure in the patient's chart.	5	_____	_____ _____

TOTAL POINTS	114		

DOCUMENTATION

COMMENTS

_____

_____

_____

_____

PROCEDURE 44-3 – PERFORMING A URINE PREGNANCY TEST

Name _____   Date _____   Score _____

Instructor _____

Task

Perform a urine pregnancy test according to the manufacturer's instructions.

Conditions

Disposable examination gloves
Patient urine specimen
Urine pregnancy test kit
Biohazardous waste container

Time: _____

Standard

In the time specified and within the scoring parameters determined by the instructor, the student will successfully perform a urine pregnancy test according to the manufacturer's instructions.

Points assigned reflect importance of step to meeting the task

Important = 1 pt.
Essential = 5 pts.
Critical = 15 pts.

Automatic failure results if any of the **CRITICAL TASKS** are omitted or performed incorrectly.

(To use a pass/fail system, instructors can record "P" or "F" in the "points earned (pass/fail)" column.)

PERFORMANCE STANDARDS	PTS	PTS EARNED (Pass/Fail)	COMMENTS
1. Washed or sanitized your hands and gathered the supplies.	1	_____	_____
2. Obtained a testing cassette or stick, reagents, and a urine specimen.	1	_____	_____
3. Following the manufacturer's instructions, performed and documented the necessary quality-control measures.	15	_____	_____
4. Following the manufacturer's instructions, applied urine to the testing cassette or stick.	15	_____	_____
5. Waited the appropriate time interval.	15	_____	_____
6. Applied other reagents if specified by the manufacturer.	15	_____	_____

PERFORMANCE STANDARDS (cont.)	PTS	PTS EARNED (Pass/Fail)	COMMENTS
7. Read the results.	5	_____	_____
8. Removed your gloves and washed your hands.	1	_____	_____ _____
9. Documented the procedure.	5	_____	_____ _____

TOTAL POINTS	73		

DOCUMENTATION

COMMENTS

Microbiology

Key Term Review   *Define the following key terms:*

1.   pathogenic   _____

_____

2.   cocci   _____

_____

3.   normal flora   _____

_____

4.   prion   _____

_____

5.   culture   _____

_____

6.   bacilli   _____

_____

7.   antimicrobial
agent   _____

_____

8.   virus   _____

_____

9.   infectious disease   _____

_____

10.   parasite   _____

_____

11.   smear   _____

_____

Key Term Review *cont.*

12. resistance _____

_____

13. incubation period _____

_____

14. fungus _____

_____

15. contagious _____

_____

Review Questions

1. Discuss three scientists and how they contributed to the field of microbiology.

_____

_____

_____

_____

2. What does it mean if an infection is contagious?

_____

_____

_____

_____

3. What are the various means of infectious disease transmission?

_____

_____

_____

_____

4. Discuss the role normal flora plays in the body.

_____

_____

_____

_____

5. List four sites where normal flora is usually found in the body.

_____

_____

_____

_____

6. List five types of microorganisms and provide two examples of each type.

_____

_____

_____

_____

7. Discuss some characteristics of bacteria.

_____

_____

_____

_____

8. What is the purpose of performing a Gram's stain?

_____

_____

_____

_____

9. Compare and contrast viruses and prions.

_____

_____

_____

_____

10. Discuss some characteristics of fungi.

_____

_____

_____

_____

11. Describe the life cycle of a protozoa.

_____

_____

_____

_____

12. What are some ways patients become infected with parasitic worms?

_____

_____

_____

_____

13. Describe the two most common methods of antibiotic susceptibility testing.

_____

_____

_____

_____

14. For the following microorganisms, indicate whether it's a bacterium, fungus, virus, or parasite (protozoa or worm):

a. _Giardia lamblia:_

_____

_____

_____

b. _Candida albicans:_

_____

_____

_____

c. *Borrelia burgdorferi:*

_____

_____

_____

_____

d. *Chlamydia trachomatis:*

_____

_____

_____

_____

e. *Enterobius vermicularis:*

_____

_____

_____

_____

f. *Ascaris lumbricoides:*

_____

_____

_____

_____

g. *Cryptococcus neoformans:*

_____

_____

_____

_____

h. HIV:

_____

_____

_____

_____

i. *Salmonella species:*

_____

_____

_____

_____

j. *Cryptosporidium species:*

_____

_____

_____

_____

15. For the following microorganisms, provide some diseases or conditions associated with them:

a. *E. coli*:

_____

_____

_____

_____

b. *Cryptosporidium* species:

_____

_____

_____

_____

c. *Helicobacter pylori*:

_____

_____

_____

_____

d. Enterobius vermicularis:

_____

_____

_____

_____

e. Varicella zoster:

_____

_____

_____

_____

f. *Pseudomonas aeruginosa*:

_____

_____

_____

_____

g. Candida albicans:

_____

_____

_____

_____

h. *Chlamydia trachomatis*:

_____

_____

_____

_____

i. *Haemophilus influenzae*:

_____

_____

_____

_____

Critical Thinking

1. Jake Owen is a 9-year-old boy who has been suffering from profuse, watery diarrhea for one week. The physician's orders read "O&P and stool culture X3." Explain to Jake's father the purpose of the specialized stool collection and how to collect the specimens.

   _____

   _____

   _____

   _____

2. As the clinical medical assistant in your practice, you receive a phone call from the hospital laboratory. The microbiology technologist needs to give you a STAT report on April Lang's blood culture. How do you handle the call?

   _____

   _____

   _____

   _____

3. Antibiotic resistance is becoming a real threat to society. How can you, as a medical assistant, educate patients on the best means to avoid bacteria from becoming resistant to antibiotics?

   _____

   _____

   _____

   _____

Teamwork Exercises

1. Divide into groups of two or three students. Using sterile specimen collection swabs, choose sites in and around your classroom to obtain environmental cultures (examples of sites include door knobs, phones, toilet handles, and water bubblers). Process your swabs onto blood agar or nutrient agar media plates and place plates in a 37°C incubator. After 24 to 48 hours, observe the plates for any bacteria growth. Describe the color, size, shape, and odor of any growth. Compare the growth from your group with the other groups. Questions to ponder include: Which environmental sites had the most growth? Which sites had no bacterial growth? If possible, refer your plates to a microbiology professor for his or her professional opinion of what the growth may be.

2. Form into groups of two or three. Your instructor will assign each group one of the following infectious diseases to research and present to the rest of the class.

   a. impetigo

   b. meningococcal meningitis

   c. streptococcal pneumonia

   d. Lyme disease

   e. syphilis

   f. gonorrhea

Note to the instructor: Procedure 45-1 and 45-4 or 45-1 and 45-5 can be assessed together.

PROCEDURE 45-1 – COLLECTING A THROAT SPECIMEN FOR MICROBIOLOGICAL TESTING

Name _____ Date _____ Score _____

Instructor _____

Task
Collect a throat specimen for culture or rapid *Strep* testing.

Conditions
Disposable examination gloves
Tongue depressor
Sterile culture swab
Label
Laboratory requisition slip
Biohazardous specimen transport bag
Biohazardous waste container

Time: _____

Standard
In the time specified and within the scoring parameters determined by the instructor, the student will successfully collect a throat specimen for culture or rapid *Strep* testing.

Points assigned reflect importance of step to meeting the task

Important = 1 pt.
Essential = 5 pts.
Critical = 15 pts.

Automatic failure results if any of the **CRITICAL TASKS** are omitted or performed incorrectly.

(To use a pass/fail system, instructors can record "P" or "F" in the "points earned (pass/fail)" column.)

PERFORMANCE STANDARDS	PTS	PTS EARNED (Pass/Fail)	COMMENTS
1. Greeted and identified the patient. Introduced self and explained the procedure.	5	_____	_____
2. Washed or sanitized hands and gathered supplies.	1	_____	_____
3. Positioned the patient in an upright, sitting position and adjusted the light if necessary.	1	_____	_____
4. Put on the gloves and mask. Instructed the patient to open his mouth widely.	15	_____	_____

PERFORMANCE STANDARDS (cont.)	PTS	PTS EARNED (Pass/Fail)	COMMENTS
5. Removed the swab from the tube. While depressing the patient's tongue with a tongue depressor, swabbed the back of the patient's throat and tonsils, taking care to thoroughly swab areas that appeared inflamed or covered in exudate. Also took care to avoid touching the patient's tongue or teeth.	15	_____	
6. Placed the swab back in the tube and crushed the transport media ampule.	5	_____	
7. Disposed of the tongue blade in the waste container. Applied the label to the culture tube and attached the completed requisition slip per laboratory policy.	1	_____	
8. Removed the gloves and mask and washed hands. Documented the procedure.	5	_____	

TOTAL POINTS	48		

DOCUMENTATION

COMMENTS

PROCEDURE 45-2 – COLLECTING A WOUND SPECIMEN FOR CULTURE

Name _____   Date _____   Score _____

Instructor _____

Task
Collect a wound specimen for culture.

Conditions
Sterile culture swab
Label
Laboratory requisition slip
Biohazardous specimen transport bag
Disposable examination gloves
Gown or laboratory coat with a zipper or button closure
Biohazardous waste container

Time: _____

Standard
In the time specified and within the scoring parameters determined by the instructor, the student will successfully collect a wound specimen for culture.

Points assigned reflect importance of step to meeting the task

Important = 1 pt.
Essential = 5 pts.
Critical = 15 pts.

Automatic failure results if any of the **CRITICAL TASKS** are omitted or performed incorrectly.

(To use a pass/fail system, instructors can record "P" or "F" in the "points earned (pass/fail)" column.)

PERFORMANCE STANDARDS	PTS	PTS EARNED (Pass/Fail)	COMMENTS
1. Assembled the supplies.	1	_____	_____
2. Greeted and identified your patient. Introduced self and explained the procedure.	5	_____	_____ _____
3. Washed or sanitized your hands.	1	_____	_____
4. Cleaned and decontaminated the surrounding skin area.	5	_____	_____ _____
5. Swabbed the infected area, being sure to swab any purulent discharge.	15	_____	_____ _____
6. Properly inserted the swab into the collection tube and activated the transport medium by squeezing the bottom of the tube.	15	_____	_____ _____ _____ _____

PERFORMANCE STANDARDS *(cont.)*	PTS	PTS EARNED (Pass/Fail)	COMMENTS
7. Labeled the culture swab with the patient's name, the date and time, and the specific site of the specimen and placed it in the proper biohazardous transport bag.	15	_____	
8. Completed the laboratory requisition slip and attached it to the specimen bag, according to facility policy. Sent the specimen to the laboratory in a timely manner.	5	_____	
9. Properly disposed of all supplies and washed hands.	5	_____	
10. Documented the procedure.	5	_____	

TOTAL POINTS	72		

DOCUMENTATION

COMMENTS

PROCEDURE 45-3 – COLLECTING A SPUTUM SPECIMEN FOR CULTURE

Name _____   Date _____   Score _____

                                          Instructor _____

Task
Collect a sputum specimen for culture.

Conditions
Sterile specimen cup
Label
Laboratory requisition slip
Approved specimen container bag
Disposable examination gloves
Face shield or mask and goggles
Gown or laboratory coat with a zipper or button
  closure
Biohazardous waste container
Cup of water

Time: _____

Standard
In the time specified and within the scoring parameters determined by the instructor, the student will successfully collect a sputum specimen for culture.

Points assigned reflect importance of step to meeting the task

Important = 1 pt.
Essential = 5 pts.
Critical = 15 pts.

Automatic failure results if any of the **CRITICAL TASKS** are omitted or performed incorrectly.

(To use a pass/fail system, instructors can record "P" or "F" in the "points earned (pass/fail)" column.)

PERFORMANCE STANDARDS	PTS	PTS EARNED (Pass/Fail)	COMMENTS
1. Assembled the supplies.	1	_____	_____
2. Greeted and identified the patient. Introduced self and explained the procedure.	5	_____	_____ _____
3. Washed or sanitized hands and applied the face shield or mask and goggles.	1	_____	_____ _____
4. Handed a glass of water to the patient and asked her to rinse her mouth.	5	_____	_____ _____
5. Instructed the patient to take two deep breathes, cough deeply, and spit the sputum into the cup.	15	_____	_____ _____

PERFORMANCE STANDARDS (cont.)	PTS	PTS EARNED (Pass/Fail)	COMMENTS
6. Made sure that no one touched the inner surfaces of the cup or lid and applied the lid and secured it snugly. Completed the label and affixed it to the specimen cup (not to the lid). Placed the specimen cup into the specimen bag and sealed it.	15	_____	_____ _____ _____ _____ _____ _____
7. Affixed the requisition slip to the specimen bag according to facility policy and sent it to the laboratory in a timely manner.	5	_____	_____ _____ _____
8. Properly disposed of all supplies and washed hands. Documented the procedure.	5	_____	_____ _____

TOTAL POINTS	52		

DOCUMENTATION

COMMENTS

PROCEDURE 45-4 – PERFORMING A RAPID STREPTOCOCCAL TEST

Name _____ Date _____ Score _____

Instructor _____

Task
Perform a rapid streptococcal test.

Conditions
Commercial rapid streptococcal test kit
Disposable examination gloves
Gown or laboratory coat with a zipper or button closure
Biohazardous waste container

Time: _____

Standard
In the time specified and within the scoring parameters determined by the instructor, the student will successfully perform a rapid streptococcal test.

Points assigned reflect importance of step to meeting the task

Important = 1 pt.
Essential = 5 pts.
Critical = 15 pts.

Automatic failure results if any of the **CRITICAL TASKS** are omitted or performed incorrectly.

(To use a pass/fail system, instructors can record "P" or "F" in the "points earned (pass/fail)" column.)

PERFORMANCE STANDARDS	PTS	PTS EARNED (Pass/Fail)	COMMENTS
1. Assembled the supplies and prepared the test kit. Ran quality-control procedures before testing the patient specimen.	15	_____	_____ _____ _____
2. Greeted and identified the patient. Introduced self and explained the procedure.	5	_____	_____ _____ _____
3. Washed or sanitized hands and put on the gloves.	1	_____	_____ _____
4. Properly collected a throat specimen, taking care to avoid touching the patient's tongue or teeth with the swab.	15	_____	_____ _____ _____
5. Followed the manufacturer's directions and placed the required number of reagent drops into the plastic testing tube.	15	_____	_____ _____ _____

PERFORMANCE STANDARDS (cont.)	PTS	PTS EARNED (Pass/Fail)	COMMENTS
6. Placed the throat specimen swab into the swab chamber of the test cassette.	15	_____	_____ _____
7. Added the extraction solution to the chamber. Fluid should have filled the chamber to the rim (approximately 10 drops). When the fluid had been added, watched for the liquid to move across the results window.	15	_____	_____ _____ _____ _____ _____ _____
8. Began timing after adding the solution.	15	_____	_____ _____
9. After 5 minutes, read the results using the manufacturer's result chart.	15	_____	_____ _____ _____
10. Disposed of the throat swab and all testing supplies in a biohazardous waste container. Documented the results in the patient's chart.	5	_____	_____ _____ _____

TOTAL POINTS	116		

DOCUMENTATION

_____	_____
_____	_____
_____	_____
_____	_____

COMMENTS

_____
_____
_____
_____

PROCEDURE 45-5 – PROCESSING A THROAT CULTURE

Name _____   Date _____   Score _____

Instructor _____

Task
Process a throat culture.

Conditions
Sterile culture swab
Tongue depressor
Sheep blood agar media plate
Sterile disposable inoculation plastic loop
Bacitracin disc
37°C incubator
Approved specimen container bag
Disposable examination gloves
Gown or laboratory coat with a zipper or button
  closure
Biohazardous waste container

Time: _____

Standard
In the time specified and within the scoring parameters determined by the instructor, the student will successfully process a throat culture.

Points assigned reflect importance of step to meeting the task

Important = 1 pt.
Essential = 5 pts.
Critical = 15 pts.

Automatic failure results if any of the **CRITICAL TASKS** are omitted or performed incorrectly.

(To use a pass/fail system, instructors can record "P" or "F" in the "points earned (pass/fail)" column.)

PERFORMANCE STANDARDS	PTS	PTS EARNED (Pass/Fail)	COMMENTS
1. Assembled the supplies.	1	_____	_____
2. Greeted and identified the patient. Introduced self and explained the procedure.	5	_____	_____
3. Washed or sanitized hands and put on the gloves.	1	_____	_____
4. Properly collected the throat specimen, taking care to avoid touching the patient's tongue or teeth.	15	_____	_____
5. Rolled the swab onto the top quarter of the blood agar plate to create the primary streak.	15	_____	_____
6. Using a sterile disposable plastic inoculation loop, spread the specimen from the primary streak into a secondary and tertiary streak.	15	_____	_____

PERFORMANCE STANDARDS *(cont.)*	PTS	PTS EARNED (Pass/Fail)	COMMENTS
7. Placed the bacitracin disc on the primary streak of the sheep blood agar plate.	15	_____	_____ _____
8. Incubated the sheep blood agar plate in the 37°C incubator for 18 to 24 hours. Did not incubate the specimen for more than 24 hours.	15	_____	_____ _____ _____
9. After 18 to 24 hours, removed the sheep blood agar plate from the incubator and read the results. If beta streptococcus group A was present, there would have been be a zone of inhibition around the bacitracin disc.	15	_____	_____ _____ _____ _____ _____ _____
10. Properly disposed of all supplies and washed hands. Documented the procedure in the patient's chart.	5	_____	_____ _____

TOTAL POINTS	102		

DOCUMENTATION

COMMENTS

Bioemergency Response and Preparedness

Key Term Review

Define the following key terms:

1. pandemic flu

2. covert event

3. bioterrorism

4. overt event

5. pandemic

6. influenza

7. bioterrorism agent

Review Questions

1. What is bioterrorism? Describe some bioterrorism events that have occurred through history.

   _____

   _____

   _____

   _____

2. Discuss the importance of bioemergency preparedness for the medical office.

   _____

   _____

   _____

   _____

3. What is the difference between an overt bioterrorism event and a covert event?

   _____

   _____

   _____

   _____

4. List the three CDC categories of bioterrorism agents, and provide at least two agents within each category.

   _____

   _____

   _____

   _____

5. Describe the importance of the laboratory response network.

   _____

   _____

   _____

   _____

6. What is the medical assistant's role when faced with a patient who may be infected with a possible bioterrorism agent?

_____

_____

_____

_____

7. Describe some guidelines when collecting a patient specimen that may be infected with a bioterrorism agent.

_____

_____

_____

_____

8. What is a pandemic flu?

_____

_____

_____

_____

9. What are some of the viruses that scientists are concerned about becoming a pandemic flu?

_____

_____

_____

_____

10. Describe the six phases of pandemic flu that the WHO has developed.

_____

_____

_____

_____

11. List some ways for a medical office to prepare in the event of a pandemic flu outbreak.

_____

_____

_____

_____

12. List some governmental Web sites that provide information on bioemergency preparedness.

_____

_____

_____

_____

Critical Thinking

1. As a member of your facility's emergency preparedness committee, you are responsible for developing a pandemic flu information sheet as well as a checklist or plan explaining to patients how to prepare for and what type of supplies to have at home in the event of a pandemic flu. Where would you look for factual information to include in this information sheet? Using the information you found, develop the patient fact sheet.

_____

_____

_____

_____

2. Research your area to find out where you can take a bioterrorism preparedness course or attend a seminar. List the agencies or institutions that offer such a course or seminar. If you find there is no such offering in your area, look online for an Internet course.

_____

_____

_____

_____

Teamwork Exercise

1. Working in groups of two or three, your instructor will assign each group a biological terrorism agent to research and give a PowerPoint presentation on.

2. Working in groups of two or three, your instructor will assign a biosafety level for each group to research and come up with a plan for their college laboratory to be able to adhere to the laboratory standards for that level.

Office Project

Prepare contact list of your local and state departments of public health, reference laboratories, hospitals, and other governmental agencies that may need to be contacted during a bioterrorism event or pandemic flu outbreak. Be sure to include telephone numbers and Web sites.

Office Emergencies

Key Term Review

Define the following key terms:

1.   protocol

2.   mock code

3.   triage

4.   automated external defibrillator

5.   recorder

6.   crash cart

7.   team captain

8.   defibrillator

Review Questions

1. What are some emergencies a medical assistant may experience in the office?

   _____

   _____

   _____

   _____

2. List six examples of emergency equipment that should be in a crash cart.

   _____

   _____

   _____

   _____

3. List six examples of emergency supplies that should be in a crash cart.

   _____

   _____

   _____

   _____

4. List six examples of emergency medicines that should be in a crash cart.

   _____

   _____

   _____

   _____

5. Differentiate between a standard defibrillator and an AED.

   _____

   _____

   _____

   _____

6. Explain the concept of triage.

   _____

   _____

   _____

   _____

7. List and describe the ABCs of basic emergency care.

_____

_____

_____

_____

8. What kinds of information should the medical assistant gather from a patient during phone triage?

_____

_____

_____

_____

9. Besides angina and a myocardial infarction, what other conditions can cause chest pain?

_____

_____

_____

_____

10. What are some advantages to using a tissue adhesive such as Dermabond to close a laceration?

_____

_____

_____

_____

11. What are some common causes for a patient to have a sudden alteration in consciousness? How should a medical assistant react to a patient who has lost consciousness?

_____

_____

_____

_____

12. What are some causes of poisoning? What are the symptoms that may accompany such types of poisonings?

_____

_____

_____

_____

13. Discuss five different environmental injuries, their signs and symptoms, and how to manage each.

_____

_____

_____

_____

14. Discuss how burns are classified.

_____

_____

_____

_____

15. Give five causes of acute abdominal pain.

_____

_____

_____

_____

16. A patient has experienced a severe injury to his lower leg. What must the medical assistant consider before applying a splint to the area?

_____

_____

_____

_____

Critical Thinking

1. You are doing your weekly grocery shopping and noticed a child who is having difficulty breathing and the mother is screaming for help. You are certified medical assistant who is trained in CPR and first aid. Describe how you would respond to this situation.

   _____

   _____

   _____

   _____

2. As a medical assistant, you are interested in becoming a certified instructor for basic life support. Research in your community where you could take such a course. Are there different agencies that offer this course? If so, compare and contrast the various courses.

   _____

   _____

   _____

   _____

3. Paula Trenton has just been diagnosed with severe bee sting anaphylaxis. She is very upset that as a mother with children who participate in many outdoor activities, her likelihood of being stung by a bee is increased and she is fearful that if it happened, no one would know what was happening to her. What are some suggestions you can give to Paula to help ease her anxiety?

   _____

   _____

   _____

   _____

4. Mrs. Jennison has called the office regarding her 15-year-old daughter's ankle injury. She had already brought her daughter to the emergency room for x-rays, which were negative, but she wants to know what she should do for her daughter since the ankle is still swollen and she is still in pain. What advice would you give Mrs. Jennison?

   _____

   _____

   _____

   _____

Teamwork Exercise

1. Divide into pairs. Role-play the following phone triage scenarios. Each student will take turns being the medical assistant and gather the appropriate patient information by asking the proper questions:

   a. Patient is experiencing sharp pains in right upper quadrant.

   b. Patient has mumbled speech, seems disoriented on the phone.

   c. Frantic grandmother is calling about grandchild who may have put a raisin up her nostril.

   d. Patient just sliced his finger while preparing dinner.

2. Divide into groups of two or three. Your instructor will assign a scenario for your group to act out in front of the class. For each scenario, your group is to determine how to correctly handle the situation.

   a. A diabetic patient has just collapsed while walking from the waiting room to an examination room.

   b. A medical assistant just administered an injection of penicillin to a patient, and he appears to be going into anaphylactic shock.

   c. A medical assistant is attending her daughter's soccer game, and a player on the field has hit her head on the goal post and collapsed.

   d. A 12-year-old epileptic patient is having a seizure in the examination room.

   e. A medical assistant is vacationing with his family in Arizona. They are in a state forest and they hear a cry for help. As they rush to a person lying on the ground, he states "I've just been bitten by a snake!"

Office Project

As a class, invite an emergency room physician, EMT, and/or paramedic to speak to your class about responding to emergency situations. Have the class create a list of questions to ask the individual/panel. Suggestions for questions may include each panel member's educational background, his or her opinions on the importance of lay people being CPR certified, and dealing with a high-pressure occupation.

Radiology and Diagnostic Imaging

Key Term Review   *Define the following key terms:*

1.   tracer   _____

_____

2.   fluoroscopy   _____

_____

3.   tomography   _____

_____

4.   cholecystogram   _____

_____

5.   dosimeter   _____

_____

6.   transducer   _____

_____

7.   claustrophobia   _____

_____

8.   contrast medium   _____

_____

9.   intravenous
       pyelogram   _____

10.   nuclear medicine   _____

_____

Key Term Review *cont.*

11.   radiolucent   _____
_____

12.   ultrasonography   _____
_____

Review Questions

1. How does the x-ray tube and the x-ray film work in combination to create an x-ray image?

2. Discuss the differences between radiopaque structures and radiolucent structures.

3. What sort of preexamination procedures must a patient take into consideration before having a basic x-ray?

4. Provide the proper positioning for the following x-rays:

    a. lower back:

b. extremities:

_____

_____

_____

_____

c. chest:

_____

_____

_____

_____

d. cervical spine:

_____

_____

_____

_____

5. Which health-care professionals are able to take x-rays?

_____

_____

_____

_____

6. Which health-care professionals are approved to read x-rays?

_____

_____

_____

_____

7. Discuss the proper care and maintenance of x-ray films.

_____

_____

_____

_____

8. What is the recommended schedule for a mammogram?

_____

_____

_____

_____

9. Discuss the fluoroscopy method of radiography.

_____

_____

_____

_____

10. List three examples of fluoroscopy exams.

_____

_____

_____

_____

11. Discuss the methodology behind ultrasound imaging.

_____

_____

_____

_____

12. Discuss the methodology behind MRI imaging.

_____

_____

_____

_____

13. Discuss five patient preparation considerations prior to having a mammogram.

_____

_____

_____

_____

14. What are some patient preparation considerations prior to a patient having an MRI?

_____

_____

_____

_____

15. Provide three reasons why a CAT scan may be performed.

_____

_____

_____

_____

16. Discuss the medical assistant's role in scheduling radiological examinations.

_____

_____

_____

_____

17. What are some side effects of radiation therapy?

_____

_____

_____

_____

18. Compare and contrast external radiation therapy with internal radiation therapy.

_____

_____

_____

_____

19. What is the purpose of a PET scan?

_____

_____

_____

_____

20. Discuss some radiation safety measures.

_____

_____

_____

_____

Critical Thinking

1. Genevieve Pierce-Gomes needs an upper GI series scheduled. Provide Genevieve the required patient preparation for this procedure.

_____

_____

_____

_____

2. Markus Stoltz is scheduled for a PET scan. After being told the procedure for the test, he expresses his concern about being injected with a radioisotope. What can you tell him?

_____

_____

_____

_____

Teamwork Exercise

1. Divide into groups of two or three students. Your instructor will assign each group one of the following procedures. Each group will develop a patient preparation guide for their procedure.

   a. MRA (not MRI)

   b. upper GI series

   c. IVP

   d. CAT scan

   e. PET scan

2. Divide the class into five groups. Your instructor will assign each group one of the following career opportunities in the field of radiology. Each group will develop a fact sheet on their career and include schools and colleges that offer such a program. In the fact sheet, make sure to include the courses within the program's curriculum.

   a. Radiology technician – hospital-based program

   b. Radiology technician – associate degree program

   c. Radiology technologist – bachelor degree program

   d. Ultrasound technician

   e. MRI technician

PROCEDURE 48-1 – PREPARING A PATIENT FOR AND ASSISTING WITH X-RAY EXAMINATION

Name _____   Date _____   Score _____

Instructor _____

Task
Prepare and position a patient for x-ray examination, label and store the x-ray, and document the procedure.

Conditions
Physician's order for x-ray examination
Patient identification card to imprint x-ray
X-ray machine and cassette with film loaded
Lead shield
Patient's medical record
X-ray processor, darkroom

Time: _____

Standards
In the time specified and within the scoring parameters determined by the instructor, the student will success-fully prepare and position the patient for x-ray exami-nation by the radiologic technologist, label and store the x-ray, and document the procedure.

Points assigned reflect importance of step to meeting the task

Important = 1 pt.
Essential = 5 pts.
Critical = 15 pts.

Automatic failure results if any of the **CRITICAL TASKS** are omitted or performed incorrectly.

(To use a pass/fail system, instructors can record "P" or "F" in the "points earned (pass/fail)" column.)

PERFORMANCE STANDARDS	PTS	PTS EARNED (Pass/Fail)	COMMENTS
1. Greeted and identified the patient and explained the examination procedure.	5	_____	_____
2. Checked the x-ray examination order.	1	_____	_____
3. Explained the procedure to the patient and obtained consent verbally or in written form, per office policy.	5	_____	_____
4. Asked a childbearing-age woman if she might be pregnant. If she was or might be, discontinued the procedure.	5	_____	_____
5. Placed the x-ray cassette in the machine.	1	_____	_____

PERFORMANCE STANDARDS (cont.)	PTS	PTS EARNED (Pass/Fail)	COMMENTS
6. Asked the patient to remove clothing and jewelry, as needed for the procedure.	5	_____	_____
7. Checked to make sure that the patient has removed all metal objects from the area to be examined.	15	_____	_____
8. Assisted the radiologic technologist with these steps, as requested:			_____
a. Positioned the patient against the x-ray film cassette.	5	_____	_____
b. Aligned the x-ray tube and cassette at the correct distance and set controls.	5	_____	_____
c. Asked the patient to hold her breath, if necessary.	5	_____	_____
9. While the x-ray machine was in use, left the room with the radiologic technologist and stood behind the lead shield.	15	_____	_____
10. Asked the patient to relax while the x-ray developed.	1	_____	_____
11. After the radiologic technologist developed the x-ray and confirmed that he does not need to repeat the procedure, asked the patient to dress.	5	_____	_____
12. Obtained the x-rays from the radiologic technologist and ensured that the films were properly named and dated.	5	_____	_____
13. Created a labeled x-ray envelope and placed the x-rays in it.	1	_____	_____
14. Documented the procedure in the patient's medical record.	5	_____	_____

TOTAL POINTS	84		

DOCUMENTATION

COMMENTS

PROCEDURE 48-2 – SCHEDULING A PATIENT FOR DIAGNOSTIC EXAMINATIONS

Name _____   Date _____   Score _____

                                           Instructor _____

Task
Schedule a patient for diagnostic examinations.

Conditions
Physician's order for specialty examination
Written instructions
Appointment card
Patient's medical record

Time: _____

Standard
In the time specified and within the scoring parameters determined by the instructor, the student will successfully explain pretesting instructions to the patient and schedule the procedure with an outside provider.

Points assigned reflect importance of step to meeting the task

Important = 1 pt.
Essential = 5 pts.
Critical = 15 pts.

Automatic failure results if any of the **CRITICAL TASKS** are omitted or performed incorrectly.

(To use a pass/fail system, instructors can record "P" or "F" in the "points earned (pass/fail)" column.)

PERFORMANCE STANDARDS	PTS	PTS EARNED (Pass/Fail)	COMMENTS
1. Reviewed the physician's order for testing.	1	_____	_____
2. Gave the patient written instructions for pre-test preparation.	1	_____	_____
3. Explained the pre-test preparation verbally to the patient.	1	_____	_____
4. Called the provider of the examination to be scheduled (hospital or radiology group) and asked to make an appointment for the examination.	5	_____	_____
5. Told the patient the available dates and times for the examination, and asked the patient to choose a date and time.	1	_____	_____

PERFORMANCE STANDARDS (cont.)	PTS	PTS EARNED (Pass/Fail)	COMMENTS
6. Confirmed the date, time, and type of examination on the phone with the scheduling personnel.	1	_____	_____ _____
7. Gave the patient an appointment card with the date and time of the examination. Provided driving directions to the examination site as needed.	5	_____	_____ _____ _____ _____ _____
8. Recorded the scheduled examination in the patient's medical record.	5	_____	_____ _____

TOTAL POINTS	20		

DOCUMENTATION

_____

COMMENTS

_____

Externship and Career Strategies

Key Terms *Define the following key terms:*

1. networking

2. skill set

3. chronological resume

4. performance evaluation

5. cover letter

6. white space

7. grandiose

8. proofread

9. externship

10. preceptor

11. functional resume _____
   _____
   _____

12. human resource _____
   department _____

Review Questions

1. What is the purpose of the medical assisting externship experience? Discuss the importance of splitting the externship experience between the administrative and clinical settings.

   _____
   _____
   _____
   _____

2. Discuss some important factors to consider during externship placement.

   _____
   _____
   _____
   _____

3. List four behaviors for students to display while out on externship.

   _____
   _____
   _____
   _____

4. Discuss some ways medical assistants use networking throughout their careers.

   _____
   _____
   _____
   _____

5. What are some general tips when interviewing for a position?

_____

_____

_____

_____

6. Discuss various job search strategies.

_____

_____

_____

_____

7. Describe the various types of resumes and why one type would be used over another.

_____

_____

_____

_____

8. Discuss some cover letter dos and don'ts.

_____

_____

_____

_____

9. What do a CMA and RMA have to offer a facility that a non-credential medical assistant does not?

_____

_____

_____

_____

10. Why is it important for a medical assistant to recertify?

_____

_____

_____

_____

Critical Thinking

1. Write a letter to your future self reminding you of how it felt to be a student in a medical assisting externship. How did you feel when you first started your hours at your site? Were you nervous, scared? What qualities did you appreciate and admire in your site preceptors? How were you treated? If your experience was not totally positive, what would you have done if you were the student's preceptor? Reflect and remember how it felt to be a student. In your letter, ask yourself to always remember what it was like to be a student so that you will treat students in your office with respect and kindness and teach them well. Make a copy of your letter and give the original to your instructor. Put the letter away and reread it a few years later and compare it to how are you treating the student externs that are at your office. (Your instructor may also mail your letter to you in a few years.)

2. Develop a job posting for a part-time medical assistant position in a women's health clinic. Include all of the qualifications you feel should be in a detailed position announcement.

3. You're reading the Sunday newspaper and see the following position advertised for a full-time medical assistant at the Overlook Medical Group, a newly opened group practice specializing in family health.

A busy family health group practice is seeking a self-motivated, experienced
medical assistant. Candidates should possess the following:
CMA or RMA certification
1–2 years experience (will consider graduate from a medical assisting program)

Send cover letter and resume to:

Cynthia Chapin, CMA
Overlook Medical Group
872 Bond Avenue
Waterford, NH 00032

Assuming you have just completed your externship and will be graduating and sitting for the
CMA exam in a few weeks:

a. Prepare a cover letter for this position.

_____

_____

_____

_____

b. Prepare a detailed resume.

_____

_____

_____

_____

Teamwork Exercises

1. In groups of two, role-play the following scenarios:

   a. A medical assisting student is externing in a medical office. The student's preceptor has asked the student to come to her office when she has finished with her patient. The preceptor wants to discuss the student's documentation techniques.

   b. The preceptor has observed the student being short and almost rude with patients today. She pulls the student aside to speak to her about her behavior.

   c. The physician catches the medical assisting student in the hallway and explains to the student that she is using the incorrect venipuncture technique.

   d. Create a scenario to role-play.

2. Divide the class into two groups. Have one group perform an Internet job search for medical assisting positions in your area, while the other group searches the newspapers for positions. Each group will create a portfolio containing information found on their searches. As a class, discuss what are some of the criteria these positions are asking for as well as the differences in the search types and benefits of both.

Office Project

If your school does not already have a bulletin board for job postings, see if you can create one either in your classroom or in a specific area of your school. Use information gathered from teamwork exercise #2 to post on the job board. If your school has a career center, see if someone will come speak to your class to discuss job hunting.

PROCEDURE 49-1 – APPLYING SKILLS FOR FINAL COMPETENCY ASSESSMENT

Name _____ Date _____ Score _____

Instructor _____

Task

Apply various skills learned throughout the clinical medical assisting course to a mock patient scenario.

Conditions

Patient's medical record

Supplies and equipment as needed for the given scenario

Time: _____

Standard

In the time specified and within the scoring parameters determined by the instructor, the student will successfully apply various skills learned throughout the clinical medical assisting course to a mock patient scenario.

Points assigned reflect importance of step to meeting the task

Important = 1 pt.
Essential = 5 pts.
Critical = 15 pts.

Automatic failure results if any of the **CRITICAL TASKS** are omitted or performed incorrectly.

(To use a pass/fail system, instructors can record "P" or "F" in the "points earned (pass/fail)" column.)

PERFORMANCE STANDARDS	PTS	PTS EARNED (Pass/Fail)	COMMENTS
1. Greeted and identified the patient.	1	_____	_____
2. Reviewed the patient's medical record.	5	_____	_____
3. Obtained and documented the patient's health history and chief complaint.	15	_____	_____
4. Demonstrated professional, therapeutic communication skills throughout the scenario.	5	_____	_____
5. Recognized and responded to verbal and nonverbal communications.	5	_____	_____
6. Identified and responded to issues of confidentiality and performed within legal and ethical boundaries.	15	_____	_____

PERFORMANCE STANDARDS (cont.)	PTS	PTS EARNED (Pass/Fail)	COMMENTS
7. Washed your hands. Followed standard precautions throughout the procedure.	5	_____	_____
8. Performed vital signs measurement and document appropriately.	15	_____	_____
9. Measured height and weight and document appropriately.	15	_____	_____
10. Put on appropriate PPEs for the procedure.	5	_____	_____
11. Prepared the patient for the procedure.	1	_____	_____
12. Performed the specialized procedure and quality control if applicable, according to the given scenario.	15	_____	_____
13. Disposed of biohazardous materials.	5	_____	_____
14. Provided patient education, including instruction on health maintenance and disease prevention. Instructed the patient according to his needs.	15	_____	_____
15. Documented the procedure and teaching in the patient's medical record.	15	_____	_____

TOTAL POINTS	137		

DOCUMENTATION

COMMENTS

_____

_____

_____